INTIMATE ENVIRONMENTS

INTIMATE ENVIRONMENTS

Sex, Intimacy, and Gender in Families

Edited by

David Kantor, Ph.D.
Kantor Family Institute,
Cambridge, Massachusetts

Barbara F. Okun, Ph.D.
Northeastern University
Boston, Massachusetts

THE GUILFORD PRESS
New York   London

© 1989 The Guilford Press
A Division of Guilford Publications, Inc.
72 Spring Street, New York, NY 10012

Printed in the United States of America

Last digit is print number: 9 8 7 6 5 4 3 2 1

Library of Congress Cataloging-in-Publication Data

Intimate environments.
    Includes bibliographies and index.
    1. Family psychotherapy. 2. Sex (Psychology)
I. Kantor, David. II. Okun, Barbara F.
[DNLM: 1. Family. 2. Family Therapy—methods.
3. Identification (Psychology). WM 430.5.F2 I615]
RC488.5.I585 1989   616.89′156   88-35802
ISBN 0-89862-748-6

To my family for their faith in
our odd ways.
   —David Kantor

To Sherman and Marcia.
   —Barbara F. Okun

CONTRIBUTORS

ELLEN M. BERMAN, M.D., Department of Psychiatry, University of Pennsylvania, Philadelphia, Pennsylvania.

DONALD A. BLOCH, M.D., The Ackerman Institute for Family Therapy, New York, New York.

MICHELE BOGRAD, Ph.D., Kantor Family Institute, Cambridge, Massachusetts.

LEE COMBRINCK-GRAHAM, M.D., Institute for Juvenile Research, Chicago, Illinois; Department of Psychiatry, University of Illinois at Chicago, Chicago, Illinois.

VIRGINIA GOLDNER, Ph.D., The Ackerman Institute for Family Therapy, New York, New York.

LARRY HOF, M.Div., Marriage Council of Philadelphia, Philadelphia, Pennsylvania; Department of Psychiatry, University of Pennsylvania, Philadelphia, Pennsylvania.

MICHAEL D. KAHN, Ph.D., Department of Psychology, University of Hartford, West Hartford, Connecticut; Department of Psychiatry, University of Connecticut School of Medicine, Farmington, Connecticut.

DAVID KANTOR, Ph.D., Kantor Family Institute, Cambridge, Massachusetts.

FLORENCE KASLOW, Ph.D., Florida Couples and Family Institute, West Palm Beach, Florida.

LAWRENCE KERNS, M.D., Institute for Juvenile Research, Chicago, Illinois.

RICHARD VINCENT MILLER, Ph.D., Private Practice, Newton, Massachusetts.

BARBARA F. OKUN, Ph.D., Department of Counseling Psychology, Special Education & Rehabilitation, Northeastern University, Boston, Massachusetts.

PEGGY PENN, M.S.W., The Ackerman Institute for Family Therapy, New York, New York.

GARY SANDERS, M.D., Family Therapy Program, Department of Psychiatry, The University of Calgary, Calgary, Alberta, Canada.

MAGGIE SCARF, Fellow, Jonathan Edwards College, Yale University, New Haven, Connecticut.

DAVID E. SCHARFF, M.D., Washington School of Psychiatry, Washington, D.C.

CARLOS SLUZKI, M.D., Department of Psychiatry, Berkshire Medical Center, Pittsfield, Massachusetts.

KARL TOMM, M.D., Family Therapy Program, Department of Psychiatry, The University of Calgary, Calgary, Alberta, Canada.

CARL WHITAKER, M.D., Department of Psychiatry, University of Wisconsin Medical School, Milwaukee, Wisconsin.

ACKNOWLEDGMENTS

During the months of gestation and preparation of this book, many people have generously contributed personal, editorial, and collegial support which has enriched this project.

I, David, wish to thank my family: Marcia, Matthew, Richard, Pamela, Melissa, Samuel, and my wife, Meredith—eight distinct and diverse voices—for making my continuing education as husband, father, stepfather, and man hard, but only as hard as it needed to be. In my own voice, as it can be discerned in the "Conversation" chapter and in my own chapter "Mythic Contracts and Journeys in Intimate Sexual Relationships," I recognize humbling lessons that I have learned from the struggles we have had as I and other family members have embarked on what I would like to think of as "searches" and "journeys" that have brought compassion and deep understanding to our family environment.

I wish also to thank two people who had a hand in the project. My deep appreciation is extended to miracle worker Jane Baskir, who has no match in making all things seem not only manageable but easy; and to Susan Bruno, whose feminist voice rescued an ailing section of my chapter when it truly needed rescuing.

I, Barbara, feel much love and gratitude toward my family, friends, colleagues, students, and clients who, over the years, have provided such rich opportunities for me to learn and grow. My special thanks to my Northeastern colleagues Mary Ballou and Deborah Greenwald for their patient readings and helpful feedback, and to Larry Litwack and Matt Luzzi for their continuous warm encouragement. Ricki Kantrowitz, Arlene Katz, Donna Raymer, and Susan Rhodes spent endless hours dialoguing with me about gender and intimacy, which helped me to clarify my thinking. My husband, Sherman, has again demonstrated endless patience and editorial acumen, which created an intimate environment in which I could love and work. My daughter, Marcia, took time from her doctoral dissertation to share with me her anthropological perspective of my work and my sons, Jeffrey and Douglas, continued to teach me about growing up male. I would also like to express my deep appreciation to the many people in my life who have been supportive and caring to me as I continue to deal with the issues addressed in this book.

PREFACE

The idea for a volume about intimacy, sex, and gender pertaining to families, family therapy, and family therapists emanated from years of our collaboration in developing and implementing a combined university and family-institute graduate family therapy training program. We wondered why love, sexuality, and intimacy are among the least addressed topics in couples and family therapy (recognizing that gender is increasingly discussed at conferences and in literature), when they may be our most important concerns. It seems to us that they clearly underlie many of the presenting problems of couples and family clients. We also mused whether or not other family therapists shared these concerns.

Just for fun, we conducted a literature search and found little, if any, adequate or substantive discussion of these issues, except in the area of sexual dysfunction or abuse. We were interested in issues of sexuality, intimacy, and gender as major components of family formation and development, not just as problems or dysfunctions, because we recognized that dilemmas over sexual and intimate matters often festered unattended amidst many of the structures that underlay the ones presented for treatment. Perhaps, we speculated, this was due to there being no theory on the role of sex and/or intimacy in family development; to therapists lacking an adequate vocabulary for dealing with sexual nuance in therapy; and to the fact that, most therapists, being human, face the same dilemmas in their private lives as do the families they treat. Thus, most family therapy writers have not reported on their personal and clinical experiences or on how their life experience has affected their clinical work.

So, in February 1986 we wrote a letter to about 25 prominent family therapists and asked them if they were interested in pursuing this further. The original responses were quite interesting. Most of the male responses were enthusiastic, and many suggested areas they would like to write about. The female responses were more guarded, asking us what we were really looking for; and many of the women wrote that, while interested, they were too committed to other work to undertake additional writing.

There was a time when we thought we would not have sufficient female respondents. But, as time went on, we found that more and more women did agree to participate and that, in fact, their chapters were submitted much earlier than many of the men's.

As our thoughts and ideas continued to evolve, we attempted to broaden our original focus. Thus, we have divergent and sometimes conflicting views presented in this volume. The contributors represent varying schools of thought and training within the field of family therapy, some of which conflict with each other. We have asked each to risk openness and frankness, to speak without fear of censure from us or from the others; and we present these contributions with respect, whether we agree with them or not.

Our contributors were each offered the opportunity to submit a "Personal Responses" addendum to their chapters, addressing the following three questions: (1) the influence of their gender and generational socialization on them as people, therapists, and writers; (2) the influence of their personal intimacy and sexual experiences; and (3) the implications of their chapter for the training and practice of family therapists. We present the material that was submitted but would like to note that many of the writers who chose not to submit additional material do provide a personal context for their views directly within their chapters.

We have organized the chapters of this book according to three major themes: (1) conceptual, theoretical discussions; (2) writings focusing on the person of the therapist; and (3) material dealing with clinical application.

In the conceptual section, David Scharff uses an object relations family therapy approach to link internal and external influences on individual–couple and couple–family development. He is particularly sensitive to the impact of parents and children on each other, the power of intergenerational issues, and the importance of sexual relationships. Next, Virginia Goldner discusses a case from psychoanalytical, developmental, and family systems perspectives and elucidates the importance of widening our conceptual frameworks. Michael Kahn uses a case to illustrate the integration of psychoanalytical and family systems theory, thereby attesting to the importance of addressing the issues of the individual in the couple system as well as reaching back to early childhood in order to understand the present relationship context. Lee Combrinck-Graham and Lawrence Kerns then provide a unique and thoughtful focus on intimacy issues of the young family. They attempt to differentiate intimacy, attachment, and bonding from one another, as well as sexuality from sensuality, within the spirals of individual development and family system patterning. They discuss how we confuse these concepts and how the intimacy capacities of the parents are influenced by their own experiences and personalities, by the infant's personality and responsiveness, and by the external environment. In doing so, they show how intricate and intertwined are these internal, family system, and external variables. In a lyrical chapter that bridges the conceptual and person-of-the-therapist themes, Michael Miller explores the sexual, intimate, and power elements of transference. He suggests that we need to deepen our understanding of the influence of these elements on the therapeutic relationship and the effectiveness of therapy in order to broaden the focus on the client's feelings about the therapist to include the importance of the therapist's loving feelings for the client. We can help clients with their intimate relationships only in the context of a loving therapeutic relationship.

The middle section of the book deals with the reciprocal influences of the personal and professional experiences and values of the therapist. Carl Whitaker, in his unique fashion, discusses the use of the therapist's personhood as the context for therapy. He is sensitive to personal and professional boundary issues, and he elucidates the dangers inherent in the therapy process when these boundaries are not respected. He also clarifies the difference between sexual and loving relationships and between intimate and performance sex. Barbara Okun next provides a conceptual framework for the reciprocal influences of personal and professional socialization on therapists' functioning, focusing on the gender-based power differential that underlies many of the intimacy and sexual difficulties therapists and clients experience and which can lead to avoidance and abuse in our personal and professional relationships. Michele Bograd then reports her findings about therapists' sexual yearnings for clients and presents a most sensitive discussion of these issues.

These personal chapters are followed by a chapter entitled "Conversations," which consists of unique dialogue among Barbara Okun, David Kantor, Maggie Scarf, Peggy Penn, Donald Bloch, and Carlos Sluzki about love, sex, and intimacy in families and family therapy, and among family therapists. In the last chapter of this section, David Kantor develops his ideas about the mythic contracts that underlie intimate sexual relationships, which were introduced in the "Conversations" chapter. He examines traditional gender arrangements, using imaginary dialogue and case examples to illustrate his points.

The final section of the book includes an expanded discussion by Larry Hof and Ellen Berman on sex therapy and family therapists. They encourage family therapists to learn to deal with sexual issues, just as they've learned to deal with other medical and nonmedical couple and family concerns. This is followed by Florence Kaslow's chapter describing the May–December marriages of the clients with whom she works in Florida. She addresses the different rhythms and intensities of male and female sex drives at different stages of life and their impact on a couple's lovemaking. Gary Sanders and Karl Tomm then elaborate the systems approach to working with sexual issues in family therapy. They provide a format for considering sexuality and sexual dysfunction as natural components of couples therapy and discuss the importance of therapist neutrality.

Our purpose in presenting these many viewpoints is to elucidate the current thinking of several leading male and female family therapists, with regard to intimacy, sex, and gender issues and how these issues and roles affect them as therapists and affect the client system(s) with which they work and the process of therapy itself. It is our hope that readers will be encouraged to think more freely and personally about these issues and begin to dialogue with others so that we can develop family therapy theories and vocabulary that reflect the existence and importance of intimacy, sexuality, and gender in our lives.

The emotional responses of prepublication readers have been unexpected. Discussions have evoked strong agreement or disagreement with the points of view presented in the book. These reactions have been largely divided along gender lines. Clearly some cords have been struck.

CONTENTS

1. FAMILY THERAPY AND SEXUAL DEVELOPMENT:
   AN OBJECT RELATIONS APPROACH   1
   David E. Scharff

2. SEX, POWER, AND GENDER:
   THE POLITICS OF PASSION   28
   Virginia Goldner

3. THROUGH A GLASS BRIGHTLY:
   TREATING SEXUAL INTIMACY AS
   THE RESTORATION OF THE WHOLE PERSON   54
   Michael D. Kahn

4. INTIMACY IN FAMILIES WITH YOUNG CHILDREN   74
   Lee Combrinck-Graham and Lawrence Kerns

5. TRANSFERENCE AND BEYOND   93
   Michael Vincent Miller

6. THOUGHTS ABOUT SEX, LOVE, AND INTIMACY   108
   Carl Whitaker

7. THERAPISTS' BLIND SPOTS RELATED
   TO GENDER SOCIALIZATION   129
   Barbara F. Okun

8. PASSIONS OF THERAPY:
   HIDDEN SEXUAL DIMENSIONS   163
   Michele Bograd

9. CONVERSATIONS   196
   David Kantor, Barbara F. Okun, Donald A. Bloch,
   Peggy Penn, Maggie Scarf, and Carlos Sluzki

10. **MYTHIC CONTRACTS AND MYTHIC JOURNEYS
    IN INTIMATE SEXUAL RELATIONSHIPS**   243
    David Kantor

11. **THE SEXUAL GENOGRAM: ASSESSING
    FAMILY-OF-ORIGIN FACTORS IN THE
    TREATMENT OF SEXUAL DYSFUNCTION**   292
    Larry Hof and Ellen M. Berman

12. **SEXUALITY IN MAY–DECEMBER MARRIAGES**   321
    Florence Kaslow

13. **A CYBERNETIC-SYSTEMIC APPROACH TO
    PROBLEMS IN SEXUAL FUNCTIONING**   346
    Gary Sanders and Karl Tomm

    AFTERWORD   381
    David Kantor and Barbara F. Okun

    INDEX   385

INTIMATE ENVIRONMENTS

FAMILY THERAPY AND SEXUAL DEVELOPMENT: AN OBJECT RELATIONS APPROACH

David E. Scharff

Throughout development the individual's unfolding sexual life takes place in the context of the family. Infants are born into relationships that are highly physical, and their first experiences of the family are through physical holding and handling, feeding, and caretaking. Emotional and physical needs cannot, in this beginning, be separated. This early unity of physical and emotional needs is not specifically sexual, but sexual relatedness grows out of it, as do all other branches of development. When in adolescent and adult sexual life, physical and emotional life are once again brought together, this joining contains echoes of the time in childhood when they were so joined. It is this fact of sexuality—that it remains the arena where physical and emotional connectedness are rejoined, that gives it a unique place in human relationships.

Sexuality has a complex relationship to family life. It sometimes seems to be at the leading edge of an individual family member's growth, as in the infant's discovery of the genitals, and again during oedipal or early adolescent phases. But a child's sexual growth also impinges on other family relationships such as the one between the parents. Having a newborn or an adolescent often interferes with parental sexual activity, but the shared joy to be had in children can equally energize sexual activity for parents. In turn, the relationships in the family at large, including the repercussions of the parents' sexual relationship, form the context in which the child grows, having a marked shaping effect on the child.

David E. Scharff. Washington School of Psychiatry, Washington, D.C.

This cycle of mutual influence can act to facilitate the child's sexual development, by shaping the sexual identity, the capacity to form relationships, and ultimately the capacity for sexual relationships. Likewise, it can act to handicap, distort, and impede these same processes.

I will begin by briefly sketching a theory of development that places sexual development in the context of psychological growth which is centered on the individual's need for relationships, that is, for attachment to primary figures such as mother, father, siblings, and other possible primary caretakers. In this general context, sexual development and sexual relating have their origin in early family relationships and can be seen, in turn, to influence the family life of an individual at every stage. This perspective allows us to understand the origin of sexual symptoms in children and adults as originating in a family context and as influencing the family in which they occur. We can then consider ways in which the sexual development and difficulties of a couple impinge on both their own relationship and the development of their children, as well as the ways in which children's sexual development has a reciprocal influence on parental lives and relationships.

AN OBJECT RELATIONS THEORY
OF INDIVIDUAL DEVELOPMENT

Let us begin with object relations theory itself, as it relates to individual development. This background is essential to understanding the role of object relations in human interactions. The most useful schematization of an object relations view, for me, has been that of W. R. D. Fairbairn (1952, 1963), a Scottish psychoanalyst who worked in Edinburgh in relative isolation from the London psychoanalytic community. His theoretical formulations compose the most durable framework for an interactional psychoanalytic theory. Fairbairn was working with children during the years he was forming his theory, which may account for the good fit between his theory and the clinical situation, as is true for two other theorists, Klein and Mahler. Fairbairn thought that the individual's psyche was organized by the internalization of the earliest interactions between mother and infant. Unlike Freud, he felt that the drives—sex and aggression—were completely organized by the interaction with the infant's caregivers. The differentiation of the baby's internal psyche occurs within the context of its being fundamentally object seeking, and this quality of the individual provides a foundation on which all developmental phases are constructed.

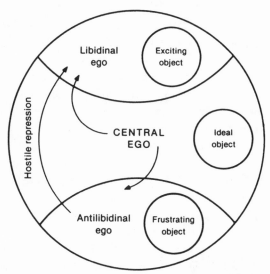

FIGURE 1.1. Fairbairn's model of psychic organization. From *The sexual relationship: An object relations view of sex and the family* (p. 217) by D. E. Scharff, 1982, London: Routledge and Kegan Paul. Copyright 1982 by David E. Scharff. Reprinted by permission.

Fairbairn's (1952, 1963) model (see Figure 1.1) holds that the infant's psyche at birth consists of a unitary or pristine, undifferentiated ego in a helpless, dependent relationship to the object of its attachment, the mother or mothering person.* To cope with the anxiety of this precarious situation of helplessness in the face of the inevitable frustration when mother cannot be perfectly depended upon, the ego defends itself from the helplessness by "splitting off" and repressing two aspects of the mother— the need-exciting part and the need-denying part—which Fairbairn called the *libidinal object* and *antilibidinal object*, respectively. Because they represent painful internal relationships, they are repressed along with the part of the self that is invested in them, namely, the libidinal and antilibidinal parts of the ego. The *affects* that in each case characterize the relationship between the part of the ego and its object are also repressed (Sutherland, 1963).

The mental apparatus, as can be seen in the figure, now includes an exciting object with its exciting or libidinal ego, a system characterized by

*By the word *mother* here I include whoever does the work of primary caretaking, definitely including fathers. I do not feel I can use the word *parent* because we are talking about the immediacy of what we call mothering. Both parents usually do this form of relating, although the differences between them are of interest (see Scharff & Scharff, 1987, Chapter 6).

the affects of excitement and painful longing; and a rejecting or persecuting object and its antilibidinal ego, a system characterized by affects of frustration and aggression. These structures are split off from conscious experience by repression. What remains is the relatively reasonable part of the infant's psyche, represented as the "central ego." The child's experiences of the dependable, caring (neither too frustrating nor too exciting) part of the mother, become internally represented by the "ideal object." Winnicott's (1965) term, the *good-enough mother* also corresponds to this object. Fairbairn associated the central ego with more conscious function. The "split off" or repressed introjected objects tend to remain relatively unmodified and unmetabolized over time. Because they are subject to repression, they tend to retain their infantile, primitive quality, even in the face of the person's later experiences.

It is because of the prevalence of these split-off systems that the excitement or frustration of intimate interactions (which activate them more easily) precipitate seemingly idiosyncratic, powerful, and abruptly changing experiences of the self and others. This happens in spite of the current experience of the real other, with whom interaction is different from that of the internalized early object relationship. As is shown in Figure 1.1, these repressed relationships deplete the central ego psychologically, as if by taking up mental space. The greater the need for repression, the less rich is the person's daily psychological functioning.

One other factor described by Fairbairn (1952, 1963) that is of interest in family life is the way in which the rejecting object system powerfully reinforces the repression of the need-exciting object by the central ego (see Figure 1.1). To understand this, I should clarify that the antilibidinal object is the frustrating sort of "bad object," the one against whom anger is felt for privation. The exciting object is not, on the other hand, the really "good object" any more than the antilibidinal object represents the useful limit-setting aspect of parental privation. The antilibidinal object is made up of the overly painful *depriving aspects of the mother* as modified by the child's elaborations on privation in its own fantasy. Just so, the libidinal object is one that *in fantasy* excites an intolerable, unsatisfiable need and compensates for the longing with an unsatisfying overindulgence. The libidinal ego attempts to induce such behavior. This unconscious system is therefore characterized by recurrent unrequited longing.

In the family, the child usually simplifies this situation by assigning the painful aspects to the same-sex parent and the alluring ones to the opposite-sex parent. In so doing, the child has "invented" its own oedipal situation; and, in trying to live out this internal situation, the child tries to modify the whole family (Scharff & Scharff, 1987).

To return to the dynamic interactions between the exciting and frustrating object systems, we can now say that rage over frustration tends to be easier for the individual to bear than painful longing. Because of this, the individual often uses rage to repress the longing further. The sense of privation spurs anger at the exciting object and at the same time motivates defenses against the pain of becoming aware of any sense of neediness. This makes the libidinal system difficult to uncover and analyze. In the clinical setting, it explains why, for instance, a couple's longing for love from each other may be covered by hate and denial. On the other hand, I have noticed that in certain adult couples and mother–child pairs a syrupy sweetness in the relationship is used to cover up underlying frustration and hostility. In these cases, the libidinal system is being used mutually to cover a sense of rejection and frustration. This is the opposite side of the coin; that is, the libidinal system lies like a blanket over the antilibidinal one, now making it harder to see and uncover (Scharff & Scharff, 1987).

Such interactions between unconscious structures—often giving a sense of an individual at war within himself—are at the heart of a theory of dynamic internal object relations. They can be seen to generate the transference phenomena in psychoanalytically based treatment. Patients act partly as if their therapists are reasonable, cooperative helpers and partly as if they are parents who excite an unpleasant longing, or are the depriving, misunderstanding part of parents, whom they hate. These transference elements are also powerful factors in family life and development, as the inner world of the growing child exerts an influence on his current external world and is shaped by new experiences in a mutual feedback system. For instance, Fairbairn (1952) notes that the oedipal situation is actually a rearrangement inside the child designed to reduce the strain of having two ambivalent relationships.

Besides Fairbairn, there are other notable proponents of object relations theory. We shall take a look here at the work of Melanie Klein (1975a, 1975b). All who draw on the British object relations theorists rely heavily on her, controversial aspects of her contribution, such as the death instinct, notwithstanding. Beginning with Freud's use of the word *object* to mean the person who is the object of the sexual and aggressive drives, she elaborated on the way the infant internalizes a good maternal object, splitting it into "good" and "bad" because, in the beginning, the infant does not have the capacity to integrate good and bad experience in the internal image of the same object. This view of what she termed the "paranoid/schizoid position" still fits what we have come to know of the infant's level of thinking in the earliest months. In addition, she postulated a later "depressive position" at about 9 months of age. This stage of the integration of good and bad experience in the internal image of the same person coincides with the growth of infants' enlarged capacity for cognitive integration late in the first year. The depressive position forms the basis for the individual's efforts at the repair of harmfully split part–objects and for the reparative functions of guilt.

Splitting of the object is an old form of thinking and relating which might also be called the earliest form of *sorting*—a less pejorative word, perhaps. Kernberg (1980) has postulated that in later development repression replaces splitting, which remains a hallmark of primitive thinking, but this is not the view of the British group in my exposure to them. They are more likely to use a combined term, *split off* (meaning split *and* repressed), to describe the fate of threatening aspects of the self and of the object.

The part of Klein's theory that I particularly want to emphasize is the importance of *projective identification* and *introjective identification*, two mechanisms that form the basis for our understanding of the interaction of two or more people at the level of their inner worlds. We might say that these two paired concepts drive the unconscious parts of an interactive engine, forming the basis for the capacity for unconscious relating. According to Segal (1973), whose explication of these concepts is particularly lucid, *introjective identification* results "when the object is introjected into the ego which then identifies with some or all of its characteristics" (p. 126). Conversely, *projective identification* "is the result of the projection of parts of the self into an object. It may result in the object being perceived as having acquired the characteristics of the projected part of the self but it can also result in the self becoming identified with the object of its projection" (p. 126). *Pathological projective identification* "is the result of minute disintegration of the self or parts of the self which are then projected into the object and disintegrated" (p. 127). Projective identification has varying aims: to avoid separation from the ideal object; to gain control of the source of danger in the bad object; to get rid of bad parts of the self by putting them into the object and then attacking it; to put the good self outside to protect it from the badness in the self; or "to improve the external object through a kind of primitive projective reparation" (pp. 127–28).

AN OBJECT RELATIONS MODEL OF INTERACTION

I would like to present now a schematic view of two people in interaction, as shown in Figure 1.2, which is an expansion of Figure 1.1. Here the two are labeled "child" and "parent," but the figure is just as accurate for two *adults* in interaction. This extension of Fairbairn (1952, 1963) to an interactive psychoanalytic theory owes everything to Henry Dicks (1967), who was the first to apply these object relations concepts to marital interaction.

Whether the dyad is composed of adults or a parent and child, when the experience of seeking and feeling rebuffed is repeated, the longing parts, the exciting object and ego, may be so thoroughly repressed that they are no longer consciously accessible to the dyad. This situation is seen clinically in couples who come to us in such a state of war that we cannot understand why they even ask for our help in staying together. We often describe such a bond as one of hopeless and pathetic "hostile dependency." But Bowlby's (1969) work, as well as the mother–infant research of the

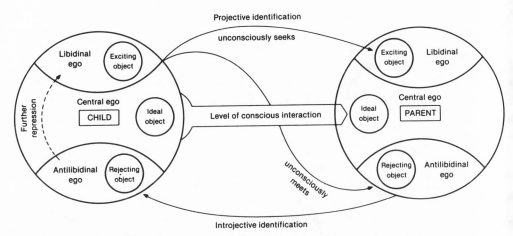

FIGURE 1.2   The mechanism here is the interaction of the child's projective and introjective identifications with the parent, as the child meets frustration, unrequited yearning, or trauma. The diagram depicts the child longing to have his needs met and identifying with similar trends in the parent via projective identification. If he meets rejection, he identifies with the frustration of the parent's own antilibidinal system via introjective identification. In an internal reaction to the frustration, the libidinal system is further repressed by the renewed force of the child's antilibidinal system. From *The sexual relationship: An object relations view of sex and the family* (p. 224) by D. E. Scharff, 1982, London: Routledge and Kegan Paul. Copyright 1982 by David E. Scharff. Reprinted by permission.

last 40 years (Stern, 1985), have sustained Fairbairn's (1952) thesis that the state of being attached to another human being is the absolute bedrock of human existence. The situation of dependency—even in the face of hostility—no longer surprises us. This situation is illustrated in the case of a child who feels rebuffed by his mother and cleaves to a hostile relationship, developing a strong aggressive bond to compensate for missing the directly loving one.

Figure 1.2 illustrates another point about the expansion from an individual point of view to an interactive one, a point which is crucial when we try to integrate individual therapy with marital, sex, and family therapy. What is split off and repressed, and therefore unconscious, in the psychology of the individual, is often alive and observable in the interactions between people. Thus, what is described as unconscious to a parent or a marital partner is alive in their communications and interactions, direct and implied, with the spouse or with a child. This fact is the basis for unconscious family sharing. It is also another way of saying that in a therapeutic relationship the transference contains, through the interpersonal interactions, tangible evidence of individual unconscious organization.

Winnicott, Lichtenstein, and Bion

Three theorists—Winnicott, Lichtenstein, and Bion—have each made contributions that flesh out a part of this theory. I will not review their work overall, but take a few elements which enlarge our specific understanding of family sexual interaction.

From Donald Winnicott (1965, 1971) I want to borrow first the idea that the mother (and parents) and infant have a psychosomatic partnership—an intense relationship that in the beginning organizes the infant through the holding, handling, and interaction with the mother. Interactive mirroring is a fundamental part of this; that is, the mother reflects the infant's condition to him usually while holding the baby in her arms as well as in her gaze. At the same time, the infant is the instrument of the mother's own unconscious needs. She leaves the stamp of a specific identity on the baby. It is the mother's place to project such an identity into the baby, and in the process of introjecting this identity the baby organizes its unformed experience (Lichtenstein, 1961).

The mother forms the "container" that Wilfred Bion (1967) described, under the rubric of an active, secure, and loving attachment which *from the beginning* also leads to a separation from the mother. We now know that separation and individuation do not begin as Mahler, Pine, and Bergman (1975) first described, as late as the eighth month. The baby is a separate being from the beginning, from his first interactions with the mother (Stern, 1985).

As the mother holds and handles the baby, she provides two basic functions (Scharff & Scharff, 1987). First she provides a context for growth and development, holding the baby in position, providing not only basic supplies but an envelope of security in which she and the baby can relate. This is her "holding function," and it sets the stage for another aspect of their interaction: centered relating. In the centered relationship, she looks into the baby's eyes, speaks to it, and provides confirmation of its experience and capacity. In this role, she provides the basic building blocks of the baby's internal objects. For the sake of our interest in the reciprocity of relationships, we must note that the baby also "holds" the mother with its body and responses and provides the building blocks for new aspects of the mother's internal object life, as mother. The relationship is mutual and reciprocal, and on both sides it includes two aspects: holding each other safely and securely, and relating centrally, an interaction at the core.

In both aspects, the beginning of the process is in the psychosomatic partnership, the relationship between parent and baby that is at the same time completely somatic and completely psychological. But as the child develops, the relationship is progressively less somatic and more psychological. The amount of time in physical contact decreases, and psychological, verbal, and symbolic interaction replace the original dominance of the somatic. For most of development, the overriding importance of somatic exchange recedes, with the exception of sexual development. We will look more closely at this later, but for now it is important to note that the somatic route to innermost psychological life, to internal objects, is established in the first weeks of life. It is therefore on this bedrock that sexual interaction is built, and it is this fundamental heritage that is drawn upon in the physical sexual exchanges of later life (Scharff, 1982).

The child also contributes to the process of its own growth. His fantasy life progresses during development. At each forward move certain distortions begin to be built in because, as the child proceeds, each new step of development tends to be taken as if the model for prior stages would still apply. Since each new stage creates something new, the old model is not quite right, and it is the parents' job as container of the child's growth to organize and correct for the new situation.

As an example of a child's distortion of meaning, let me cite the 3-year-old girl who announced to her mother one day that her "bottom" was an alligator with big teeth, clearly an early formulation of the vagina dentata. She based her understanding of her vulva on the model of her mouth. Without making this interpretation, it was possible for the mother to act as an organizing container by suggesting a softer fantasy likeness and encouraging the little girl to make her model of her body less threatening. In doing so, the mother contributed to the girl's body identity not through a physical exchange, but through providing a holding relationship of understanding and tolerance, inside which she took in the girl's concern and reflected back something more accurate. She provided modified building blocks for the girl's self-image.

The Contributions of Masters and Johnson

Masters and Johnson (1966, 1970) have described for us the literal aspects of sexual action and interaction. Their behavioral treatment format is grounded in the bodily experience of two people in intense interaction, in an adult psychosomatic partnership. Using this treatment format allows us to get much better descriptions of what actually happens between people. Aside from physically caused disabilities, most of these sexual difficulties, viewed from an object relations perspective, are not really dysfunctions in the sense of a mechanical failure. Rather, they are what I have called "disjunctions," or failures in internal object relations as expressed somatically (Scharff, 1982). To translate these interactions into object relations language, we retrace the path to earlier versions of the psychosomatic partnership. If we assume that sexual interaction represents the physical expression of primary emotional bonds, a role inherited from parent–infant interaction, then it follows that adult physical experience will reawaken and reverberate with the emotional aspects of this earliest set of relationships. However, sexual life also absorbs currents from relationships after childhood—from latency, adolescence, and adulthood.

FAMILY INFLUENCE ON SEXUAL DEVELOPMENT

At certain points in development, genital sexuality leads the developmental push. This occurs in all the familiar ways, such as during the development of masturbation, during oedipal development, and during puberty. Here a push from inside the individual "sexualizes" experience; that is, it leads to the expression of object-related issues in sexual "language." This understanding is, of course, the contribution of psychoanalytic drive theory, as first beautifully described by Freud in 1905 in "Three Essays on the Theory of Sexuality."

Unfolding individual sexual development occurs, however, within the context of the relationship to parents, family, and, later, the successors to these original primary objects. These relationships begin with the original psychosomatic relationship and are then extended into the realm of more psychological relating. However, the fact that the origin of sexual development blends somatic and psychological relating means that the sexual development of the individual must always be understood in the context of relationships with both external objects and internal objects. It is the interaction of internal and external object relationships that forms the study of the individual in the family.

With regard to sexual development, it is crucial to understand that, if early experiences of object loss occur during one of the periods of heightened genital urgency, the symptoms of loss are apt to take sexual form. Moreover, the family sets the *context* for development. For instance, in certain families, the parents stimulate the sexualization of relationships because they, at their relatively more advanced level of development, use sexual interaction as an overriding language for all emotional interaction. They provide a sexually excited or libidinized context for general development. Other families minimize the importance of sexuality in development and in relationships by engaging in a kind of antisexualization that denies sexual significance to even those aspects that are obviously sexual, such as the child's masturbation, the 4-year-old girl's excited love for her father, and adolescent bodily sexual development. These families provide an antisexual context for sexual development, encouraging excessive repression of sexual issues in the growing child.

The minimization of sexual exchange is part of the repression of the libidinal system and results in inhibitions of sexual life or in the excision of parts of ordinary sexual function. Hysterical patients who say they would be happy with their marriage if only no sex were ever required are often expressing the result of this kind of family influence during their growth. There are also those who have a split form of sexual repression, as exemplified by one genitally responsive woman who forbade her dependent husband to touch her breast, saying the skin was "irritable." For her the unconscious meaning of his touching her breasts had come to be that she would be turned into a mother who would be sucked dry and abandoned, a fear that echoed what she felt had happened to her own mother.

A familiar example of a family that sexualizes the general development of its children is that of parents who have a sense of having missed something in their own sexual lives and who pass on to their budding adolescent children this unconscious longing for sexual acting out (Johnson & Szurek, 1952; Szurek, 1974). While feeling sexually deprived themselves, these parents encourage the children to form an introjective identification with the parents' excited longing for sexual expression. The children then act out something sexual on behalf of the parents.

Case Example: Penelope

In the following case history, we will see how early experience with objects affected the adult sexual functioning of a woman I will call Penelope. This case drew on the reconstruction of early experience in the treatment of an adult.

Penelope was a reserved 40-year-old mother of three who was fond of her husband and her family. She could masturbate to orgasm but "felt no arousal" in sexual encounters with her husband Richard. "I don't feel any warmth *from* him; he just can't get it across to me," she said on repeated occasions. In sex therapy, she was able to progress to the point of experiencing orgasm by clitoral stimulation in Richard's presence, but she could not bear for him to watch her do so. She also began to complain more bitterly that "he gave off no warmth."

Richard was a very reserved man, but as treatment progressed he was increasingly enabled to express warmth for Penelope. She had originally chosen him largely because he did not pose the risk of what to her was an intolerable amount of closeness. The larger part of the failure was Penelope's inability to receive and react to his warmth and to his caring glances, both to feel them internally and to reflect them to him. She contended that the coldness came solely from *his* inability to feel and reflect warmth. In turn, Richard felt rejected by Penelope's insistence that he could never care warmly enough.

Penelope remembered her parents as distant and cold, even beyond the norm of the taciturn and isolated Vermont culture from which she came. She specifically recalled that her parents repeatedly quashed any expression of hurt, sadness, or anger on her part with the insistent rejoinder, "Nonsense! You don't feel angry. You feel fine." Or, "Don't cry! It doesn't hurt!" Penelope was able to describe, after some time, withdrawing from her parents in order to preserve quietly any sense of what she actually felt.

The adult needs for kissing, smiling, and physical caring in lovemaking and at other times have their origins in the shared gazing, touching, holding, and vocal babbling of infant and mother. In adulthood, as in infancy, the response of each partner to the other is required for a sense of continued well-being in marital life. Failures of mirroring in infancy often lead to what Winnicott (1965) called "false-self" problems, in which the "real" core of the self is hidden behind the shield of a false-self, and the individual tries to act as she thinks the other expects—often resenting doing so. These false-self problems make it difficult to recreate the mirroring experience in adult marital and sexual life. Without the capacity for mutual, interactive mirroring, which has its origins in the original psychosomatic relationship, gratifying sexual exchange is severely hampered, becoming instead a rejecting antilibidinal exchange.

Penelope's experience, as we grew to understand, represented the internalization of her experience not just with a repressive culture—for I do not think that this alone is a sufficient explanation for sexual repression—but also with unresponsive parents whom she experienced as frustrating objects, inducing in her a "false-self" identity based on denying what she felt. The result was that she learned to distance herself from her external objects to protect an embattled core. She picked Richard, who was also very distant, relating to him partly through a continuing bond of mutual frustration. When he did try to respond to her needy side, she grew more frightened and fortified the physical wall between him and herself. The antisexual feelings arose in response to the threatening, awakening sense of neediness. Responding to Richard would have meant to her unconsciously that he would replace her parents in telling her how to feel, thus taking control of her feelings and invalidating her as the person who received and controlled sensations from her own body. He would have been taking her over at her core. For her, the battle was between risking loss of her "self" to him or taking the less threatening risk of merely losing him.

Penelope demonstrated the way the lack of adult reciprocity echoes early failures in mirroring and identity formation. Her need to defend a core "true self" dictated a defensive detachment from her adult primary object. Her adult inability to tolerate mutual arousal stemmed directly from the way she had internalized the early experience of not being understood by her parents. She felt they had provided an unsafe holding context for sexual relating and for the shared expression of neediness. Sexual arousal with Richard penetrated her defenses, threatening to expose her needy core self. She reacted by bolstering the repression of that neediness and shunning Richard.*

---

*Although Penelope decided on a separation from Richard, she agreed with the recommendation for intensive psychotherapy in order that these issues not spoil future relationships.

Case Example: Debbie

Whereas in the preceding example childhood experience had to be reconstructed, in this case we will take a closer look by examining the development of a single child whose parents' situation was observed clinically. This example shows how a girl's development was sexualized through her parents' use of unconscious projective identification at certain crucial moments in her growth. In turn, this child's development sexualized the subsequent course of the family.

Debbie M came at age 4 for evaluation because of diffuse anxiety and a clinging, ambivalent attachment to her mother. Frequent uncontrolled masturbation in front of parents and strangers was a particularly striking symptom. When Debbie seemed to sense her parents taking note of her masturbating under a blanket, she would "look guilty but rub even harder." She was frequently unable to stop unless her parents held her gently on their lap.

The family history provided four converging lines of family contribution. The first came from the couple themselves. Mrs. M, the mother, had grown up largely abandoned by her own mother, given over to her grandmother. However from time to time, Mrs. M's mother would take her back, creating an alternating cycle of seduction and abandonment. While she was with her mother, she had been sexually abused by a neighbor, threatened sexually by a stepfather, and tantalized by her own mother. In summary, Mrs. M grew up with threatened and sexualized primary relationships. From all I could discover, Mr. M, Debbie's father, had consistent, safe parenting on the whole, but he had been indulged in a generally overstimulating way by his parents.

In the marriage, Mrs. M was unable to respond sexually to her husband, enacting a cycle of sexual rejection that exacerbated Mr. M's heightened longing for love and care. But Mrs. M also felt rejected and threatened. Her own fear of sex made her long for a holding relationship that would provide safety by not insisting on sex. When Mr. M expressed his mounting sexual frustration, she felt him to be like her stepfather, who threatened incestuous sex. And when Mrs. M refused in fright, she felt Mr. M to be threatening abandonment like her own mother.

Thus, Mr. M's indulged background made the sexual frustration especially difficult for him, while Mrs. M's experience of alternating abandonment and sexualization made sex feel like a threat to life, even though she exhibited a seductive quality, too. Their resulting cycle of sexualization, frustration, and threatened abandonment made for a painful marriage. This marital constellation had affected Debbie. Mrs. M felt too guilty to set limits on Debbie and, moreover, identified with the longing expressed in Debbie's masturbation and in her sexualized appeal for love.

The second line of parental contribution began when Mrs. M went to work full time when Debbie was 6 months old. Mr. M had already been so completely devoted to his work that he was basically unavailable to Debbie and, in many ways, to his wife. While early substitute child care was adequate and loving, at age 2½ Debbie was suddenly placed in extended institutional day care when her first sitter left. Thus, Debbie's handling of separation–individuation issues was in all probability hampered, as she was removed from a primary attachment figure just when she should have been consolidating her toddler's capacity for autonomy. It is common to see deprived infants and toddlers regress and turn autoerotically to their own bodies for self-gratification in these situations of early loss.

In this setting, the parents added a third factor to the sexualization of Debbie's development, which was their propensity to sexualize experience in general. Mrs. M did so by fearing sexuality while at the same time expecting it would inevitably erupt. Since her early experience had been sexualized, she had a way of anxiously sexualizing relationships herself. Mr. M's early family experience had included a moderately sexually exciting mode of interaction, which he also passed on to Debbie.

Finally the fourth aspect of sexualization erupted when both parents turned to Debbie for their affectional needs. Mr. M, feeling deprived by his wife's sexual withholding, unconsciously turned to Debbie for love. Although there was never any hint of sexual abuse, they did have an overly physical interaction during her childhood from the age of 2½. Mrs. M, in her sexual retreat from her husband, also turned to Debbie for a safer kind of affection, which recreated the clinging kind of relationship she had grown up with, when she had slept in the bed with her parenting grandmother. Thus, in this fourth powerful mode there were specific projections of sexualization onto Debbie, which she internalized from each parent and which came as each parent tried to compensate for the failed sex in their couple relationship. As Debbie continued to grow, all later developmental periods were sexualized as each of these four factors continued to exert influence—some because they had become part of her internal object world and others because they constituted continuing factors in Debbie's family experience.

INTERACTION OF THE FAMILY
AND SEXUAL DEVELOPMENT

The last aspect of the family and sexual development to be illustrated is the way the child's continuing development influences the family. This is true in normal families, but a family such as the one just discussed allows us to see ordinary things writ large. Thus, we will continue to refer to Debbie's case in the discussion in this section. Generally, as the child's own development proceeds through periods of heightened sexuality, the parents' sexuality is stirred up in turn. Thus, when Debbie expressed an overly sexualized version of oedipal development, her parents' vulnerability came under increased assault. It happened again during her adolescence when, despite considerable improvement from treatment, the family was once again in distress. Debbie's bodily sexual growth and excited sexual interests, for instance, rubbed salt in the wound of her parents' marginal sexual relationship.

The interaction of the family and sexual development, well illustrated in Debbie's family, can be summarized as follows:

1. Each parent's sexual failure is partly a result of, and partly contributes to, difficulty in his or her own internal world. It is a major factor in their mutually frustrating interaction.

2. Through mutual projective identification, the parents establish a relationship that represents a balance between satisfactory and unsatisfactory object relationships. While unsatisfactory sexual life is partly the result of such factors, it also contributes to a cycle of frustration and longing that magnifies this aspect of the parental relationship.

3. In the beginning, it is not the parental sexual failure that causes the child's developmental difficulty. Rather, the same internal object issues of the parents that influence the parents' sexual difficulty also influence their relationships to their children. From one perspective, their sexual difficulty and the child's developmental difficulties are independent results of the same internal object issues. The child takes in, as the stuff of her internal world, the object relations issues with each parent, which, when operating between the parents, have been part of their sexual difficulty.

4. The same elements of an antilibidinal inner world are present in the parents' sexual failure and in the child's development, even though these are not congruent expressions of the antilibidinal issues. While parental sexual failure per se does not cause the child's developmental difficulty (except in the case of overt incest), it does contribute to the feelings that form the external psychological context for her growth. The

child lives and grows in an environmental envelope largely determined by the parents. The sexual frustration and sense of rejection shared by the parents color their relationship. Part of what the child takes into her internal world is an imprint of the quality of the relationship between the parents. The difficulties in their relationship create a climate that tends to push a child toward symptomatology, but, even more important, this sense of parental difficulty is internalized by the child and becomes an inner factor.

5. Some families contribute their own tinting of sexualization to general experience pushing the children either toward the sexualization of experience or toward minimization of sexual expression. Debbie's masturbation and the subsequent sexualization of her development also reflected her parents' shared tendency toward a generalized sexualization of experience, which was spurred by the failures in their sexual relationship.

6. The child's continued growth has a reciprocal effect on the parents' object relations and sexual life. As Debbie passed through phases of normally heightened sexual development, the parents experienced renewed assaults on their shaky marital and sexual adjustment.

ASSESSMENT AND TREATMENT: A CASE HISTORY

The following case history chronicles the assessment and treatment of a family I followed over an extended period, from the time of the couple's initial sexual difficulty to the birth of their children several years later. This span afforded me a view of the effects of internal object relations on the individuals, the couple, and the widened family. "Kim," their young child, experienced diffuse anxiety which crystallized, like Debbie's, into the symptom of uncontrollable masturbation. Although this symptom was superficially the same as Debbie's, the meaning, treatment, and outcome were different.*

I first met this couple, whom I will call Bill and Peggy Noonan, when I began treating Peggy with twice-weekly psychotherapy for depression and poor self-esteem, which began when she felt sexually rejected by Bill. Because there had been almost no sex in the marriage, I also saw Bill and Peggy together, to assess their sexual relationship and Bill's inhibited sexual desire. These sessions occurred while Bill's mother was dying.

---

*This family has been reported in earlier publications, from the standpoint of individual development (Scharff, 1982) and regarding the use of play in family therapy (Scharff & Scharff, 1987).

Bill had two important dreams. In the first, a woman was crucifying him by nailing him to a wall. He thought in the dream that he was going to die. As he awakened, he thought of the woman as Judas and heard the phrase, "You will betray me before the cock crows." In the next dream, his landlady was a whore who offered fellatio, saying, "Do you want me to help you out, to make you feel good? I did it to your father recently. He really liked it." As she performed fellatio, he reached for her breasts. In describing the dream, Bill reported Peggy's observation that the landlady looked like his mother. These two dreams captured the quality of profound threat and excited craving he felt about his internal maternal object, an ambivalence that made sexual feeling for his wife impossible. Because of Bill's profound difficulty not just in regard to sexual desire but in developing any intimate personal relatedness, I referred him for individual psychoanalysis.

Peggy continued her twice-weekly sessions with me for several years, confronting the hostility she felt for her own mother over early absences and compensatory idealized overinvestment in her father. She had a fullblown oedipal idealization of her father, supported by denigration and anger at her mother, both for absences necessitated by her mother's employment and for being, as Peggy had then thought, a disapproving rival for her father. Her father had died when Peggy was 12, and her blocked grief had focused on her mother during adolescence.

Peggy's treatment was successful, and her depression cleared. Her self-esteem grew as she discovered a loving empathy in her adult relationship with her mother. She terminated individual treatment, feeling that she would give Bill the additional time he needed to try to change but, if he could not develop more intimacy and renew a sex life, she would be able to leave her marriage. Eventually, Bill's analysis was also successful and the couple began to enjoy their marriage, which now included active sex.

Despite the fact that they were still in their twenties, the couple then had some fertility difficulty, which was another source of shared sexual anxiety. They were finally able to conceive, and I received an announcement of Kim's birth 5 years after I had first met them. But their cherished child's sleep difficulty at 9 months once again brought Peggy back to consult me. In retrospect, it was a mistake on my part not to see the baby together with her two parents, given our long working relationship. I referred them instead to an infant psychiatry team, but the work sputtered and was only marginally helpful. The sleep difficulty cleared up eventually, but an anxious quality remained between Kim and Peggy.

When Peggy once again called me, Kim, then 2¾, was having temper tantrums and masturbating excessively at home and in public. I had recently met with Peggy for a history of Kim's development and of the current state of her marriage. Bill was fully involved in the marriage and was sexually functional, but Peggy had become withdrawn sexually. She found herself resenting the years of his sexual disinterest, even though she felt he had worked hard to change. Consciously she wanted to be able to respond to him. With these two difficulties now spelled out, we agreed to take a look at the overall family situation, to understand better the connection between Peggy's lack of sexual interest and Kim's distress.

The First Family Session

As I entered the waiting room to greet them for their first family session, Bill was reading loudly and energetically to Kim, who was on his lap. He smiled slightly sheepishly, seeing me after all this time with such changed circumstances. Peggy sat alone across the room. As they sat down, Kim stayed close to Bill. She climbed on his lap, and there was a bit of quiet roughhousing.

During the first few minutes the parents talked about their concern with Kim's touching her genitalia; while they did so, I was making friends with Kim. She was only slightly reticent, smiling from between the knees of both parents. Her parents indicated that she liked puppets, so I brought over a rabbit puppet and offered to let her have it. She said she also had a rabbit and showed it shyly but easily to her parents. Bill said she related more easily to men and would not warm up to a woman in this way. I noticed that Kim mostly stayed at home base with her parents and came forward to me only very slowly.

In the next few minutes, Bill teased Kim intermittently while he took the lead in discussing their concern with her masturbation. He cited his own lifelong concern with the adequacy of his genitals. Apparently without being aware of it, he touched his genital area frequently as he talked. He said he had grown up in a family that was not only distant emotionally but discouraging of sexuality. He reminded me that he had felt completely rejected and threatened by his cold, forbidding mother and that his father had preferred his sister to him. I thought of those dreams of Bill's from many years ago, which had been so striking that I had never forgotten them. They had revealed the threat sex held for him, as well as the sexualization of his wish for a caring mother. Now Bill was saying that he was uncomfortable when Kim touched herself, even when he was changing her, and far more so when she masturbated in public. They had taken baths together "only until Kim was 1 year old," but she still ran for the bathroom when she heard the sound of him urinating. Peggy confirmed that Kim was very excited about this event: "Oh yeah. She really races for it. It's hard to keep her out of there!"

While the parents told me about these matters, Kim climbed on Bill's lap and jumped off the couch. She focused on her father while casting glances at her mother and me. She showed her parents a series of two- and three-block towers made of cylinders, play which I speculatively linked with Bill's sexualizing.

Bill went on to say that he found himself doing things that were uncomfortably similar to behaviors of his own father which he had always disliked. For instance, he would lose his patience with Kim during her temper tantrums. Peggy said his reaction was not too bad, but she knew he found it frustrating. He said he would also like help with their renewed sexual difficulty, and would like to make himself a better father than his own father had been to him. Peggy looked up from playing with Kim on the floor at this point and agreed that they needed help with both areas. "But I don't think things are awful, Dr. Scharff," she said. "Really, they're pretty good." "Oh, that's true," agreed Bill. "You know, there are tears coming to my eyes right now. If you knew the change in the quality of our life. . . . There's no comparison. Now I can love somebody!"

In this family assessment session, I limited my comments to the possible relationship between the couple's sexual difficulty and their concern with Kim's masturbation. I drew silently on my observations of the overexcitement in Kim's interaction with her father, which I had felt from the first moment of the interview and which had been confirmed by the history of sexual excitement between them. I felt Bill was deeply invested in an exciting relationship as a compensation for his fear of being a rejecting parent, as he felt both his parents had been to him. But I felt unsure about how to discuss this without injuring Bill's vulnerable sense of fathering and perhaps seeming to side with Peggy against him. So I elected to wait to comment on the excited aspects of the relationship until a later interview, when I might have confirmation of my hunches, a more solid footing with the couple, and perhaps more easily understandable material from a session to share with them.

I noted during the session that Kim was much calmer while playing with her mother, much less excited. Although this kind of difference between play with a father and a mother is often true, I felt there was an exaggerated edge to her play with her father that left Kim overly excited. Peggy's observation that Kim raced to the bathroom to see Bill urinate confirmed this feeling. Peggy's half-knowing tolerance of this excessive excitement seemed to constitute both a projective identification and a masochistic surrender. She was encouraging a premature oedipal relationship between Kim and Bill because of her unconscious investment in vicariously reliving her own familial pattern in which she had turned excitedly to her father and away from her mother, whom she felt to be rejecting. Thus, she was putting herself in the position of being the mother who was taken for granted and subtly abused, possibly doing herself out of being a loved mother by encouraging a sexualized and therefore guilty oedipal phase. These matters seemed to be relevant to Peggy's current sexual withdrawal. They had not come to light years earlier in her own treatment because the possibility they might occur was masked by Bill's sexual withdrawal. But, just as important, Peggy's sexual withdrawal at this phase of family growth also illustrated the way in which the developmental phase of the child introduces newly sexualized elements into the family, which may trigger sexual symptoms in other family members.

Later Family Sessions

In the second family session, I noticed that Kim was much calmer. She played more with her mother and displayed a less excited manner with her father than previously. At this point, I was still unable to understand the origins of the temper tantrums, but I did give some guidance on managing them with firmer limits. This allowed more material to emerge about them in the third session. It turned out that they were also linked to the sexual difficulties in the family. The tantrums frequently occurred when Kim was in bed with her parents in the morning. Bill would read to her and then get up, leavng her in bed with Peggy. At one such juncture that week, Kim threw a fit aimed at Peggy, over the correct arrangement of the bedpillows. It became possible for us to see the parallels between Kim's masturbation and her tantrums, namely, her anxiety about her relationship with her parents. She was troubled both about her mother and about managing her disappointment when the excited situation with her father inevitably ended.

In the fourth family session, the pattern of relationships was the same. Kim showed a consistently excited relationship with her father and played in a calmer, more organized way with her mother. Bill had been away for a few days, and Kim had spoken repeatedly of missing him. Bill reported that he was glad to see her when she greeted him at the airport. "She couldn't stop kissing and hugging me," he said. "I got a bit of a sexual rush. Not in my genitals, just in my chest. It was such a relief to have such a strong feeling after being away. I can't get over it." I could then understand how his relief at finding these feelings fueled his own excited joy at being a loving parent.

By then I felt our working together was on a solid enough footing that I could comment on the observations I had made concerning the overly excited relationship between Kim and Bill, and the way Peggy, in her investment in that kind of relationship from her own past with her father, supported it despite reservations. She said, "I've asked Bill about getting so wound up with Kim, but he says, "Relax. We're just having fun." She had bowed to his insistence.

I said that, while nothing definitive had happened yet, I could see the set of relationships converging toward a repetition of what Peggy had with her own parents and what Bill longed for with his. "I remember, Peggy, what a crush you had on your father, who could do no wrong, while your mother could do no right. I'm worried that you may have started down a path of encouraging Kim to feel something similar about the two of you. And Bill, you long for this even at the cost of your marriage, because it was so painfully missing for you growing up."

Both Bill and Peggy looked startled and upset. As we talked, I was able to show them evidence I had been collecting from our sessions and to connect it to their own misgivings. Even as I was talking to them, Kim had begun to play with the family of flexible dolls, putting twin baby dolls in a bed with the parent dolls. She had done this before in a random way, but on this occasion I noticed that the play of the babies snuggling with the parents got more forceful as I talked with Bill about his investment in a warm, exciting relationship with Kim. The play was not specifically oedipal, I thought, because the mother stayed in bed with the group, but it was excessively animated.

Then I turned to talking about Peggy's reluctance to set limits on Bill because her unconscious identification with her own denigrated mother led her to support a sexualized relationship between Bill and Kim. Kim's play changed abruptly. Suddenly the mommy doll sent the babies to their room for playing in the sink. The mommy doll became firmly rejecting of excitement. I joined Kim on the floor, took the daddy doll from the bed where it still lay, and had the daddy say, "Mommy, maybe the babies would like to play with me." With that the babies ran from the scene with the mommy and jumped onto the daddy and began an excited romp. I said, "Sometimes the babies like to see Daddy when Mommy is mad at them." Kim said, "I like to have my daddy come home all the time. But sometimes my mommy really gets mad at me!" She smiled at Peggy and said, "Don't you, Mommy?"

The shift in Kim's play enabled me to demonstrate to Bill and Peggy that Kim clearly had internalized and magnified the split between them. She had taken in the shared projective identifications from early in their relationship, now restimulated by her growth. In her individual relationships she assigned the painful, rejecting side to Peggy and sought the exciting side with Bill. The point sank home for them as I reviewed the play, which they had also seen but not understood, and they looked at each other with new understanding.

Kim's play demonstrated that she had two individual relationships which split excitement onto her father and inhibition onto her mother. In one sense these patterns were simply exaggerated forms of the usual difference between a child's relationship with mother and father. The very exaggeration of this split, however, showed both that Kim had incorporated something of the couple's relationship to each other and also was starting to impose her internal object relations back onto them. Her growth, especially as it veered toward the emergence of sexual issues in the phallic and oedipal phases, was restimulating old and previously settled parental liabilities. And, of course, Kim's forming self was affected by the impact she was having on her parents, including the anxiety it engendered, her mother's increased depression, and the excitement with her father.

Within a few days after this session, Peggy's interest in sexual relatedness with Bill returned, to their mutual relief. Over the next weeks, Bill and Peggy brought in examples of their shared tendency to foster an anxious sexualization of the relationship with Kim. Both parents became stauncher in their capacity to set limits with Kim, and Bill drew back from the overly exciting aspects of the interaction with her, while still maintaining his interest and performance as a father. The issues behind the family's pattern emerged for a reworking, which went quickly because of their extensive previous therapies.

Long-Term Family Development

I was lucky to be able to follow this family over the next couple of years after this intervention. Therapeutic work remained to be done with Kim on aspects of the early family constellation that she had already internalized. In addition, it emerged that she had some constitutional difficulty in staying organized when aggression threatened. So I saw her in play therapy for these residual difficulties, and I saw the parents periodically. I was still seeing Kim when her mother became pregnant, when Kim was 4, and saw Kim's mild regression in therapy. She would order me to build houses and towns of blocks for dolls. Soon, repeated fires would threaten entire villages of dolls and animals. The fire brigade would assemble outside the walls, and then the action would stop. The pregnancy seemed to threaten her with disaster, which she could not allow me to discuss. At home, however, and consciously with me, she was thrilled to be getting the baby brother she had been hounding her parents to have.

When Peggy gave birth to a healthy boy, Kim showed up for her next session hopping like a rabbit, anxious to show off her own prowess, telling me why she could do more than her new brother, Alex. Then she sat on the couch, her legs spread apart, scratching an area of her labia at the edge of her underpants, looking at me as if daring me to speak about it. This was the first time I had even seen Kim, now 4¾, masturbating. Her parents had reported that the symptomatic masturbation had ceased long ago, so this was a regression triggered by the birth of her brother. Overcoming my own reluctance to talk to her about it, I asked Kim about touching herself near her vulva.

"It's baby eczema," she explained impatiently.

I said, "Oh, I see. It's itchy eczema you get from having a baby in the family."

"No! I like having the baby. And when Mommy's feeding Alex with her breast, Daddy reads to me."

"Yes, it can be fun," I said. "But it can make you wish you were the baby getting Mommy's breast. And you might wish you were the mommy and had a baby yourself."

Kim was silent for awhile, scratching the inside of her thigh absent-mindedly. Then she said, "Alex won't get Mommy's breast when he grows up. And I'll have a baby someday myself. Now, come on! Build a house for my dolls."

Over the next weeks, we built many houses, which were bustling with family activity as Kim worked on the theme of always being older than Alex, on how she would maintain her parents' love by caring for him, and on how that would help her to be ready to have babies herself.

THE CYCLE OF MUTUAL INFLUENCE

My experience with the Noonan family illustrated certain intergenerational sexual issues, from their initial appearance in couple's therapy to their transmission to their child, and to the child's reciprocal influence on parental sexuality. Even though psychoanalytic and psychotherapeutic treatment had moved the couple past their initial difficulty with issues of sexuality and intimacy, they retained a vulnerability that became exacerbated by the birth of their children. The skills they had developed in previous therapy, however, allowed them to work through the new developments quickly. If it had not been for Kim's constitutionally determined vulnerability, she might not have needed further individual work herself. But since it seemed useful for her to have it, I was there to observe her brief regression to sexual symptomatology during the family stress of the birth of her brother, and to watch her hard at work on her reaction formation.

The Noonan case gives an unusual view of the interaction between individual and family sexual development. Parents bring their own object relations to the marriage, and the unconscious aspect of their sexual relationship is determined by their joined object relations. Parents later influence their children, both by the individual relationship each parent has with a child and by the kind of couple relationship they present to a child. The child internalizes these elements—a relationship to each parent and to the two of them combined—and splits off the painful parts, modifying her internal world in complex ways as this occurs. The internal object relations thus formed determine the child's emotional path through subsequent developmental stages. In turn, however, the child modifies her family from the time of arrival, introducing challenges to the family at conscious and unconscious levels and becoming a new primary object for the parents. As they also internalize experience with the child, individually and as a couple, their own internal worlds are forever altered. At times this alteration produces strains that may result in sexual symptomatology, which in turn have a further effect not only on the couple but on the family as a whole, including the children. The cycle of mutual influence of family development and sexuality is endless.

When we are presented clinically with sexual symptomatology, the determination of an appropriate intervention rests on whether the internal object relations of a single family member pose the predominant difficulty, or whether mutual projective identification characterizes a couple or family. If we are seeing a single individual without a partner or a current nuclear family, individual or group therapy are our only options. In circumstances where there is a partner, spouse, or family, the question of how to balance the intervention is more complex. Many modes of intervention are mutually compatible in an object relations approach, including individual, couples, family, group, and sex therapy. When we are working with the family and couple, then we are working with their capacity to provide shared holding for the growth of relationships and of individual family members. When we work with the individual, we look together at the internal object relations difficulties. In conjoint sex therapy, a symptom the couple shares is used as a vehicle to look both at the failure of their mutual holding capacity and at strains in their internal object relations. The specifics of these approaches have been elaborated elsewhere (see Scharff, 1982; Scharff & Scharff, 1987).

In families and patients with sexual difficulties, what we are after is the linking of the sexual symptoms with the currents of development, that is, the uncovering of the object relations issues that have impaired the individual and family capacity to love and support each other. When we are able to do so, we provide a context in which sexual symptomatology can be traced to its original components, enabling the individual and family to relate in richer ways. They long to do so. Each of them yearns to be loved and to be able to love. The sexual symptomatology represents a failure of this wish. When therapeutic endeavors are successful, our patients are freed to love and to be loved in return.

REFERENCES

Bion, W. R. (1967). *Second thoughts*. London: Heinemann.
Bowlby, J. (1969). *Attachment and loss. Vol. 1: Attachment*. London: Hogarth Press.
Dicks, H. W. (1967). *Marital tensions: Clinical studies toward a psychoanalytic theory of interaction*. London: Routledge & Kegan Paul.
Fairbairn, W. R. D. (1952). *Psychoanalytic studies of the personality*. London: Routledge & Kegan Paul. (Also published in the United States as *An object relations theory of the personality*. New York: Basic Books, 1954.)
Fairbairn, W. R. D. (1963). Synopsis of an object relations theory of the personality. *International Journal of Psycho-Analysis, 44,* 224–225.
Freud, S. (1905). Three essays on the theory of sexuality. In *The standard edition of the complete psychological works of Sigmund Freud* (Vol. 7, pp. 124–245). London: Hogarth Press, 1958.
Johnson, A. M., & Szurek, S. A. (1952). The genesis of anti-social acting out in children and adults. *Psychoanalytic Quarterly, 21,* 313–343.
Kernberg, O. (1980). *Internal world and external reality: Object relations theory applied*. New York: Jason Aronson.
Klein, M. (1975a). *Envy and gratitude and other works, 1946–1963*. London: Hogarth Press and the Institute of Psycho-Analysis.
Klein, M. (1975b). *Love, guilt and reparation and other works, 1921–1945*. London: Hogarth Press and the Institute of Psycho-Analysis.
Lichtenstein, H. (1961). Identity and sexuality: A study of their interrelationship in man. *Journal of the American Psychoanalytic Association, 9,* 179–260.
Mahler, M., Pine, F., & Bergman, A. (1975). *The psychological birth of the human infant: Symbiosis and individuation*. New York: Basic Books.

Masters, W. H., & Johnson, V. E. (1966). *Human sexual response.* Boston: Little, Brown.

Masters, W. H., & Johnson, V. E. (1970). *Human sexual inadequacy.* Boston: Little, Brown.

Scharff, D. E. (1982). *The sexual relationship: An object relations view of sex and the family.* London: Routledge & Kegan Paul.

Scharff, D. E., & Scharff, J. S. (1987). *Object relations family therapy.* Northvale, NJ: Jason Aronson.

Segal, H. (1973). *Introduction to the work of Melanie Klein* (new, enlarged ed.). London: Hogarth Press.

Stern, D. N. (1985). *The interpersonal world of the infant: A view from psychoanalysis and developmental psychology.* New York: Basic Books.

Sutherland, J. (1963). Object relations theory and the conceptual model of psychoanalysis. *British Journal of Medical Psychology, 36,* 109–124.

Szurek, S. A. (1974). Concerning the sexual disorders of parents and their children. *Journal of Nervous and Mental Disease, 120,* 369–378.

Winnicott, D. W. (1965). *The maturational processes and the facilitating environment: Studies on the theory of emotional development.* London: Hogarth Press.

Winnicott, D. W. (1971). *Playing and reality.* London: Tavistock.

2

SEX, POWER, AND GENDER: THE POLITICS OF PASSION

Virginia Goldner

Family therapists are not trained to think about sex in its own terms. We tend to leap over its irrational, individual, and body meanings and metaphors, because we are looking for the "couple metaphors" from which we can locate sexual issues. This habit of mind makes sex the same as money, communication, housekeeping, or any other arena of relationship struggle. This parsimony is often just the right antidote for a couple's tendency to inflate the importance and meaning of their sex life and its disappointments. However, it is too often too narrow a focus, especially if there are sexual problems that go "deeper" than the "she's not turned on because she's secretly angry at him" variety. Because sex is simultaneously internal and relational, we need a theory that incorporates both levels of experience and does not reduce one to the other.

In this chapter, I attempt this kind of theoretical integration in my discussion of a couple for whom sex was just "too good." The following is a minimally edited transcript of an initial interview I conducted with a couple at the Ackerman Institute for Family Therapy in 1986. I have reproduced it practically verbatim because I wanted to recapture the experience of hearing the protagonists, Dan and Sarah, tell their story. Although the storytelling is obviously guided and shaped by the therapist, the story is the thing, as you will see.

THERAPIST: I'm meeting you for the first time, so I know nothing about why you're here or whose idea it was to come here, so anywhere you want to start is fine with me.

Virginia Goldner. The Ackerman Institute for Family Therapy, New York, New York.

SARAH: Whose idea was it, mine or yours?

DAN: Yours.

SARAH: Yeah, I think I decided we should break up, Dan said if we stayed together we could see a counselor, I said on those terms we could stay together. Is that it?

DAN: I think so.

THERAPIST: (*to Sarah*) What made you feel *you* wanted to break up?

SARAH: I was unhappy . . . in the relationship, in my life. I believed if I changed that I'd feel better.

THERAPIST: You felt unhappy in a lot of places and thought if you made a change with Dan it would help you generally?

SARAH: Careerwise.

THERAPIST: How did you think if you broke up with Dan it might help you with the rest of your life? That's an interesting . . .

SARAH: Cause I felt that . . . (*looks around at cameras*) It's hard . . . (*therapist nods*) I felt that careerwise I would spend more time thinking about my career if I wasn't spending all my time thinking about how the relationship wasn't working (*laughs*) . . . and I think it's important at this time . . . I want to be a singer and an actress, mostly a singer, and I felt if I was alone, just not in any relationship with any man, alone by myself, I could figure out what I was going to do and do it and not spend any time thinking about a relationship at all.

THERAPIST: How old are you?

SARAH: Twenty-one.

THERAPIST: And you?

DAN: Thirty-one—a generation gap.

THERAPIST: Yeah, I was thinking along those lines . . . I'll come back to that; I'll ask you what that age difference means to each of you . . . So you had this idea that, if you were not in a relationship with a man, you would be really free to think about your career and what your next move would be . . .

SARAH: And also I remember a couple of years ago I wasn't in a relationship and I felt like I wasn't exactly happy, but I felt like I was more into my career when I wasn't into a relationship. I *remembered* that and I thought maybe if I was alone that would happen again. I'd start thinking about my career, not only my career, but think about myself, who I am and what I want in life. I get lost in other people, I just lose myself.

THERAPIST: Other people, or the men you fall in love with?

SARAH: Men I fall in love with. Men I'm attached to.

THERAPIST: With your friends or family, do those relationships also lead you to lose your bearings?

SARAH: No. Just men.

THERAPIST: Romantic attachments.

SARAH: It's happened before.

THERAPIST: A similar pattern . . . (*turning to Dan*) When she told you this, did it come as a surprise, was it out of the blue, did you expect it, had you talked about it?

DAN: We'd been having difficulty for quite some time. (*sketchily summarizes sequence of fighting, breaking up, seeing each other on a part-time basis*) When she said this to me, it was in the heat of an emotional argument. I said let's wait to talk about it. So the next day we talked. I understand being a career-oriented, very driven person. I understand someone's need to consume themselves with their ambition. I tried to find out what I was doing that was in her way, and she said, "If I woke up in the morning and didn't have anyone to concern myself with, I'd have more time to dedicate to . . . I'd be so unhappy, so miserable that I'd be *forced* to go out into the world."

THERAPIST: That's an interesting way to go into the world.

SARAH: (*laughs*) When I was alone I remember waking up feeling so lonely that last time that it *made* me have to go out and do things with other people, rather than feeling comfortable.

THERAPIST: (*to Dan*) What do you think of this idea?

DAN: I understand, but as I said, there's also a tremendous value in having a security blanket, or a security pad, too, in this very turbulent entertainment business.

(*Couple reviews in somewhat more detail the process of defining their current relationship as one where they see each other just on weekends.*)

THERAPIST: Whose idea was that?

SARAH: We agreed together.

THERAPIST: (*turning to Dan*) Why did that arrangement suit *you* best?

DAN: I have a lot invested in Sarah emotionally. It's a very difficult and crazy relationship and a lot of other things that I suppose stem from dependency and selfish need on my part.

THERAPIST: What do you mean by that? I'd like to understand— dependency? selfish need?

DAN: There are times I feel I *need* her, I need somebody. I'm sort of a lonely person, I have a lot of acquaintances, superficial friends, very, very few people I can open up to, so weekends suited me better because it would still keep me in contact with . . . this need. I felt it as a need . . .

We're starting in on the outside of these problems . . . and eventually we'll work our way *in.*

THERAPIST: You mean we three at this point? (*Dan nods*) Of course.

DAN: We've had a lot of difficulties we're equally responsible for . . . I don't want it to end, if it *has* to end, the way it seemed to be headed. I want a *creative* separation, working it out with someone else, the fact that we're here. Also, it's very hard to be with me. I'm not strong enough to maintain my equilibrium in the business I'm in. I'm very high when I'm working, very low when I'm not. I take it out on who I'm with.

THERAPIST: How?

DAN: I'm very black, melancholy, brooding. I'm difficult and unpleasant to be with, and I was drinking when I wasn't working, causing and perpetuating a difficult situation.

SARAH: I didn't say anything, even though it bothered me.

DAN: I'm no alcoholic, I would drink till I didn't feel the pain, numb myself. I wouldn't be responsive, go to the movies and have fun. I'd just want to sit and brood.

THERAPIST: How did that aspect of the way Dan copes affect you?

SARAH: It was a drag. . . . That's a mean thing to say.

THERAPIST: Mean?

SARAH: That someone is a drag. If Dan is in a bad mood, I don't even exist. If I'm in a good mood, I want to go out dancing, to the movies, but with him, the whole weekend, there's a weight on me. It's heavy on me to deal with him all the time. I want to be light and funny, sometimes it's important just to have a good time.

THERAPIST: Sarah seems a light, somewhat cheerful, sunny sort of person. Is that so, is that what drew you to her?

DAN: I suppose so, when you first meet her. But that's not what drew me to her. She was much less sunny, she was very unhappy. What drew me to her is she has a tremendous intellect, and I was living with someone at the time, for 6 years. With Sarah I felt I found someone with whom I could share intellectual observations. Aside from the fact that I was physically attracted, but that wasn't the most important thing. She was someone who understood *pain* in a very intelligent way, and could understand *joy.* I still feel that very strongly. She's not like theater people. She has tremendous insight into life itself, even though I am much older.

THERAPIST: Would you say you found in her qualities you most value in yourself?

DAN: *Not* in myself. She helped me find them in myself. I would say they are probably there, since I feel much more intellectually capable now, and that has a lot to do with her.

THERAPIST: I'm interested in how your relationship started. Is it safe to say you fell in love with each other? Not all romances start that way.

SARAH: He fell in love with me first. (*laughs*) No.

THERAPIST: That could be so. (*to Dan*) She's good at protecting you, even though she wants to get out of that role. (*back to Sarah*) So, is that so, he fell in love with you first, and brought you along?

SARAH: It was great. He was so different from anyone I'd met. Guys want to sleep with me right away, but he wanted to talk and talk. He had another relationship. I never wanted to take him away from that girl. I totally wanted him to stay with her. I hate to see anyone break up, and he was going through hard times. I wanted to help him. I would always say, "Whatever happens, I want you to stay with her." Also, I didn't want to get too serious with anyone. I wanted to think of myself and my career.

THERAPIST: How long had you been out of a relationship?

SARAH: Six months.

THERAPIST: It was the aftermath of that relationship that gave you the idea that you were truer to yourself when you weren't in a relationship?

SARAH: When I split up with my last boyfriend, it was devastating. But after a month, I started finding out who I was again. I had no idea who I was with him. It was scary. But with Dan, he really listened. We thought on the same wavelength. I could tell him almost anything, and he wouldn't be shocked. Any fantasy, any weird thing I would want to do. Anything I'd done, anything I'd want to do. And he wouldn't go "Oh my God." Nothing would shock him.

THERAPIST: Like what?

SARAH: Getting up and dancing around. There was no pressure to be normal.

THERAPIST: Had you felt that with anyone else? To be really understood and show all the parts of yourself and feel they were good?

SARAH: With other girlfriends and my sister. Not guys.

THERAPIST: (*to Dan*) You look skeptical.

DAN: When I start thinking, I must look like I'm going to kill somebody! It's a very deceiving appearance.

THERAPIST: (*to Sarah*) So that's how he looks, when he's black and brooding, that look I thought meant . . . .

SARAH: That, or like he's not there, like he's off into space, and I feel like shaking him!

THERAPIST: So you find in each other things that are very rare and unusual. And it works very well until it doesn't. Would you try now to remember together how it was good and how it then unraveled, so we can trace this? Collaborate together on the plot line.

DAN: I was on Broadway. You saw me act the scene of that guy in love. I was so happy that you were so happy. And I was playing music at clubs.

SARAH: That was the best. When we'd write songs together in clubs and perform together. I probably wouldn't have thought to be a singer/songwriter if it weren't for that.

DAN: I told her mother, "I'll marry her and have her child." She said, "She is only eighteen!" But I didn't care. I was *totally* in love with her. And then I got this movie I was filming in California. I was going to be away 6 months.

SARAH: I figured that was it. I gave him this ring that night because I was totally sure it was over. I thought, "Okay, maybe it'll be better for me. It's good for me to be alone, to know myself better." That was the idea even then—"good for me to be alone." But then he started calling me, like once or twice a day.

DAN: I *didn't* have the idea that it was over. I called her *twice* the first day. I spent over $1,200 in phone bills!

SARAH: If it wasn't for that, it would be over. He called so much.

THERAPIST: Did you call him?

BOTH: I/She couldn't afford it.

SARAH: We'd talk endlessly on the phone.

DAN: I'd try to reassure her.

THERAPIST: Is that what it meant? Reassurance?

SARAH: Yes.

DAN: And then one night after 2 months, I said, "I'll call you at 10." I wanted to tell her I was there with all these women and it meant nothing. All I saw was her. Every song reminded me of her. I wanted to see *her* dance, listen to *her* sing. So I called her, and she wasn't home. I called every half hour until 3 A.M. I was worried. She lives in a very bad neighborhood. I inherit this from my mother; I am a worry artist. I worry about everything that everyone else does.

THERAPIST: What do you mean?

DAN: I fantasize they'll get killed. In a perverse fashion, it's an intense form of prayer to protect people.

THERAPIST: You mean, if you worry the worst thing, it protects them from the worst thing?

DAN: Yes. So I had a few friends holding me together. When we had a rehearsal, I even had the secretary of the movie company calling to see if she was okay. When she came out to visit me, I found out that she'd slept with someone that night. And that was the beginning of a lot of problems. I'm not trying to be blameful, because . . .

SARAH: He was gone for 6 *months*! I spent *so* many nights alone, I don't feel that guilty about it.

THERAPIST: Why did you tell him?

SARAH: Why did I tell him that night?

THERAPIST: Why did you tell him at all?

SARAH: First of all, the time he was gone I lost 20 pounds, for *him*. All I could think of was exercising so I could look really good when I got off the plane for *him*. I wasn't into any other guy. And then one night . . . it was just a fluke. All the time I was thinking of him, because when he started calling, I thought I had a really strong relationship on the phone . . . (*turning to him*) Why did I tell you?

THERAPIST: Why are you asking him? Do you sometimes feel he knows your mind better than you know it yourself?

SARAH: No, I just don't want to tell you why I told him (*they all laugh*)

THERAPIST: (*turning to Dan*) Why doesn't she want to tell me?

DAN: She's embarrassed.

THERAPIST: Is she embarrassed for herself, for you, or for both of you?

DAN: Both of us . . . I have been working through some bizarre sickness where I would get sexually turned on by things Sarah did with other men. I started making love to her the first night she was there, and I started interrogating her. The first half of her sexual encounter was then revealed to me. A couple of nights later, when I was doing the same thing, the rest of the sexual encounter was revealed to me. So, after I had an orgasm, even though I got off on it in fantasy, the reality would set in and I became like a crazy man. I don't remember feeling so betrayed in my life, and fucked over. I felt very much in love with her, but I felt this is what's going to happen with this girl. Every time I go away, she's going to fuck someone else. All these things came up in me. The feeling of the "mother figure" in my life not being there when I needed her. That night put me through so much agony, and she was out getting fucked! That, on top of the guilt I felt for having gotten off on the experience, was the beginning of a number of problems sexually which we've had.

SARAH: Now I wish I hadn't told him.

THERAPIST: Something that worked for both of you sexually turned terrible that night.

SARAH: Because it was *reality*.

THERAPIST: You must have had the feeling when you told him that this was part of a sexual game you had been evolving that pleased both of you, and you were shocked when it wasn't.

SARAH: Yeah, during sex he'd say, "What did you do?" over and over again. I tried not to tell him, but he'd say, "Tell me, tell me," and he'd make it that I'd *want* to tell him because he'd get really turned on. Afterwards, he'd hate me, after he had an orgasm. I'd be lying there, and he'd push me away, and I'd think, Why did I tell him?

THERAPIST: Do you mean this one time? Or in the past, when you would tell him?

SARAH: I'd tell him things I did before I met him. He'd have that reaction a little bit, but . . .

DAN: It all began one night when we both knew I'd be going away. We got coke and danced. We went back to my apartment, and she told me she'd once slept with two men. That fantasy had never occurred to me in my sexual existence as a man. I got very into it, and I proceeded to always want that to happen.

SARAH: It started when we were making love and Dan asked, "Let's get Ruthie—my roommate—to come in, too." I said, "No, why don't we include a guy?" He was furious. I didn't really mean it. I just wanted to show him how it felt to have him ask to have another girl there. I just didn't want to get jealous. That's how it all started. He didn't like that at all.

DAN: Then I got off on it. I began to feel, Maybe she *deserves* two men; she's a beautiful girl. Eventually I got over the effects of that incident, when she really had screwed someone else.

THERAPIST: (*to Sarah*) How long were you with him in California? How did you spend your time?

SARAH: It was nice not having to work, being taken care of. But it wasn't great for my career. Then we were getting along well, after you got over it.

DAN: But it was always gnawing at me—the *pain* of it.

SARAH: But every time in bed he asked me to talk about the same thing.

DAN: That's why I can't . . . justify my pain or anger. I not only induced it but unconsciously encouraged it.

SARAH: I feel that.

THERAPIST: You encouraged her to do that . . . that one night. So what's confusing you both is, even after the pain, it still became something that worked between you sexually but made a terrible rift between you emotionally. It works in bed, but not out of bed.

DAN: It still does.

THERAPIST: Still . . .

SARAH: Him wanting me to sleep with other guys.

THERAPIST: Wanting her to do it in reality?

DAN: Yeah, with me there.

THERAPIST: Have you done it? . . . How was it for each of you?

DAN: We were on coke and totally numb. It was very exciting, sexually weird and fun in a dark, secret, sexual way. It felt strange, since we see the guy often. But it wasn't that bad, since he never made love to her. He was too stoned to get it up. But we did . . . please her a great deal. She had a lot of fun. But it was the same type of thing. It caused tremendous excitement in bed and difficulty out of it.

THERAPIST: A big aftershock.

SARAH: I didn't want to do it at the beginning of the night. I said, "No coke, no sex." I took a stand. But he got so determined, I knew I had to get away from him that night, otherwise something would happen.

THERAPIST: Because when he is very determined, his will is stronger than your will?

SARAH: Yes. I feel that. He's so persistent. I want to do it so he'll stop bothering me. And I knew he was in that mood. I thought, What am I going to do to get him not to want to be with me that night, or maybe ever? I felt totally trapped, confused. I wanted to get away. So I told a lie. I said, "I'm seeing someone else." He asked me, "Are you sleeping with him?" I said, "Yes." He freaked out and punched me in the stomach. While he was hitting me, a guy on the street told him to stop, and he went to call the cops. I thought, Oh my God, I have to get Dan away from this. I don't want the police to get him. So we went to do coke, and I said, "I don't want to do any." And then he talked me into getting dressed in black lace stockings and gloves, makeup, and a really tight black dress.

THERAPIST: How did he talk you into it when it was not what you wanted? Or was your mood changing?

SARAH: After he hit me, I was upset. And then we laughed about it. I didn't want not to be with him. I was upset, and I wanted him to be normal. Somehow, I started losing my will. I remember I was feeling really angry, but not strong enough to say, I'm not going to do this, and go home. And he got me to dress up. I said no, but he talked me into it. We go to this place and he wants it to be Ralph. He tells me to flirt with him. I say no. But finally we come back to Dan's apartment, and I say to Ralph, "I don't want to do this," and he said, "I don't either," but Dan had more will than both of us put together. He wanted it so badly, nothing was going to stop him. We must have wanted it a little bit, but if it wasn't for Dan it *definitely* wasn't going to happen.

THERAPIST: (*to Dan*) Do you experience yourself as bending people to your will?

DAN: When I want something, nothing stops me. That's why I've been a success in this business. But I misuse it.

THERAPIST: When you're in that mood, is there anything she could do to turn your will around? She thinks not.

DAN: No, there's not. It's up to me.

SARAH: Just to leave, be strong enough to go.

THERAPIST: If you're with him, you're with him on his terms. The only way to reset the terms is if you actually leave?

SARAH: Otherwise the whole night is a war. We're *at* each other: No! Yes! I say, Forget it, it's not worth the fight.

DAN: Yeah, but she said in the middle of that night, "I don't know why I fought you. This is what I wanted, too." I don't think that I'm this Charles Manson type character, hypnotizing people into what they want. There's something in Sarah, too.

THERAPIST: (*to Sarah*) You must have thought about that. That some part of you wants to do it. What is it that he wants from you, that part of you wants to do?

SARAH: Like that other night. The idea of sleeping with two men, that's nice. You get a lot of attention. It's doing coke, having him angry at me after it's over. I like sleeping with two men, except it bothers me that *he* wants me to. The two men is sort of intriguing.

THERAPIST: So how did that experience and the sexual motif between you lead to the kind of problems that brought you here and seem insurmountable?

SARAH: After that happened, he was totally distant and cold. I felt totally abandoned. I felt he wanted it *so* badly. He was going to get it. And then he HATED me for it. I couldn't take it for him to be that different. That's when we broke up.

DAN: There is definitely something in me. I've been in therapy before. I'm quite aware that I have a very empty part of my personality because I got very little attention from my father. I had to compensate by being this overachiever, because of this lack of male affection. I've wondered if I'm working out homosexual tendencies vicariously through her. Or is it that I'm willing to take what Sarah wants anyway to its fullest extreme? A little of both. She has a *tremendous* need for male affection . . . She says she didn't flirt with that guy that night when I asked her to. That's true, but she has since flirted with that guy when I didn't want it to happen.

SARAH: After that night, I felt close to that guy. I wanted to talk to him.

DAN: Which, she knows, makes me upset. But she does it anyway. I try to block it out, but I don't think it's fair play.

SARAH: He says, "Flirt with him *now*," and then I flirt. Another night, he says, no, I can't. I don't want him to have such control.

THERAPIST: You want to feel that, if there's a game you both play, there should be two script writers. (*to Dan*) When she wants to write the scene, you feel there's something unfair about that.

DAN: I wish I never had this problem. Then Sarah got pregnant and had an abortion. That was probably the most traumatic experience I've ever had on this earth as a man. It was certainly traumatic for her.

SARAH: Dan said, "I want you to have my baby. Our genes are good for each other." What happened made me feel that what he said and what he felt were two different things, when it really came down to it.

THERAPIST: (*to Sarah*) So, for you, it felt like the sex game. He wanted you to play this with him, but the reality had a different meaning. Was this a baby you wanted?

SARAH: No, but I wanted him to want it, to want *me* and it. To prove to me that he really meant it, not just saying it. I'm happy that I don't have a baby, but . . .

DAN: The sexual fantasy was in bed every night after the abortion.

SARAH: One of the reasons he didn't want me to have the baby was that he couldn't say any of those things to me in bed when I was pregnant. He was so nice and gentle towards me because I was pregnant.

THERAPIST: Did you like the lovemaking better this other way?

SARAH: Yes, and I liked *him* better.

DAN: After the abortion, I'd been out of work for 3 months. I had a very good chance to get the lead in a Broadway show. I supported both of us. Sarah wasn't working. We were living extravagantly. Then one night I was preparing for this Broadway audition; it was the third callback. I wanted to go to bed early and work on my script. So I pulled the same shit. I fucked her, got off on my fantasy, and rolled over to work on my script.

SARAH: I felt very unhappy and used. I went into the bathroom and cried. I felt he didn't care about me.

DAN: I had this audition primarily on my mind. So she went out dancing, did cocaine, slept with someone else, and didn't come home. I thought, Oh my God, what happened? I called her sister because I was so worried.

THERAPIST: Worried that she had betrayed you sexually, or that something had happened to her?

DAN: That something had happened. She would have called me. She knows I worry. But she was very involved with that other guy. But her sister laughed at me. That put me in a violent state of mind. I had a rough childhood. She called later and lied about where she was. Then she called to say she had lied. I was infuriated. I hadn't slept. When she showed up at 10 AM, I threw her out. But, again, at the door, she seduced me into getting off on her having fucked this other guy, which I DID, and then I became even more angry, and kicked her out.

SARAH: I did it because I had to do something so bad, that he'd break up with me.

THERAPIST: You didn't feel you could leave on your own two feet?

SARAH: No, I couldn't just say, Dan, I don't want to break up, but I have to for myself—because his will is . . .

DAN: When I came home that afternoon, she was lying in my bed.

SARAH: I got so freaked out, I had no place to go. I'd been kicked out and I was totally alone, thinking, How could he kick me out? I live here, too. I regretted what I did, so I went back.

DAN: I said, Forget this, I've been totally fucked over. So I threw her out again. I didn't care. How could she do this the night before my big audition, and she does this to me. I feel like such a victim!

The story this couple tells invites a variety of readings. Least familiar to family therapists, but crucial to my understanding of Sarah's and Dan's experience, is a psychoanalytic reading of the transformation of bonding into bondage, which is at the core of the couple's narrative. In this regard, the classic work of Massud Khan (1979) and more recently of Jessica Benjamin (1988) inform my point of view.

Another equally essential psychoanalytic perspective is to be found in Robert Stoller's (1979) deliciously nasty take on sexual excitement as the eroticization of hostility. By arguing that "good sex" is good precisely because it is *bad*, that is, "dirty," sinful, and sexily hostile, Stoller lifts sex out of the transcendent realm and puts it back in the gutter. This brings all of us morally and psychically closer to the couple in question, which is what makes their story, for all its painful absurdity, surprisingly erotic.

It "works" pornographically because, in its sheer extravagance, it demonstrates how the eroticization of gender clichés remains fundamental to sexual passion. Dan's and Sarah's gendered, sexualized scripts reciprocate so that his male training in forbidden looking meshes with her female knowledge of herself as someone who is secretly to allow what she must appear to forbid. Given their competitive natures, the ad might read: MALE VOYEUR SEEKS FEMALE EXHIBITIONIST FOR CONTROL GAME. Given the elements of circularity in this game-without-end, the copy could also be reversed: FEMALE EXHIBITIONIST SEEKS MALE VOYEUR.

The "game" metaphor is important here because the problem, as it emerges in the session, is not the sex game itself but the collapse of the distinction between the game and the reality. Inside the frame of "play," the mutual debasement of the sex game "worked," in Stoller's (1979) sense. The hostility that drives the erotic impulse, he argues, is an attempt, repeated over and over, to undo the childhood traumas and frustrations that threatened the development of one's masculinity and femininity. Since these patients were not in analysis, it is not possible to reconstruct the historic origins of their gendered vulnerabilities (except to add a crucial piece of Sarah's history that, when she was 3 years old, her father caught her mother in bed with another man and promptly divorced her).

However, even without the analytically retrieved early material, Dan and Sarah's sex script seems written for Stoller (1979). It contains all the dramatic elements he lists that, when stitched together, produce a surge of sexual excitement, hostility, mystery, risk, illusion, revenge, reversal of trauma, and dehumanization of the other. Looking only at the reciprocal processes of objectification in the sex play, it is easy to see how the game could provide a pseudosolution for the narcissistically damaging aspects of their relationship.

For Dan, the game reversed the narcissistic injury of his sense of sexual exclusion and masculine insufficiency (maybe she DESERVES two men; she's a beautiful girl). As long as Sarah was *his* object to dominate and possess, he could transform his sexual humiliation into a sexual triumph by putting himself into the scene as the pornographic director, pacing the action for his maximum arousal and release.

For Sarah, the game was her only starring role, the one sphere in which she was figure and he was ground. In the real world, she was an unemployed, untrained unknown, tenuously attached to a working actor who was 10 years her senior and one callback away from a major Broadway or film role. But in bed, she could reverse the humiliation of her invisibility and marginality. There, it was Dan who was both the debased groupie and the enraptured audience, and it was Sarah whose every move filled the screen.

So what was the problem? If the sex provided a playful counterpoint to some of the painful realities of their situation, why did it lose its playfulness, take on a life of its own, and ultimately take over the relationship?

I think the game turned grim and pathological for a number of reasons. Going back to its beginnings, well before Sarah took the first step in making it "real," we can see that, for Dan, the masculine fragility that made the game necessary also made it impossible for him, even then, to protect the boundary between play and reality and between past and present. Once his orgasm subsided, he had no way to protect his masculine and sexual self-esteem from the threat of Sarah's sexual past, so that she, who a moment before had been his sexual playmate, then became the object of his hatred.

Dan's inability to use sex playfully and reparatively demonstrates the complex structuring of sexual excitement. Again, in Stoller's (1979) terms, passion requires a sense of mystery and secrecy. The secret is the knowledge, held in one part of the mind, that the erotic story is contrived, that the daydream is manufactured, that the partner is pretending. One part of oneself must know the script is an illusion so that the experience is safely under control, while another part must operate as if it does not know the secret. This is the part that convinces the genitals that the story is real. But when excitement subsides, the secret is out and the illusion ends, and the truth can bring disgust, lethargy, and estrangement. Given Dan's narcissistic frailty, there was no transitional space between spheres. He was either on one side of the looking glass or the other.

But even if Dan were not handicapped by his exaggerated sense of masculine inadequacy, the game was bound to be corrupted. This is because, once the game was used to solve the problem of power in the relationship, it could no longer be "recreational." Control of sex became a metaphor for control of the relationship.

Framing the problem in these terms sets the stage for another kind of commentary, one informed by the systemic perspective. A systems reading of Sarah's and Dan's dilemma would begin with Haley's (1963) presumption that they, like all couples, were involved in one primary struggle—a contest for power over who defines the relationship. Establishing who's in charge, and of what, takes many forms: Who will dominate? Who will be taken care of? Under what circumstances? How openly will the couple compete for position? and so on.

When conceptualizing the issues involved in establishing the balance of power in a relationship, I have found Bateson's (1958) distinction between "complementary" and "symmetrical" power arrangements to be consistently useful. As a quick reminder, in complementary relationships, each partner exchanges "opposite" behavior, so that if one is "up," the other is "down." Gender divisions are inherently complementary, so if he is "logical" she must be "emotional," if he is "strong" she must be "weak," and so forth. In symmetrical relationships, the partners exchange the same type of behavior, so that both give orders, both try to get taken care of, and so on.

Each of these arrangements has its consequences. In a complementary division of labor, the couple operates to maximize differences and minimize (*overt*) competition. Each partner appears to provide what the other lacks, in what constitutes the yin/yang view of the gender dichotomy. The other side of the truth, of course, is that, eventually, neither can understand the other's experience.

In a symmetrical division of labor, differences are minimized, since both partners want the same thing. But, while they may understand each other better, they must also compete more ferociously, since only one of them can occupy a particular position (giving the orders, being taken care of) at a particular time.

Sarah's and Dan's relationship, like most couples', can be conceptualized as containing a mix of complementary and symmetrical elements. What we shall try to understand is how the sex game, which began as a complementary equalizer, became transformed into a symmetrical, escalating battleground for control of the relationship as a whole. In slowing down their sequence, I shall try to map the means whereby sex became power and bonding turned to bondage. Given the conditions of male domination under which all men and women in our culture fall in love and have sex, my discussion will focus on how Sarah's participation can be understood as simultaneously a form of resistance to and collusion with the structure of patriarchal romance.

Let us begin our analysis of this extravagant and painful relationship by locating the protagonists in hierarchical space. This will require stretching Bateson's (1958) circular view of complementarity to include the idea that the positions of up and down are not strictly a matter of perspective, which means that they are not necessarily eternally reversible. Many social hierarchies are inscribed in the social order and cannot be changed until the world changes. These include age, sex, and class hierarchies.

For this couple, comparing their social position in the world at large, Dan is up and Sarah is down. He is 10 years her senior, a man well launched in his acting career and capable of earning "good money." Sarah is a young woman, barely out of adolescence, with no training, no professional contacts or role models other than her boyfriend, and no money.

Moving the lens in closer and looking at the organization of their relationship, another unequal but complementary organization comes into focus. This involves their division of emotional labor. In the terms of their system, Dan is figure while Sarah is ground; Dan is subject while Sarah is faciliating environment:

> SARAH: I just lose myself [in romantic relationships]. If I . . . didn't have anyone to concern myself with, . . . I'd be . . . so miserable that I'd be *forced* to go out into the world.
> DAN: There's . . . a tremendous value in having a security blanket . . . in this very turbulent entertainment business.

Sarah is tending the relationship; Dan is being tended. For him, the relationship *is* a security blanket, where love facilitates work. For Sarah, love compromises work; she must choose one or the other.

> DAN: I have a lot invested in Sarah. . . . dependency and selfish need. . . . Weekends suited me because it would still keep me in contact with this need. . . . It's very hard to be with me. . . . I'm very high when I'm working, very low when I'm not. I take it out on who I'm with.
> SARAH: If Dan is in a bad mood, I don't even exist. . . . The whole weekend, there's a weight on me.

Dan's primary relationship is with his career. When he is working, he is happily obsessed, when he's not he's morbidly preoccupied. Sarah's subjectivity is not a part of their relationship. Dan's *defines* it. To find herself, she must leave him. If she leaves, it is not "her" he has lost, but the "need satisfier" that he can keep contact with on weekends.

What is sad and interesting about this arrangement is that, looking back, we can see that things were not always so skewed. This standard gendered arrangement of male subject and female facilitator evolved out of a more genuinely reciprocal exchange. Indeed, in the early phases of their relationship, we can find evidence of a fragile mutuality—the provision of reparative empathy and mutual idealization:

> DAN: Sarah helped me find [valuable qualities] in myself. . . . I feel more intellectually capable now, and that had a lot to do with her.
> SARAH: He was so different from anyone I'd met. . . . He really listened. . . . I could tell him almost anything. . . . There was no pressure to be normal.

But the language, even early on, betrays their tendency to subvert reparative empathy into exhibitionism, voyeurism, and domination. Let's look first at the way in which both partners "misuse" Sarah's empathy:

DAN: What drew me to her is she has a tremendous intellect . . . I
was physically attracted, but that wasn't the most important
thing. She was someone who understood *pain* in a very intelligent way. . . . She has tremendous insight into life itself.

As Sarah articulated Dan's pain, he felt freer to idealize it and then to
idealize her as the vehicle through which his morbidity was to be elevated.
It eventually became an ideal unto itself.

DAN: I wouldn't . . . go to the movies and have fun. I'd just want to
sit and brood.

And for Sarah's side, we can see, even in the session, how she protects
Dan's self-esteem at the cost of the truth and of her own narcissism:

SARAH: He fell in love with me first (*laughs*). No. . . . It's a drag [to be
with him when he wants to brood]. That's a mean thing to say.

Looking now at the subversion of Dan's empathy, we can begin with
Sarah's memory of that early period.

SARAH: I could tell him almost anything, and he wouldn't be shocked.
Any fantasy, any weird thing I would want to do. Anything I'd
done. . . . [Like] getting up and dancing around.

Dan's acceptance of her playful, body-exuberant narcissism became transformed by both of them into material for sexploitation, so that his
provision of a "maternal environment" became voyeuristic, and her self-
expression became exhibitionistic. A motive for her can be found in the
line, "Sometimes he doesn't seem there, and I feel like shaking him."
What had been, for a short while, a reciprocal arrangement of
positions, each being a subject to the other's empathic, appreciative mirror, became a rigid, mutually objectifying process. Sarah eventually cooperated in becoming a sexual object, and Dan ultimately transformed
himself into the split-off, dissociated voyeur that Khan (1979) and Benjamin (1985) write about so evocatively. As Benjamin puts it, "The male
posture, whether assumed by all men or not, prepares for the role of
master. He is disposed to objectify and control the other . . . in order to
deny his dependency. The female posture disposes the woman to accept
objectification and control in order to flee separation . . . (the experience
of) aloneness and self-assertion. He asserts individual selfhood, while she
relinquishes it" (p. 63).
This mutual process of alienation of the experience of self and other
was already in place in Sarah's and Dan's description of the height of their

romantic period, where performance had already replaced personal experience. In describing their "best time," they recalled:

> DAN: I was on Broadway. You saw me act the part of that guy in love.
> SARAH: That was the best, when we'd write songs together in clubs and perform together.

Situated in this emotional and social context, it is not surprising that the threat of separation could destabilize the couple's fragile equilibrium. Moreover, although they don't think about it in these terms, once Dan had left for California, the power differential between the two lovers became even more exaggerated, which added to the strain. Dan was in California shooting a movie. Sarah was left in New York with nothing particular to do and without any money, not even enough to call him when she wanted to. Dan's calls, framed as "reassurance," were actually a means of controlling her. By calling her twice a day, he prevented her from being and feeling alone.

Dan's control strategy works. Sarah remembered feeling relieved when Dan first left, thinking, "Okay, maybe it'll be better for me, . . . good for me to be alone, to know myself better." But instead, Dan insinuated himself into her solitude so that everything in her mind and life became geared to *her* one big scene: "Getting off the Plane":

> SARAH: All the time he was gone I lost 20 pounds, for *him*. All I could think of was exercising so I could look really good when I got off the plane for *him*.

Sarah was no longer a subject in search of herself, but had transformed herself into a subject-as-object.

This construction of Muriel Dimen's (1986) captures the truth of Sarah's situation: "Women are not men's slaves, but they know, as subjects, that they are treated as objects, into which they must sometimes also transform themselves" (p. 5). For Sarah, this knowledge organized her will and became her subjectivity.

Sarah's one form of rebellion (not independence) was to fuck someone else. She struck a defiant tone in the interview, saying, "I don't feel that guilty about it," but, in truth, Sarah was compliant, even in her rebellion. Her behavior was no more than a pseudoindependent act already cast in terms of the game. She did not try to free herself from Dan by devoting herself to theater classes, auditions, or even some form of structured self-observation like therapy. Also, as she revealed by way of proving her "good faith," she was thinking of Dan all the way through her one-night stand, not her lover or herself!

Finally, we can see this act as Sarah's move from complementarity to symmetry, since it contains a competitive impulse. She had to know Dan would "catch" her, since he had said he'd call at 10 that night. She also was, even if she was unaware of the feeling, chafing against his control and her obsession with his affirmation. So part of her motive was to derail him, just as she had been derailed. For that one night and part of the next day, Sarah had arranged it so that Dan would be thinking of her—not only when he felt like it, like at night, at a club, or when he was into seduction, but when he was trying to sleep, or rehearse, or hang out with his friends.

In objectifying her subjectivity by acting out her resistance to Dan within his categories, Sarah lost her personal voice and "spoke" only in Dan's language. We saw this in an earlier stage of the game, when Dan insulted and challenged her during sex by saying, "Let's get your room-mate." Sarah countered, "Why don't we include a guy." In talking to me, she explained, "I didn't really mean it. I just wanted to show him how it felt to have him ask to have another girl there." Instead of giving voice to her own particular experience of Dan's request, Sarah mimicked him in order to make her point. And this was how their game went. Ultimately, this escalating mimicry became a dangerous "game without end."

It is also important to see in this anecdote that there was already a presumption of differential entitlement to narcissistic protection from sexual or gender injury in this couple. When Sarah mimicked Dan by suggesting they get another man, he got furious. Dan's freedom to hide his masculine vulnerability in rage, and rage about being reminded of his vulnerability, once again constituted him as the subject and star of this melodrama. Sarah's form of self-expression was restricted to analogy.

Sarah's use of her sexuality as a substitute for speech and independent action is to be found again in the incident that Dan remembers as starting the game:

> DAN: It all began one night when we both knew I'd be going away. We got coke . . . and she told me she'd once slept with two men.

Here, one can speculate that the impending separation, which threatened each of them in different ways, created the need for a ritual and the sex play provided the material.

For Sarah, we can imagine that Dan's leaving her in order to do a Hollywood movie trampled on her narcissism. It shattered the illusion of the romantic twinship—of the two songwriting performers on their way to the top—and dumped her back into the reality of being a 21-year-old untrained, unemployed unknown. Her only remaining forum for stardom was sexual, with Dan cast as her enraptured audience. So she used her exhibitionism, which until then had been a shared activity with Dan, *against* him, to put him in his place. She let him know she had been a star *before* she knew him, a sex star, with two *other* men adoring her.

For Dan, we can say that Sarah's revelation, to borrow Stoller's telling metaphor about the sudden, unexpected ways that eros strikes, "stabbed him with excitement" (1979, p. 15).

> DAN: That fantasy had never occurred to me in my sexual existence as a man. . . . I proceeded to always want that to happen. . . . I began to feel, Maybe she *deserves* two men; she's a beautiful woman.

A process unfolded by which Dan turned humiliation to triumph. What he described as a fantasy that had never occurred to him in his sexual existence as a male was in truth not fantasy. It was fact, and it was two *other* men who had slept with *his* lover. By proceeding to "always want that to happen" in bed, Dan got Sarah to undo his sexual exclusion and emasculation. By casting himself as a slave of love, he orchestrated his humiliation and sexual subjugation ("maybe she *deserves* two men") and, via his erotic domination, neutralized his enemies, since he was then directing a pornographic scene starring his girlfriend and a couple of extras.

Beyond the sexual repair of his masculinity, we can see the fantasy as also solving the separation problem generally. Dan did not want to suffer what he called "the mother figure in my life not being there when I needed her," so he arranged it so that Sarah would always be at the other end of a phone line. Since his calls were framed as reassurance that Sarah was still his sexual ideal, Dan could deny the humiliation of his dependency and *his* need for reassurance—reassurance that he would not be abandoned.

At that point, the mutual, symmetrically competitive uses of the sex game were in place and each subsequent move would inspire a counter-move in a dangerous, escalating spiral. The next move took place when Sarah arrived in California. Dan wanted to play the game again, to reassure himself and reestablish to her that she belonged to him. Sarah had a sexual secret but could not resist telling him, since her sexual potency was her only source of self-assertion, power, and revenge in the relationship:

> SARAH: I tried not to tell him, but . . . he'd make it that I'd *want* to tell him because he'd get really turned on.

But the problem that the sex game was supposed to solve was not solved, because once the erotic spell was broken Dan had to face the reality of Sarah's betrayal, and with it the realization that he truly could not control her, no matter how hard he tried:

DAN: So, after I had an orgasm, even though I got off on it in fantasy, the reality would set in and I became like a crazy man. . . . I felt very much in love with her, but I felt this is what's going to happen with this girl. Every time I go away, she's going to fuck someone else.

Since Sarah's escalation was "real," it could not be symbolically nullified by being taken into their bed. But we also know that Dan's narcissism was sufficiently damaged that he could not even tolerate the knowledge of Sarah's having any sexual past that did not include him:

SARAH: I'd tell him things I did before I met him. He'd have that reaction. . . . He'd hate me, after he'd had an orgasm. I'd be lying there, and he'd push me away.

If Dan was compelled to rewrite Sarah's sexual history every time they made love, then how would he undo the actual exclusion of her sleeping with another man now that he *was* in her life? This could only be done by a symmetrical escalation:

DAN: It was always gnawing at me, the *pain* of it.
SARAH: But every time in bed he asked me to talk about the same thing.

Clearly, it was no longer sufficient for Dan to reestablish his authority by controlling Sarah via an *acted in* sexual fantasy, the "talking game" in bed. Since Sarah had *acted out* the scene without him, in the real world, Dan's next move was inevitable. He had to cast and direct the scene himself, in the real world. Sarah, however, was ready with a countermove. Interestingly, once again she could only assert her subjectivity and her will not to play Dan's game on Dan's terms:

SARAH: I didn't want to do it, . . . but he got so determined, I knew I had to get away from him that night. . . . I thought, What am I going to do to get him not to want to be with me that night, or maybe ever? . . . So I told a lie. I said, "I'm seeing someone else." He asked me, "Are you sleeping with him?" I said, "Yes."

What was significant about Sarah's escalation was that not only had the categories of play and reality been corrupted by the struggle for control, but even the distinction between lies and truth had lost its meaning. This bizarre escalation was constructed out of the revelation that Sarah had slept with another man even though Dan had *not* gone away (one step worse than his worst fear), only it was *not true*.

We can see the reasons for this "fraudulent" maneuver in Sarah's view of her options. Both she and Dan agreed that, in a direct battle of wills, Dan would prevail. Sarah's only alternative to submission was to leave the field, which, because of her gendered commitment to romantic attachment, she could not do without the help of therapy. As she scanned for a way out, she could only think of how she could get Dan to reject her. The idea that *she* could walk out was not even in her thinking.

Given his resolve, her passivity, and their proclivity for erotic solutions, it is not surprising that they eventually acted out an oedipal drama in which no one was excluded. As could be expected, for Sarah this attempt to repair the oedipal catastrophe of her mother's indiscretion (which led to her father's precipitous departure when Sarah was age 3) turned out no better. Dan, when the night was over, once again constituted himself the victim of Sarah's sexual potency and emotionally abandoned her:

> SARAH: After that happened, he was totally distant and cold. I felt totally abandoned. . . . He wanted it *so* badly . . . and then he *hated* me for it.

With the sex drama having taken over their lives and their relationship, Sarah's next move was the ultimate bid for control. She began to compete for authorship of the script:

> SARAH: The idea of sleeping with two men, that's nice. . . . It bothers me that *he* wants me to. . . . I don't want him to have such control.
>
> DAN: She didn't flirt with that guy that night when I asked her to. . . . but she has since flirted with that guy when I didn't want it to happen . . . which, she knows, makes me upset. But she does it anyway . . . I don't think it's fair play.

At this point, we can say that there was no longer even an analogical separation between sex and power. The struggle for control over the definition of the sex game *was* the struggle for control of the relationship. Fantasy had lost all its interiority. What was once repressed or suppressed had become spoken, acted-in, and acted out, and it eventually absorbed the protagonists and some innocent bystanders, including a fetus. The destruction of boundaries led to a circumstance where Dan wanted the fetus aborted so that he could continue to live out his fantasy, and Sarah, who said she didn't want the baby for itself, still wanted it because it represented external proof of her value to Dan as an object of desire.

> SARAH: I wanted him to want [the baby], to want *me* and it. . . . I'm happy that I don't have a baby.

In the final sequence, we can see all the elements in the competition playing out at fast-forward. Dan has to restore his authority after Sarah started up a friendship with the other man in their one-night trio, so he played the talking sex game with her while preparing for a Broadway audition:

> DAN: I pulled the same shit. I fucked her, got off on my fantasy, and rolled over to work on my script.

Then it was Sarah who was jolted out of the erotic spell by the insult of being nothing more than a 5-minute study break. She retaliated with the next possible escalation: acting out the drama of betraying and excluding him in reality, in the present, while he was in town, and on the night before his big audition. (She also made sure he got no sleep by calling twice in the middle of the night.) Thus, Dan was finally provoked into ending the game, a step Sarah could not take:

> SARAH: I had to do something so bad, that he'd break up with me.

But even then Sarah couldn't let go. Using Dan's strategy, she stopped him from kicking her out the next morning by eroticizing her betrayal. She seduced him right at the door into getting off on it. Dan lost his resolve, fucked her, and then, in the aftershock, flew into a rage and kicked her out. Somehow, as was always the case between them, Dan got the last word and managed to claim for himself the victim position.

> DAN: How could she do this [to me] the night before my big audition? . . . I feel like such a victim!

Because this is a chapter about sexual passion and power, and not about therapy, I will not discuss at length how my colleague, Jorge Colapinto, and I treated this case.* Suffice it to say, we considered the couple's erotic struggles to be a melodramatic diversion from the central issues in each of their lives. Most significant was the fact that Sarah (which we learned in the second session) had run away from home at the age of 14. In the wake of her semibreak up with Dan, she had, for the first time in 8 years, moved back in with her mother. By elevating the importance of the newly evolving mother–daughter relationship, we helped the couple move toward a more face-saving separation, or as Dan had asked for in the first session, a "creative separation."

---

*While the therapy was partly conducted by Jorge Colapinto and myself, only I was present during the initial interview.

The following short excerpt from the end of the second session illustrates how we positioned ourselves in relation to this couple, in order to shift their center of gravity.

THERAPIST (Colapinto): You, Dan, would like this therapy to work so that you and Sarah can remain a couple, so that Sarah will stay. You, Sarah, want this therapy to work so that you can leave without his being angry at you, and so that you can have a friendly goodbye. (*They both nod.*)

THERAPIST (Goldner to Colapinto): It just occurs to me now, Jorge, that if Sarah were to choose Dan she would be leaving her mother alone again after all these years.

SARAH: (*nodding*) She feels obligated to take me back because she feels so guilty.

THERAPIST (Goldner): What does she feel guilty about?

SARAH: Because our family, for the second time broke up when I was 14, and I ran away from home. I had to take care of myself, but I really wasn't grown up at all. I was a kid.

THERAPIST (Goldner to Colapinto): So you see, by coming back she gives her mother a chance to repair this, and if she chooses to move back in with Dan, she deprives her mother of the chance to make up for all that lost time between the ages of 14 and 21.

DAN: And I could be in the way of that. I could just be in the way. I'm *glad you said that*, because I feel less, uh, *angst* about the situation now that you said that I could be in the way of something that she's trying to complete with her mother. And that has nothing to do with me. I am *not* . . . I did wrong by her, I have hurt her badly and I've done a lot of things that are possibly irreparable. I don't know, that's what I'm trying to find out. But that aside, if I didn't do *anything*, if I was the greatest guy in the world, if I never hurt her once during the 3 years I've known her, I could still, possibly, just simply be in the way of her completing something with her mother, which I would have never thought of if you didn't make that point. And I appreciate that. I don't know if it's of any use to Sarah, but it's useful to me. . . . I think you're *onto* something that is bigger than both of us and our problems.

PERSONAL RESPONSES

Like many others of my generation (those who came of age in the 60s), this year—1988—invites reminiscence, reflection, and the inevitable comparison with that historic watershed year 1968. In my case, and in relation to this chapter, 20 years ago I was living in Cambridge, Massachusetts, having dropped out of graduate school in order (in the language of the period) "to work full-time in the women's movement." (This now quaint phrase captures the hidden truth of that revolutionary moment since "working full-time" did not refer, as it does now, to paid employment, and I have absolutely no idea how I supported myself in that heady year.) At any rate, my politics, even then, gravitated toward the written word and the psychological, and so I became involved in writing the chapter on sexuality for the original *Our Bodies, Our Selves* (Simon & Schuster, 1973).

I wrote then as a young woman in my twenties, claiming for my generation and my sex the right to define, assert, and interpret our own sexuality, which meant taking it back from the male-medical and psychiatric establishment. Now, as a middle-aged family therapist, I often meet young women like "Sarah" who could have been me back then. And I can't help but wonder whether the sexual freedom she now takes for granted (but which she owes to the militance of my generation) isn't bondage by another name. Sarah's mother, a woman of my age who chose sexual liberation over domestic security, ended up at 40 still preoccupied with sex and men and no better positioned financially and professionally than her 23-year-old daughter.

The lesson from history seems to be stark. Freedom to enjoy and elaborate the possibilities of a regressive experience like sex creates an illusion of potency that lasts only as long as the erotic moment. For Dan and Sarah, the illusion of sexual liberation masked the reality of their existential bondage, just as the apparent fluidity of their complementary positions masked the fixity of the underlying gender hierarchy.

These two young people are casualties of the sexual revolution that my generation fought to accomplish. Their freedom to pursue pleasure, fantasy, and variety is constrained by the structures of domination that organize their relationship and define the contours of their imagination. Their pleasure cannot be playful because it has become the medium through which their gendered struggle for power is enacted.

As long as sex is hyped-up as an expression of creativity, true love, emotional maturity, existential transcendence, political rebellion, or whatever other grandiose metaphor applies, and as long as we therapists somehow share the illusion that sex is larger than life, we will all collude in making Sarah and Dan's drama the only genre that can play. Unless the world becomes a fairer place, which will require confronting the disquieting truths about gender inequality, the use of sex to gain and maintain power will remain a central motif in all of our lives.

REFERENCES

Bateson, G. (1958). *Naven* (rev. ed.). Stanford, CA: Stanford University Press.

Benjamin, J. (1985). The bonds of love: Rational violence and erotic domination. In H. Eisenstein & A. Jardine (Eds.), *The future of difference* (pp. 41–70). New Brunswick, NJ: Rutgers University Press.

Benjamin, J. (1988). *The bonds of love: Psychoanalysis, feminism and the problem of domination.* New York: Pantheon.

Boston Women's Health Book Collective. (1973). *Our Bodies, Our Selves.* New York: Simon & Schuster.

Dimen, M. (1986). *Surviving sexual contradictions.* New York: Macmillan.

Haley, J. (1963). *Strategies of psychotherapy.* New York: Grune & Stratton.

Khan, M. (1979). *Alienation in perversions.* New York: International Universities Press.

Stoller, R. (1979). *Sexual excitement: The dynamics of erotic love.* New York: Pantheon.

3

THROUGH A GLASS BRIGHTLY: TREATING SEXUAL INTIMACY AS THE RESTORATION OF THE WHOLE PERSON

Michael D. Kahn

It was dusk. The apartment was empty except for the two of them. As they lay entwined in a warm embrace, this room, this bed, was the universe. Aside from the faint sounds of their tranquil breathing, they were silent. She stroked the nape of his neck. He nuzzled her erect nipple, first gently with his nose, then licked it, tasted, smelled and absorbed her body odor. It was a hot and humid August day, and they had been perspiring. Slowly he caressed her one breast as he softly rolled his face over the contours of the other. He pressed his body close against her, sighed, and, fully spent, closed his eyes and soon fell into a deep, satisfying sleep. Ever so slowly she slipped herself out from under him, lest she disturb him, cradled him in her arms, and moved him to his crib. Having completed his 6 o'clock feeding, the 4-month-old had also experienced one more minute contribution to his further sexual development.*

In 1905, Freud stated, "No one who has seen a baby sinking back satiated from the breast and falling asleep with flushed cheeks and a blissful smile can escape the reflection that this picture persists as a prototype of the expression of sexual satisfaction in later life" (p. 182).

Michael D. Kahn. Department of Psychology, University of Hartford, West Hartford, Connecticut; Department of Psychiatry, University of Connecticut School of Medicine, Farmington, Connecticut.

*The original author of this paragraph is unknown, but grateful acknowledgment is made to Paul Reid and Sandra Scantling, who made it available to me.

These opening quotations illustrate what is both obvious and elusive to most people: the human yearning for a sensual experience which reinvokes the sexual satisfaction previously experienced in infancy. For too many adults, such experiences occur infrequently or are lost or obliterated in their sexually intimate relationships, whether they have one exclusive partner or many partners. While reading this passage, we can experience the moment-by-moment nature of sexual life—the sensual, immediate, and concrete sensations detached from outer concerns, consequences, history, or future. What we cannot experience is the awareness the participants have of each other's psychological being, how each appreciates the dialectical interchange between them. The baby, a boy, is active—taking, feeding, domineering whereas the mother is passive—giving, existing as an object for the other. The surprise element is, of course, the abrupt shift in our understanding of the passage: What first appears to be a description of two adult lovers is in fact one of a mother and an infant.

I believe that this admittedly and purposefully titillating passage illustrates the central dilemma of sexual relatedness in the human species. We all begin life as self-centered creatures, seeking only self-gratifying experiences, taking for granted the caretaker and expecting that person to be loving, always available, satisfying, and capable of meeting our biologically driven needs for excitement, soothing, sensory stimulation, and attachment. Yet, adult sexuality is often flawed by the inability of two individuals seeking self-satisfaction to mutually satisfy each other.

As a therapist, I find it unusual for any couple, regardless of their presenting complaints, to have a perennially stable, always mutually satisfying sex life. Although such notable sex therapists as Masters and Johnson (1966, 1970), Kaplan (1974, 1979), and Offit (1981) profess that such a mutually satisfying sex relationship is not difficult to obtain, it appears that millions of people cannot achieve it. Or, if they have such a relationship, they often lose it for a myriad of reasons such as external stress, boredom, habit destructiveness, insensivity, or internalized fears. A follow-up review of Masters and Johnson's pioneering study *Human Sexual Inadequacy*, in which an improvement rate of 80% among treated couples was reported has been called into serious question by Zilbergeld and Evans (1980). They cite numerous methodological flaws, reporting errors, and criteria confusion, and suggest that the symptom remission rate, given the special population and conditions involved, may have only approached 50% (and even that level was suspect).

What is missing? If we know what we want, why can't we have it? What goes wrong? What interferes with the important mother/child bonding or what replaces it? Is it necessarily true that much of what becomes elusive in the realm of adult sexuality has its origins in early childhood? With these questions in mind, this chapter will explore the theoretical concepts that have contributed to my integration of self psychology and family systems approaches to problems of sexual intimacy.

PROFESSIONAL BACKGROUND

Similar to most family therapists of my middle-aged generation, I was trained in individual models of psychotherapy based on traditional developmental, personality, psychopathology, and psychoanalytic theories. This training was augmented by an undergraduate major in English, a personal psychoanalysis, and a general education in psychology, all of which emphasized the self and the vicissitudes of personality formation.

During the late 1960s, when I was first introduced to the intriguing ideas of family systems theory held by Haley, Bateson, and Jackson, I became disenchanted with traditional psychoanalytic concepts, finding them rooted in a linear epistemology and a biologically deterministic framework which had little room for general system ideas and concepts from 20th-century social science. With the burgeoning of the family therapy literature and with training opportunities becoming richer and more available to clinicians, I, like many others, found systems therapy and psychoanalysis to be seemingly irreconcilable. Because they are conceptually and pragmatically of such variance, it was almost impossible to reconcile, much less integrate, the two perspectives.

By 1970, when I had begun to teach family therapy and provide training to other therapists, I was puzzled as to how to combine what I felt to be two rich ways of describing human experience: the world of the self and the world of the system. Nor was I particularly helped by my peers and mentors: Psychoanalysts ignored family therapy, family therapists mocked psychoanalysis, and neither group seemed to adequately describe how it treated people with sexual difficulties. (It would be tedious and distracting to summarize all of the descriptions of this tendentious split; simply stated, during the 70s, each group viewed the other as either simpleminded, arrogant, presumptious, immoral, or some combination of the above.)

THEORETICAL INFLUENCES

In the past two decades, many young and seasoned family therapists, who were hearing about sexual problems in their practices, remained ignorant of the huge conceptual advances taking place in psychoanalytic theorizing and practice. For too many of these family therapists, psychoanalytic thinking had been peremptorily written off. But psychoanalysis was no longer a monolithic entity. A serious split was occurring within psychoanalysis between the drive-dominated classical metapsychology of early Freud and his champions Fenichel, Jacobson, Brenner, and, some would say, Kernberg and the object-relations advocates of the more interpersonal psychology of later Freud, Sullivan, Hartman, Horney, Guntrip, and Fairbairn. The classical group emphasized instincts and a topological psychology of id, ego, and superego and ignored or totally subordinated the influence of external factors on the developing child's psyche. As Modell (1985) said, classical psychoanalysis offered us a one person psychology. The interpersonal view, referred to as a two person psychology by Modell, contained a more environmentally attuned developmental framework in which biological drives were gradually superseded or were, at the infant's birth, secondary to the child's primary need for a satisfying relationship with a gratifying object (i.e., person). Hence, the name "object relations" was used for this school of thought.

What was also occurring (and hopefully the reader will bear with this necessary, brief synopsis since its relevance to issues of sexuality will become readily apparent) was an examination of the fertile ground of preoedipal relations. Early parent–child relationships during the beginning stages of infancy had been explored in the controversial and seemingly outrageous writings of Melanie Klein in the 1920s, 1930s, and 1940s and were now being systematically and vigorously expanded by the epoch-making contributions of Margaret Mahler (1967, 1968) and her collaborators (Mahler, Pine, & Bergman, 1975).*

Separation–individuation was considered a central construct by Mahler, who emphasized the child's need during its first 3 years of life to emerge from a symbiotic phase of primary narcissism, in which fantasies of self and object are fused, to a more fully developed stable sense of the self. According to Mahler, the infant's most satisfactory movement toward individuation is buoyed by the inner representations of "an ordinary devoted mother" and cognitive representations or schemata of the vicissi-

---

*I am purposely limiting my exposition of certain psychoanalytic theorists to a few key concepts. For a more expanded exposition of the developmental emphasis in psychoanalytic metapsychology and the relevance of drive-dominated and object-relations concepts, the reader is urged to consult two excellent comprehensive sources, Greenberg and Mitchell's *Object Relations in Psychoanalytic Theory* (1983) and Eagle's *Recent Developments in Psychoanalysis: A Critical Evaluation* (1984).

tudes of the adaptive process by the child to that mother. Sexuality in the
child is seen as a biological given which propels the child to seek narcissistic gratification. This narcissistic gratification is sustained and organized
as a bodily and psychological experience for the infant primarily by the
mother, whose reliable presence helps neutralize overwhelming feelings
in the child and lays the groundwork for satisfying fantasies and more
elaborate inner representations.

Mahler's contributions encouraged me to begin thinking about just
how to adopt a soothing, comforting, "maternal" position toward adult
patients, particularly toward those—and there seemed to be many—who
could speak about their early deprivations of such comforting maternal
experience. Although unable, in the context of once-a-week psychotherapy, to significantly recall their experiences before the age of three, these
adults sufficiently described their parents' behavior during their child and
adolescent years to justify some retrospective deductions on my part about
what those earliest years actually entailed. Thus, I could begin seeing the
developmental shortcomings in these individuals' backgrounds by understanding their descriptions about current sexual intimacy. Their sexual
symptoms included chronic dissatisfaction with their partner, compulsive
needs to have sex or to win at the game of sexual dominance, perversions
or distortions of usual object choice, as well as such usual sexual dysfunctions as vaginismus, premature ejaculation, impotence, retarded ejaculation, and orgasmic inhibition. The link between problematic sexual symptoms and issues of maternal deprivation or disruptions in maternal
soothing seemed plausible; particularly because both are manifestations of
the need for an unbroken blending of self needs and other needs. When I
began to interpret judiciously along these lines to my patients, it seemed
to help eliminate some of these symptoms.

Two other figures loom large as seminal thinkers in the revisionism
of psychoanalysis in the 1970s: Donald Winnicott and Heinz Kohut.*
Their ideas play an important role in guiding my approach to dealing with
sexual problems. Winnicott (1958, 1965a, 1965b, 1971) wrote not only
about the importance of a constant maternal "holding environment," but
also about the emerging ability of the infant to tolerate being alone (an

---

*Mahler, Winnicott, and Kohut all began publishing their contributions in the 1940s, but it
was not until the 1970s (which says something about the all too familiar problem of how
long it takes for resistance to new ideas to fade and for science to allow long cherished
concepts to be replaced by newer ones) that their concepts began to be widely deliberated
in psychoanalytic circles. In addition, Mahler and Kohut didn't publish their most extensive
works until the 1970s, reflecting some of their own processes of creative maturation.

extension of Klein's concept of the depressive position) and to experience comforting solitude and quiescence under the aegis of a nonintrusive mother. The child's capacity to create a solacing medium for himself or herself, a hallucinatory sense of omnipotence by imagining and fantasy, is the beginning of transitional experience and is the foundation for creativity arising from the tension between attachment and separation (Horton, 1981; Scharff, 1982). The "psychosomatic partnership" between infant and mother, as Winnicott called it, refers to the moment-by-moment transactions between an attentive parent and a child who is becoming attuned to his or her body's responsiveness, his or her loss and attainment of boundaries, his or her experiences of tension and release, his or her rhythms of satisfaction and frustration, all leading to the emergence of what Winnicott called the "true self." Winnicott considered the possession of "false self," in contrast, to be the unhappy and inevitable consequence of a child living with a mother who precipitously and unpredictably withdraws her attentiveness to her child's voracious demands for gratification. The more extreme and unreliable the maternal attempts are to meet these demands, the more likely the child will need to protect his or her true self from the experiences of loss, annihilation, and disintegration. The child will then become cognitively hyperattuned and hypervigilant to environmental shifts and external clues and will try to stay clear of murky, emotional waters. During the 1960s, psychologists called this cognitive style "field dependency."

In the sexual arena, I began to see evidence of the false self in patients who demonstrated excessive problems with jealousy, control, and fear of orgasmic release. The true self needed to remain hidden behind the patient's verbiage, pat stories, or a too-readily proclaimed certainty in order to avoid anticipated scorn or ridicule. In addition, individuals, who too readily suffered excessive shame and humiliation or who needed to withhold orgasmic release, had, upon my inquiries in therapy, precisely the kinds of erratic experiences with their mothers that Winnicott described. When I asked about masturbation experiences, I found that these individuals had an excessive need to control their own bodies. They preferred masturbation because it lacked the threat of a potential (from the partner) replication of maternal withdrawal.

I also began to become attuned, in couples and individual patients, to what Winnicott referred to as the absence or presence of the spirit of play. Those who could not easily play at home had, of course, difficulty with playful elements in therapy sessions. Even though the pressure was on to be "serious," a good, productive session often occurred when I was able to be less controlling of tempo and content. This more spontaneous occurrence would emanate from the dynamic interplay between the patient's thoughts, fantasies, or associations and my thoughts or fantasies (not always spoken, of course). Winnicott, and later Carl Whitaker (1976) in a very different way, had urged therapists to relearn their childhood experiences of playing. Because we've all been urged to relinquish this type of transitional mode of relatedness with maturity, the therapist often responds to the typically constricted patient without playfulness. Winnicott said "Psychotherapy has to do with two people playing together. The work done by the therapist is directed towards bringing the patient from a state of not being able to play into a state of being able to play" (1971, p. 38). And what better way is there for two adults to be introduced to play than through the vehicle of language.

Symbol formation, with its emphasis on the creative aspect of transforming remembered experiences into descriptive words, is one way of playing involving a prelogical fusion of subject and object. Playing, therefore, includes the making of puns; seeing paradoxes; and telling parables, myths, and analogs from other patients' lives. (When you have been in practice a long time, it will probably occur to you sometime as it did to me, somewhere between the twelfth and fifteenth year, that you have been accumulating a rich storehouse of tales of what it is like to be human.) I began to reevaluate and rediscover how language is a symbolic way station between objective reality (what we cannot have) and subjective reality (what we fantasize and wish we could regress to and hold on to forever). I began asking couples and individuals to describe in more detail just how, what, and where they experienced sexual intimacy. Their words were often empty, barren, pseudoscientific, or just plain meaningless. When I pushed for more clarity, I often began hearing a mix of past and present sensient experience. They often felt some embarrassment, then relief, that someone was finally getting to the core of their intimate life. We sometimes chuckled over how difficult it was for adults to articulate what should be the most natural of events. This was particularly true when they could recall how important, meaningful, and soothing a sexual ritual had been to them in childhood.

Winnicott's concepts that there are transitional objects of all kinds (not just symbolic words) and that there is transitional relatedness which serves as the bridge upon which one grows in confidence and sense of security became key for me. The dynamic tension in transitional space of having and not having, oscillating between what Bruce Lackie (1987) has called the center and the edge, is what seems to have the potential to either overwhelm or sustain individuals. The sexual experience, it is clear, is one domain where people seem to feel such tension through the extremes of terror and belonging, and the abyss of abandonment and the exhilaration of merging. In their therapy sessions, some patients were able to give me minute details of their sexual experiences. And I became more adept at asking questions about microexperiences of shame, of guilt, of hurt, of letting go, of holding on, of becoming excited, of feeling let down, etcetera.

By the early 1980s, nourished by colleagues such as Paul Horton (1981, 1988) who was thinking about solacing experiences throughout the life cycle and Jill and David Scharff (1987) and their colleagues at the Washington School of Psychiatry who work in object-relations family therapy, I felt encouraged that my own thinking was on the right track. Most importantly, the individual patients and families I was seeing were getting better. I was learning how to help individuals, couples, and families to develop a more sustaining, adequate holding environment for themselves. I was providing more support and using interpretation, patience, humor, playfulness, dream-work, and much less directiveness. I realized that therapy for sexual problems was in fact therapy to help restore the whole person. As patients began to feel more intact, more integrated, more knowledgeable about themselves, and less ashamed, many of their complaints about sexual problems diminished and, in some instances, disappeared.

The final key theorist/therapist in my synthesis of influences is Heinz Kohut (1971, 1977, 1984). Originally a classical analyst, Kohut departed markedly from drive theory in his theory about the self and the individual's lifelong need for sustaining relationships. Several of Kohut's key concepts are relevant to this discussion. He perceived sexual relatedness and other forms of intimacy to be the narcissistic strivings of the individual for unbroken connections to either an idealizable other (the idealized selfobject) or to someone who could mirror the grandiose needs of the self (the mirroring selfobject), not just as drive-discharge or object-directed libido. Requiring both of these kinds of selfobjects and, as Greenberg and Mitchell (1983) have stated, seldom getting enough of either, individuals develop narcissistic defects in their core sense of self. These defects, stemming from frustrations and disappointments with the original self-objects—the parents—lead to character rigidities, fixations with sex or food or anality, compulsive rituals, and obsessiveness.

It is the therapist's responsibility, under such circumstances, to restore the individual's optimal sense of narcissistic entitlement by being an attuned selfobject (White, 1985), available during the course of treatment to provide effective, noncontingent mirroring and, during other phases of therapy, to allow idealization by the patient. This therapy has to be experience-near, empathic, at a level in which the patient's meanings can be felt and understood. The therapist has to be sensitive to when not to say

something, to speaking too much like an expert, and to allowing the patient
to structure the description of their own intimate experiences (mirroring).
Interpretation should be used to clarify, demystify, or soothe (idealization).
The rhythm of when to switch from one dimension to the other can only be
understood by being tuned in to the subtle shifts in the patient's voice, body
language, tone, content, etcetera. For me, originally trained in phenomenological psychology and existential philosophy, Kohut's formulations corre-
sponded to my own appreciation for the individual's striving for a cohesive
sense of self despite my earlier therapeutic reliance on concepts of identity
formation (Kahn, 1968–1969). Now, the tie between the self and the
individual's selfobject(s)—those relationships in which healthy development can be seen as open-ended opportunities for mature interrelatedness
began to stand out as an all-important configuration.

As Stolorow (1986) noted, "'selfobject' does not refer to an environmental entity or caregiving agent. Rather it designates a class of psychological functions pertaining to the maintenance, restoration and transformation of self experience. We refer, in other words, to a dimension of
experiencing an object in which a specific bond is required for maintaining, restoring or consolidating the organization of self experience"
(p. 274). Without such self–selfobject bonds, an individual might engage
in, for example, compulsive sexual acting out or experience panic reactions to an affair or desertion by a partner. I began to see beyond the basic
headlines of sexual relatedness or sexual symptomology. Breaks or separations from the person's selfobjects meant a fragmentation of the self,
annihilation fears, or a disintegration of the holding framework for some
people at their deepest level of being. I began to find my traditional moral
position on certain sexual matters more strained. Increasingly, much of
what I was hearing seemed to be oriented to the individual's striving for
survival and personal cohesion. Sexual pursuing, sexual withholding, fet-
ishes, and certain ways of becoming excited were all often outcomes or
precursors of the individual's deeply felt sense of personal dissolution or
attempts at feeling complete. The challenge for me was how to fit all of
this into a larger systems way of thinking.

FILTERING PSYCHOANALYTIC CONCEPTS
THROUGH A SYSTEM LENS

Family therapists have typically dealt with sexual issues using two main
theoretical frameworks, both explicitly behaviorally and environmentally
based. The first, sex therapy, originally derived from the pioneering

fantasy → arousal as attempt at feeling complete

influences of Masters and Johnson (1966, 1970). It taught us the inestimable benefits of utilizing behavioral practice, prescription, sensate focus, and noncontingency contracting with couples. Although I do not consider myself a sex therapist per se, I, like many others, use some elements of this approach in my own work. These sex therapy techniques are quick, to the point, sometimes effective, and, even when they fail, revealing of something important about the inner life of each individual. The other principal influence for family therapists has been the family-of-origin approach in which multigenerational familial influences upon the individual, readily recalled, informs us of previous issues of grief, loss, fusion, disengagement, conflict, pathology, etcetera. Previously developed familial patterns often become covert rules for all kinds of behavior including sexual behavior. Feelings of shame and guilt about the body or sexual excitement or sexual rules can often be directly traced back to the readily ascertained dictates, morals, values, and actions of parents, siblings, grandparents, aunts, and uncles.

In most cases, however, I find that I must go beyond what can be immediately recalled or initially prescribed. Whereas family therapy has focused on technical innovation and change, psychoanalysis has emphasized understanding and insight. To separate these two approaches, using exclusively either the technology of family therapy or that of psychoanalysis, is to engage in dualistic thinking. This dualistic thinking splits the inner and outer worlds of intimate experience into what, on one hand, is felt, imagined, and fantasized and, on the other hand, how and in what ways things are done.

If we are ever going to understand anyone's notion of shame or of ecstasy, we must attend to a synthesis of the individual's ways of behaving and feeling. In treating sexual intimacy, this entails a move from the issues of three generations and the couple's or individual's day-to-day interactions to the deeper issues of self-development (see also Kahn, 1986; Nichols, 1987; Sander, 1979; Scharff & Scharff, 1987; Slipp, 1984 for similar philosophical approaches). Generational issues are generally easier for people to speak about and such material often contains a safer, reality-oriented, often rehearsed quality which usually elicits a similar, equally plausible and equally justifiable response from the partner. We have used the term "complementarity" to describe this match or fit of stories. I do need to initially hear this material, however. It creates the necessary background and opens up the opportunity for the individual's self-experience to then be more clearly articulated and contextually understood. This material of self-experience is usually expressed in a more tentative, vague, and uncertain manner and the therapist's empathic skills and tolerance for incomprehensibility is usually more severely tested at this point in the therapeutic process.

Most people make love wordlessly. We, as therapists and individuals, do not have an adequate language, either personally or professionally, for this most intimate of experiences—the derivative of early-in-life transitional relatedness, and neither do couples. When I ask an individual to speak about any of the following sexual dimensions: fantasies, control, excitement, pleasure, shame, or tension, I also ask the partner to be a mirroring selfobject by becoming sensitive to the nuances of the other person's feelings and how they relate to that person's family-of-origin experiences. During this phase of the therapy, I somewhat control the agenda by pushing the couple or individual beyond that with which they feel familiar or comfortable. This is a technical necessity. Because most clients cannot afford daily therapy, entering into this world of highly charged, intimate experience with the partner listening intently requires a modification of technique from that of the highly rarified four or five sessions a week of psychoanalysis. The therapist must listen for each person's discomfort or evasions and, with an empathic stance, ask about the innuendos of attachment, holding, sensation, mounting-need excitation, arousal, satisfaction, playing, fantasies, and inner reality. Sometimes, I will mention my own discomfort at hearing some of this intimate material. This is said with humor or an expressed understanding of the universality of it all in order to relieve some of the tension or embarrassment the patient is feeling. This can occur only *after* I am certain I am being viewed as an idealized selfobject. After all, I am asking people to discuss issues usually never before acknowledged to themselves much less shared. If I see evidence of shame and embarrassment, I will often ask the couple to hold each other at night and speak to each other about their fantasies of each other's bodies and their own feelings about themselves. They are instructed to do this both before and after lovemaking. Then, if able, they are asked to talk about their experiences in subsequent therapy sessions.

It also is important to interpret a patient's developmental failures. Most people do not understand and appreciate how nascent and vulnerable one's psychological structures are in the first 3 years of life. It helps for people to know and understand where, when, and what was going on with their family during that period. As the therapist, my responsibility is to figure out how these experiences contributed to breaks in the patient's holding experience, which now get repeated in the intimacy of adult sexuality. I stay particularly attuned to signals of breaks in the continuity of experience. This weaving together of past and present, large systemic experience with microexperience, primitive past with the articulate and mature present gradually strengthens the individual. Individuals become less embarrassed, more accepting, less grandiose, and more empathic of why their partners respond as they do. Kohut called this weaving and strengthening of structures "transmuting internalization." In other words, it is a process through which one builds a cohesive, less fragmented sense of self.

It is also important to interpret, always in a balanced way so as not to prejudice either of the partners, the amount of projection, projective identification, and collusion that occurs between people. Collusion always exists in any relationship where there is more to lose by leaving than by staying. Individuals who have experienced serious breaks and disruptions in their holding framework while growing up, often project unresolved issues onto their intimate partner. This partnership is, after all, the latter-day representative of the psychosomatic partnership of old.

What are the sexual issues and problems of sexual intimacy I find myself dealing with? The list seems to be endless: exhibitionism, sado-masochism, inhibition, shame, anxiety, premature ejaculation, frigidity, vaginismus, impotence, transexualism, transvestism, homosexuality, heterosexuality, bisexuality, aggression, promiscuity, fear, compulsivity, voyeurism, fetishism, eroticism, excitement, masturbation, object choice, pedophilia, rape, pornography, hermaphrodism, nudity, body boundaries, fantasies, scoptophilia, fear of touching, onanism, etcetera. No matter what the behavioral and contextual interventions I choose to use with a particular problem, ultimately my end goal is to help the individual, as we keep working with him or her, to restore his or her cohesive self. The case I have selected to describe in detail illustrates this basic point. There are many other situations where the working principles I have described are very much the same.

NANCY AND ROGER: ALONE TOGETHER

Nancy, a 37-year-old high school teacher, was referred for therapy by her husband's ex-therapist one week after becoming married. Her husband Roger was a 38-year-old business executive. There was no mention of a sexual problem. The difficulty had to do with "family." Nancy's wedding had been purposefully tiny. No family or friends had been invited lest her family rift be exposed to the world. Although the couple, particularly Nancy, had been raised as staunchly Catholic, the marriage ceremony was performed by a justice of the peace. The couple, who had always maintained separate apartments, had been engaged for one and one-half years, but Nancy's family, consisting of mother, father, and a sister 3 years older, ignored the engagement, never sending a card or saying anything. Roger's parents and five siblings were a bit more effusive; they made a few phone calls and sent a check as a wedding gift. But they, too, separated by 600 miles, seemed reluctant to celebrate Nancy and Roger's marriage in spite of the fact that the couple had dated each other exclusively for 14 years! Nancy was furious, especially at her own family. Roger's family was slightly "better" than hers and could be "forgiven" for their "ignorance" since they were "blue-collar" and "unsophisticated." Her family, however, should have known "better." It was evident how hurt and unappreciated Nancy felt for what she saw as their betrayal of her filial loyalty.

Nancy had always been exceedingly compliant with her parents. Like her mother, she was a teacher; she had waited to marry until age 37, as her mother waited until age 36; she had seldom gone out as a teenager as her family never went out; and like her mother, she had married a Catholic. Roger, like Nancy's father, had relatively little to do with his siblings. Roger was educated, whereas they were not. Nancy's father had left Ireland as a teenager, and only acknowledged his family's existence by sending them clothes annually, never calling or writing them. Nancy's father seldom mentioned his father, and Nancy had no idea of how many aunts or uncles she had on his side or how or when her grandparents had died. Her mother was an only child who, Nancy said, had been "spoiled." But from the description I heard of the maternal grandmother with whom Nancy had grown up, the mother was unquestionably a hostage, rigidly bound to her family.

By the second session, it was apparent that Nancy had grown up in an enmeshed, depressed, and rigidly arranged household. Nancy's father had married her mother upon the death of the mother's father and had moved into the depressed, matriarchically dominated home. Nancy's grand-mother would just "sit" in her own space, controlling everybody, and dictating rules for intimacy and communication. It sounded as if the grandmother was malignantly paranoid, agoraphobic, and harsh. When I expressed the idea that Nancy's parents were victims, rather than persecu-tors, Nancy looked startled. This hypothesis that everyone was deprived and living pinched lives made Nancy question her feelings of hurt, anger, and self-righteousness over being the only deprived one.

I suggested, and Nancy acknowledged, that she tried to "get back" at her parents and sister by having a solitary, disappointing wedding thereby branding the family as ingrates. Nancy, too, could act vindictively! By the third session, a congratulatory card from the parents along with a three thousand dollar check had arrived. Nancy saw it as a "token." She said she had never been interested really in marrying as it was "the end of the line, a living death." She seemed to have a vague impression that her mother had once been a vibrant person. Had marrying and having children killed her spirit, we jointly wondered? I pressed on with my developmental inquiry and discovered that the year before Nancy's birth the parents had had another baby who had died shortly after birth. The family had mourned briefly; Nancy's mother covered her grief by immediately becoming pregnant. Had Nancy attached properly to her mother? The barrenness and depression of the family was becoming more contextually framed: The family never enjoyed themselves; Nancy and her sister had no toys; Nancy shared a room with her grandmother (who never went out and then died) and her sister until twelve years of age; no visitors ever came to the house; the parents constantly watched their pennies and lived only to work; her mother said the novena faithfully and the rosary daily; and her father worked the second shift and weekends. Thus, absent, hardworking, and exhausted, Nancy defined him as heroic for sacrificing himself for the "good of the family." I offered the interpretation that if a child receives little gratification from one parent, she will turn emotionally to the other but mythologize the latter as the good parent, even if that one is detached and unavailable. Given this information, it was not surprising that Nancy had married Roger. He, too, was unavailable, staying alone 2 to 3 days a week in the far away city of his employment. In my mind, it seemed inevitable that he, too, would ultimately become a source of disappointment and frustration for Nancy. Nancy confirmed my impression. I then offered my opinion that Nancy's mother could do nothing with her grief, anger, sadness, and pain but project it onto and into her children. By the fourth session, Nancy was opening up. She called her mother mean, critical, self-denying, dogmatic, complaining and bombastic. Nancy said she hated her home, but she couldn't say she hated her mother. I then asked Nancy if she had been held as a child, hugged, or kissed. She responded that neither parent was affectionate.

Did she have sex with Roger? The answer was inescapable, obvious. The last time they had had sex was one and one-half years previous on the night of their engagement after many years of sexual inhibition and malaise. In 14 years, they had had sex only 8 or 10 times. She no longer wanted any sex. It was always disappointing; the couple would argue, then ignore the problem. Nancy seemed to be reliving with Roger the barrenness of her childhood—no play, no hope, and no fun. There was no transitional relatedness. The amount of projective identification, on the other hand, was intense. In Nancy's view, Roger was as "limited" as she was. He, too, had lived a pinched life. If there was no expansiveness in their lives as children, she wondered aloud, what right did either of them have to expect excitement and pleasure as adults? If she could never aspire to anything, how could sex and love become possible?

Nancy started the next session by saying that she had never before realized she had had a sexual problem. She had always blamed Roger. We spent the next three sessions getting a more detailed sexual history, interwoven with more of the details of her background. The isomorphism of deprived family life and self-inhibition in which she could not be her own soothing selfobject was striking. She clearly had an inhibition of sexual desire, as Roger plainly did. She was nonorgasmic and had never consciously masturbated as an adolescent or adult. She could become excited, however, by rubbing her thighs together which was often accompanied by thoughts of men making love to her, although these fantasies had not occurred in a long time.

Sexual desire often seemed to "switch off." Her first sexual experience occurred after college, at age 23, with an "inappropriate man" (an encounter unconsciously designed, I thought, to fail). Immediately thereafter she met Roger and all other dating stopped. As Nancy spoke, she acknowledged that it was difficult to continue with this topic. She was anxious, at times coquettish and fidgety, but she wanted help with this problem. When I asked her to start masturbating at home in order to achieve orgasm and to monitor her fantasies, she agreed.

By the ninth session, Nancy had tried masturbating, but her desire and interest would "switch off" or plateau. I instructed her to talk with Roger about her feelings and experiences. She reported that he was interested, then aroused, and the couple had sex for the first time in one and one-half years. It wasn't that satisfactory. She held back her excitement, but did acknowledge that she didn't want to give in to an old temptation to pay Roger back and retaliate for past hurts. She again repeated her astonishment that she had a sexual problem. I instructed her to vary her masturbatory style and interpreted how she had probably imprinted sexuality at an unsatisfactory level. At this point, Nancy "switched off," changing the conversation to Roger and his mother. I learned that Roger's mother was a prude, and that his parents never touched or talked about sex in that house either. Later on, Roger told me that he too slept in a bedroom with an adult—his father—until he was twelve, and that mother slept alone on the living room couch. In the tenth session, Nancy announced that she and Roger had had great, exciting, and repeated sex, although it was still a nonorgasmic experience for Nancy, and masturbation, which she continued, had little in the way of accompanying sexual fantasies. By the eleventh session, the couple agreed that repeated sex was a goal worth pursuing. But Nancy described Roger as feeling claustrophobic with this increased "togetherness," and stated that she had fallen asleep frequently that week when he appeared disinterested in her. The couple was collusively aligned, afraid to progress further. It was time to start the next phase of treatment, couple therapy.

Roger came in gladly with Nancy and expressed his own frustrations. He admitted that he could be passive–agressive and was an isolator, an obsessive–compulsive, and a conflict-avoider. That week he had punched a hole in the wall after Nancy criticized him for ignoring her. He explained that his seeming disinterest was really fear and confusion about how to approach Nancy and please her. We were able to establish a therapeutic alliance, and Nancy acknowledged that, even though she regretted losing her individual therapy (I had become an idealized selfobject), she wanted very much to get closer to Roger. During the next six sessions (numbers twelve through seventeen), the couple was encouraged to keep having sex, to report their fantasies to each other, and to explore each other's bodies in a sensitive way. In sessions, however, they spent the time describing their isolation, their deprivations, and their common backgrounds. At one point Nancy said, "We're the same, Catholic; we both had repressive, peculiar parents; and we're both last borns." Roger began describing his own inhibitions. He had never enjoyed sex either. There was a pervasive sense of guilt about the whole matter.

By session eighteen, Roger was not retreating as much. We were able to start seeing the patterns of withdrawal and pursuit used by each of them. I seemed to have gotten them sufficiently engaged with each other so that only one would be sexually detached at any one time. They now had intercourse on the average of four times a week, but I still had to help them overcome their contingency thinking. Each believed he/she had no right to manipulate the other's body or needs. Roger, particularly, was too adept at sensing Nancy's ambivalence. If she wasn't interested or aroused, then he couldn't maintain his interest because that would mean he was "selfish." He had reacted in this way with his own mother, whenever her moods had fluctuated. It was only by the fortieth session that the couple began to accept their biological differences. Roger could allow himself to become sexually aroused faster than Nancy. We laughingly referred to this as his needing to "prime the pump," whereas Nancy, once aroused, could maintain sexual interest and excitement much longer. As she put it, "Once I get hungry, I want to have three meals, not just one!"

During the twentieth to thirty-eighth sessions, we concentrated on the microexperiences of their relationship. Neither of them had ever had much autoerotic experience. With my encouragement, they began to talk more about their fantasies. Roger was able to increasingly detect his sadness when he was apart from Nancy, and he set out to change his work schedule so as to be home every night. She was becoming his holding environment. He was dropping his false self. Nancy was now aware of how unavailable her father had really been. When I asked in what way they felt they were becoming a couple, Roger said, "We're now having sex and making love." They began making plans to have a first anniversary celebration which they planned to invite all their friends to this time. I ventured that we might pause for a while. At this point, they, in effect, said that they weren't ready: Sex was now mechanical and too compulsively determined. Roger feared losing control. Obviously, they said that they still needed me.

This couple clearly was becoming concerned that they needed and depended upon each other too much. They were quite isolated from family, community, and friends. Mechanisms of introjection and projection which had developed over 30 some odd years can keep a couple bound together and do not magically disappear after 40 hours of psychotherapy. I saw Roger and Nancy for what turned out to be 50 more hours of therapy during the next 18 months. They needed the extra push and permission from me to learn more about sex from books I recommended, from a few soft porn movies they rented, from the adventure of wearing more risqué clothes to bed, and from the excitement and relaxation that occurred during the vacations they now began taking. But, above all, they needed sensitivity and a new language of subtlety to become attuned to each other. They were accomplishing this and were pleased with their progress. Nonetheless, there were plenty of occasions when they would backslide. They had been so deprived for so long that sex, which was now reliable, available, and anticipated, would sometimes become too important, evident by Nancy's saying, "I want it all now." Because they had been loyal and compliant children, they had little problem attaching to me but this time it was in the service of their own needs. They seemed to benefit from hearing my reassurances, words of support, and empathy for what they had been through.

Sex, which all along, had been a metaphor for the barrenness and emptiness of their earlier lives, now was a symbol of the transitional relatedness of life itself. The couple became aware that things change, that the "center cannot hold" (Yeats's "The Second Coming," quoted in Lackie,

1987), that things ebb and flow. Roger was emotionally available for Nancy when her father died of a myocardial infarction. For three months, through the forty-second to the fifty-fifth sessions during the acute mourning stage, there was little sex. But Roger was there for her, as an empathic mirroring selfobject, holding her and touching her. After that period, during which Nancy's concerns about her parents and the obligation of caring for her mother dominated the sessions, Roger began speaking more of his dawning realizations about his own thwarted sexual development. Roger had just never thought of himself as a sexual person. He had masturbated very little, had never had fantasies, and had never felt emotionally or physically held. His mother, who took green "nerve medicine," his father, who was "simple" and expected little of life, and his siblings who were disengaged had never given Roger a sense of family. He and Nancy were, he ruefully acknowledged, made for each other. It was no wonder that this couple did not expect to have children—their expectations of an expanding future had always been thwarted. But they now were sexually intimate and more alive. Nancy was orgasmic; Roger more able to tolerate breaks and discontinuities in their relatedness without retreating or feeling irretrievably damaged; and they now had a language to express excitement, loss, hope, and shame.

The last phase of therapy concentrated on how to include in their lives the community and friends. If they could be a couple at home and in bed, they now could be a couple in the larger world. They began to entertain friends, set up a social calendar, and sought social contacts in the community. We terminated after 90 sessions on a cautious note of optimism. The couple seemed ready to be on their own.

CONCLUSION

This case illustrates many of the principles of an integrative self psychological, family systems approach to difficulties of sexual intimacy. I believe that by addressing the issues of the whole person, by reaching back to early childhood, to the present context of the person's interactions, and then on to the future realization of what a person would like to become, we can restore a sense of vitality in individuals and in couples. We need the technology of sex therapy to help people make necessary changes, but we also need to understand the deepest recesses of the individual's experience and the nature of the families in which they have developed in order to create a synthesis, a balance, and a restoration of that person's potential. If

72   KAHN

we are sensitive to those essential themes, the attainment of a genuine
sexual intimacy, among other things, is bound to follow.

REFERENCES

Eagle, M. N. (1984). *Recent developments in psychoanalysis: A critical evaluation.* New-
    ford: McGraw-Hill.
Freud, S. (1905). Three essays on the theory of sexuality. In L. Strachey (Ed.). The standard
    edition of the complete psychological works of Sigmund Freud (Vol. 7). London:
    Hogarth Press.
Greenberg, J., & Mitchell, S. (1983). *Object relations in psychoanalytic theory.* Cambridge:
    Harvard University Press.
Horton, P. (1981). *Solace: The missing dimension in psychiatry.* Chicago: University of
    Chicago Press.
Horton, P., Gewirtz, H., & Kreutter, K. (Eds.). (1988). *The solace paradigm: An eclectic
    search for psychological immunity.* Madison, CT: International Universities Press.
Kahn, M. D. (1968-1969). The adolescent struggle with identity as a force in psychother-
    apy. *Adolescence, 12*(3), 395-424.
Kahn, M. D. (1986). The self and system: Integrating Kohut and Milan. In S. Sugarman
    (Ed.). *The interface of individual and family therapy* (pp. 50-64). Rockville: Aspen.
Kaplan, H. S. (1974). *The new sex therapy: Active treatment of sexual dysfunctions.* New
    York: Brunner/Mazel.
Kaplan, H. S. (1979). *Disorders of sexual desire and other new concepts and techniques in
    sex therapy.* New York: Brunner/Mazel.
Klein, M. (1964). *Contributions to psychoanalysis, 1921-1945.* New York: McGraw-Hill.
Kohut, H. (1971). *The analysis of the self.* New York: International Universities Press.
Kohut, H. (1977). *The restoration of the self.* New York: International Universities Press.
Kohut, H. (1984). *How does analysis cure?* Chicago: University of Chicago Press.
Lackie, B. (1987). *Catch a falling kingdom: A meditation on King Lear.* Unpublished
    manuscript.
Mahler, M. (1967). On human symbiosis and the vicissitudes of individualism. *Journal of
    the American Psychoanalytic Association, 15,* 740-763.
Mahler, M. (1968). *On human symbiosis and the vicissitudes of individuation* (Vol. 1).
    New York: International Universities Press.
Mahler, M., Pine, E., & Bergman, A. (1975). *The psychological birth of the human infant:
    Symbiosis and individuation.* New York: Basic Books.
Masters, W. H., & Johnson, V. E. (1966). *Human sexual response.* Boston: Little, Brown.
Masters, W. H., & Johnson, V. E. (1970). *Human sexual inadequacy.* Boston: Little, Brown.
Modell, A. H. (1985). The two contexts of the self. *Contemporary Psychoanalysis, 21*(1),
    70-91.
Nichols, M. P. (1987). *The self in the system: Expanding the limits of family therapy.* New
    York: Brunner/Mazel.
Offit, A. K. (1981). *Night thoughts: Reflections of a sex therapist.* New York: Congdon
    and Lattes.
Sander, F. (1979). *Individual and family therapy: Toward an integration.* New York: Jason
    Aronson.

Scharff, D. (1982). *The sexual relationship: An object relations view of sex and the family.* London: Routledge & Kegan Paul.

Scharff, D., & Scharff, J. (1987). *Object relations family therapy.* Northvale, NJ: Jason Aronson.

Slipp, S. (1984). *Object relations: A dynamic bridge between individual and family treatment.* New York: Jason Aronson.

Stolorow, R. (1986). On experiencing an object: A multidimensional perspective. In A. Goldberg (Ed.). *Progress in self psychology: Vol. 2* (pp. 273–279). New York: Guilford Press.

Whitaker, C. (1976). The hinderance of theory in clinical work. In P. J. Guerin (Ed.). *Family therapy theory and practice* (pp. 154–164). New York: Gardner Press.

White, M. T. (1985). The rediscovery of intergenerational continuity and mutuality. In A. Goldberg (Ed.). *Progress in self psychology: Vol. 1* (pp. 228–239). New York: Guilford Press.

Winnicott, D. W. (1958). *Through pediatrics to psychoanalysis.* London: Hogarth Press.

Winnicott, D. W. (1965a). *The maturational process and the facilitating environment.* New York: International Universities Press.

Winnicott, D. W. (1965b). *The family and individual development.* London: Tavistock.

Winnicott, D. W. (1971). *Playing and reality.* Middlesex, England: Penguin.

Zilbergeld, B., & Evans, M. (1980). The inadequacy of Masters and Johnson. *Psychology Today, 14,* 29–43.

4

INTIMACY IN FAMILIES WITH YOUNG CHILDREN

Lee Combrinck-Graham and Lawrence Kerns

The shape of the family with very young children is ideal for the practice of intimacy. Regardless of how the family of young children is situated ethnically, socioeconomically, or psychologically, interpersonal forces will draw individuals together into caretaking and closeness. During this period of family life, the capacity for intimacy is established for the first time in the children, through holding and the intense responsiveness of their caretakers. The capacity for intimacy is also reworked in this phase of family life by the adults in the family. Simply being close physically, however, does not itself engender a healthy capacity for intimacy. It is also necessary to have clear role differentiation in order that the process of intimate exchange can be unambiguously recorded in the system.

Intimacy means intense involvement and responsiveness between individuals. The term *intimacy* derives from the Latin, *intimus*, referring to the inner or inmost regions, such as the innermost parts of an organism. In the family, intimacy refers to the innermost workings or the private interior of the family. In relationships between individuals, intimacy becomes the goal of the relationship, the joining of innermost feelings and qualities, an emotional closeness and knowledge of each other that is deep (as opposed to superficial) and is mutual or reciprocal. In this sense it differs from attachment, which describes only one half of and one direction of a relationship between two people. In the same sense it differs from bonding, which is used to describe parental behavior. An individual

Lee Combrinck-Graham. Institute for Juvenile Research, Chicago, Illinois; Department of Psychiatry, University of Illinois at Chicago, Chicago, Illinois.

Lawrence Kerns. Institute for Juvenile Research, Chicago, Illinois.

may have the capacity for intimacy, but no one can be intimate except in relationship to another. Intimacy is a characteristic of interpersonal behavior.

Sexuality, on the other hand, is an attribute of individuals. Sexuality is a function of individual psychology comprised of the attitudes, beliefs, behaviors, and affects of individuals that can be directed toward others and are associated with both erotic feelings and reproductive functioning. Sexuality relates to the individual's interest in the sexual act and can be expressed in self-stimulation activities or in relationship to other individuals. In defining sexuality this way, we are deliberately turning away from the general and, we believe, confusing use of the term to describe a range of pleasurable and intimate feelings that are not specifically associated with either sex or reproduction.

Love, though defined as a fundamental drive in Freudian metapsychology, is so abstract that we believe it belongs with philosophers and poets and should not be treated as a clinical subject.

CONFUSION OF SEXUALITY AND INTIMACY

Ever since Freud labeled some feelings of parents toward their children as sexual and discovered fantasies of children about their parents which he similarly labeled as sexual, there has been a confusion of intimacy with sexuality. Certainly one short essay will not straighten out 80 years of thinking this way, but we can describe how this confusion came about and some of the places we think it has led us, as we try to examine the intimate context of the young family.

Since Victorian sexuality was understated, Freud's publications and formulations of his discoveries about human sexuality seemed to have a liberating effect, as seen by the way the subject became a pervasive, explanatory metaphor. As Ellis wrote in 1900,

> The erectile nipple corresponds to the erectile penis: the eager watery mouth of the infant to the moist and throbbing vagina, the vitally albuminous milk to the vitally albuminous semen. The complete mutual satisfaction, physical and psychic, of mother and child in the transfer from one to the other of a precious organized fluid, is the one true psychological analogy to the relationship of a man and a woman at the climax of the sexual act. (Cited in Kagan, 1984, p. 84)

The exuberance for an erotic metaphor for human behavior reflected in this quotation was historically determined. Freud's language unleashed sexualized perceptions that had long hovered under the surface of Victorian society.

Now, however, it seems to be time to move beyond the sexual metaphor as a way of describing human behavior and interaction. For the worst seems to have happened. The metaphor has become so reified that there is serious confusion about what is sexual and what is not, a confusion that has prompted the development of some very strange ideas and practices. Men cannot be intimate with other men, because intimacy implies sexuality and intimacy with men therefore implies homosexuality. A similar confusion is creeping into women's relationships with each other. In an era of virtual panic about child sexual abuse, a father who caresses his daughter has to wonder about the boundary between intimacy and sexuality. Parents avoid expressing passion for one another in front of their children, lest the children be traumatized. Children are tucked away at night, alone in their cribs and beds, while parents have each other's company.

A case in point is the 7-year-old daughter of divorced parents who was characterized by her father in a custody battle as masturbating publicly. He believed that this was a sign of her emotional difficulties, particularly those associated with the issue of sorting out the households of her two parents. Neither the child's mother nor her teachers had observed public masturbation. The father took her to a psychiatrist, who characterized her physical activity, especially the way she swung her legs when excited, as masturbating. The father admired his daughter's physical courage and coordination when she taught herself how to ride a two-wheeler, but his concern about her sexuality led him and his second wife to hold her at arm's length, watching this physically expressive child with horror at what they experienced as primitive and poorly controlled sexuality. At her mother's, the same child's physical expressiveness was read as a sign of enthusiasm, involvement, and energy. The child was frequently hugged, kissed, and wrestled with by her mother and stepfather, the latter taking courage by his wife's example. At her mother's, the child slept long and well; at her father's, she was fearful and sad. Here is an example of how the interpretation of behavior as sexual led a father to hold back necessary comfort from his daughter.

Some have observed that sexuality expressed outside of the marriage but within the nuclear family represents the formation of a cross-generational coalition, which is purported to be the most disturbed kind of family process. We must ask, then, "Are all families of children in the oedipal period disturbed because of the shared fantasies of the child's union with the parent of the opposite sex and the expulsion of the same-sex parent?" No, this has gone too far. We believe that cross-generational sex within families is exploitative and does interfere with the development and well-being of the child, in particular, and the rest of the family, as well. If oedipal fantasies were really sexual, then these serious disturbances would characterize relating in all families of preschool children. We believe that oedipal fantasies are relational (as we shall discuss further, later) and that these longings of the child to be closer to a parent are aspects of the practice of intimate relating in the young family.

Since the early family experience of the young child is the first opportunity to experience healthy intimacy, it is necessary to clear up some of these misconceptions by which intimacy is confused with sexuality, so that the young family can prepare all of its members for the ongoing practice of intimacy and the timely experience of sexuality.

THE SHAPE OF THE YOUNG FAMILY
IN THE FAMILY-LIFE SPIRAL

Combrinck-Graham (1983, 1985) has said that the family-life spiral is the ecology of individual development, and she has constructed a model that demonstrates the overlap of individual developmental lines within evolving characteristic family shapes (see Figure 4.1). Looking at a span of three generations of family life, she proposed that the family shape oscillates between being closely knit and diffused, depending on whether it is dominated by centripetal or centrifugal forces in the relationships. Combrinck-Graham characterized the families of young children as primarily nonpathologically enmeshed and held together by centripetal forces that draw the family members toward intimate relating.

Enmeshment is usually thought of as an extreme and dysfunctional family organization. When Wood (1985) tried to characterize enmeshment in terms of the two organizational dimensions of hierarchy and proximity, she presented scales of organization on each of these dimensions. Although a high degree of responsiveness and interpersonal resonance within the family is characteristic of proximity, the healthy family in the centripetal period also has elements of clear differentiation of function, similar to what Wood refers to as hierarchy. The dimension of proximity includes physical and emotional closeness, while hierarchy denotes levels of power, in Wood's view. We believe that it is more useful to think of hierarchy as role differentiation, represented abstractly by the concept of interpersonal and intergenerational boundaries.

Although there is a predominant emphasis on intimate relating in the young family, the movement of all of the individuals in the family

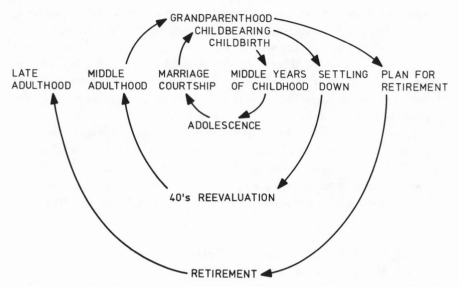

FIGURE 4.1. Family life spiral. From "A Developmental Model for Family Systems" by Lee Combrinck-Graham, 1985, *Family Process, 24,* p. 142. Copyright 1985 by Family Process, Inc. Reprinted by permission.

toward more differentiated functioning is an important dynamic which constantly reshapes the family. But, even at the most diffused centrifugal period of family life, closeness and intimacy have their places. Thus, if we apply the dimensions of proximity and hierarchy, as we have defined them, a healthy family stays meshed but oscillates between emphasis on proximity in the young family and on hierarchy in the older family.

Because of the atmosphere of closeness, resonance, and recriprocity of the very young family, it is ideal for the learning and practice of intimacy, not just for the young child but also for other family members, including the older siblings and the parents, grandparents, and other relatives.

CENTRIPETAL FORCES IN THE YOUNG FAMILY

Bowlby's (1969) studies of infant attachment were conducted with families in their centripetal period. He carefully observed attachment behavior and defined it as any form of behavior that results in the infant attaining or maintaining proximity to her caretaker. He emphasized the biological function and adaptive, survival advantages of what he viewed as species-characteristic behavior patterns. The concept of attachment is also consistent with and perhaps even necessary to our scheme for the development of intimacy. Physical closeness (high proximity) of parent and child is a necessary condition for the development of emotional closeness and mutual responsiveness. Indeed, Bowlby (1982) later went on to enlarge his concept of attachment to include the propensity of human beings to make strong affectional bonds to particular others, and he explained love relations, separation anxiety, depression, and mourning as derivatives of attachment and loss. Combining Bowlby's theories about infant attachment behavior with later theories about caretakers' attachment behaviors (bonding), we find a good foundation in individual behavior theory for understanding the atmosphere in the centripetal-period family that is crucial to the development of intimacy.

Equally crucial to an understanding of the developmental origins of intimacy are the concepts of reciprocity (Brazelton, Koslowski, & Main, 1974) and fitting together (Sander, 1980). Both terms refer to the mutuality of the early parent–child relationship, the recognition by infant researchers that parent and infant are reacting to and relating with each other, are accommodating to each other, and are both learning about their relationships simultaneously. Parents influence the child, and the child influences the parents, in terms of how they respond both to the child and to each other (Minuchin, 1985).

The child's development of the capacity for intimacy thus occurs in the context of the parents' rediscovery and reworking of their own intimate relating, both with the child and with each other (Benedek, 1959). Adults feel "bonded" to the child; the child forms a reciprocal attachment to the adults. Although the focus of attention is usually on the child, important adjustments and modifications are taking place within those who are adapting and accommodating to the child's development. Mahler, Pine, and Bergman (1975), for example, recognize the mother's significant role in the child's movement through the phases of separation and individuation. They do not, however, explicitly address the corresponding changes in the mother. Stern's (1985) studies of the development of self suggest that Mahler and associates' propositions about an autistic phase are probably not accurate, but the importance of Mahler's contribution for our presentation is that she recognizes the mutuality of the evolution both of attachment and separation. Kramer* suggests that, when the child attains a certain degree of separation in the "practicing" subphase, the

*S. Kramer (1978), personal communication.

parents' relationship with each other also shifts. The child's rapproche-
ment with the mother may actually be stimulated by the father's reclaim-
ing of the mother.

These kinds of patterns are plausible in societies where nursing small
infants is a primary activity of their mothers, and where, once the infant is
weaned, the reproductive cycle may begin again. With the varieties of infant
formulas, child-care arrangements, and reproductive controls available in
our society, this proposition is probably too simplistic. But it does address
readjustment and accommodation in different levels of the family system.

We don't know what "causes" the family to be intimate like this.
People who have been present at the birth of a baby know what a
powerful and moving experience it is. Klaus and Kennell (1976) assert
that everyone present at the birth bonds immediately to the infant. This
suggests that infants stimulate intimate behavior. On the other hand,
there is the generativity (Erikson, 1968) of the parents, which is the
developmental context in which they are producing babies. Infants are
usually the product of sexual intimacy, so the closeness between the
parents generates the intimate atmosphere of the family with young
children. Some individuals have babies in the hope of creating an intimate
relationship. How often we have heard it said, "Maybe if we have a baby
our marital relationship will improve." Pregnant teenagers often express
the desire to keep the baby on the basis of wanting someone to love and to
love them. So perhaps the act of becoming pregnant and carrying a fetus
to term determines the intimate context of the young family.

We do know that the life of the family with infants and toddlers is a
palpably close one, starting with the birth itself and with breast feeding or
holding the baby cradled in the arms to feed. There is encompassed
holding for soothing, rocking, comforting, and bathing, and these actions
of physical closeness are infectious, so that older children crawl into
parents' laps to be "babied" and parents hold each other close. As the
infant grows older, the close physical relationship continues to be the
primary way in which he relates and is related to, through physical
teaching, as in games such as "pat-a-cake"; in restraining, disciplining,
appreciating, and rewarding actions; and in putting-to-sleep rituals. A
toddler's shaky first explorations require a physical presence, his frustration or pain requires a scooping up, a holding close, a kiss to make it
better. These are the facts of life with young children that bring about the
atmosphere of close physical relating that is a substrate for intimacy.

It may be a biological necessity for the family to be so closely knit. It is
a matter of survival, not just of the individuals and particularly the

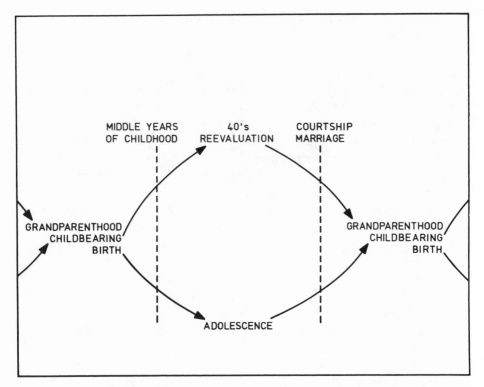

FIGURE 4.2. Oscillation of the family system. From "A Developmental Model for Family Systems" by Lee Combrinck-Graham, 1985, *Family Process, 24,* p. 143. Copyright 1985 by Family Process, Inc. Reprinted by permission.

vulnerable infant, but of the family itself. Without physical care, the infant dies; without intimacy, the infant fails to thrive; without reciprocal intimacy, the family fails to thrive.

Another view of the intensely intimate atmosphere of the young family is seen in the metarhythms of the family-life spiral proposed in Combrinck-Graham's (1985) model. As shown in Figure 4.2, this suggests an oscillation in family shape between the intimate, centripetal atmosphere discussed here and a more differentiated, centrifugal atmosphere characteristic of families with adolescents. Thus the degree of intimacy may be determined as a part of a larger pattern of human interactional experience.

MULTIGENERATIONAL CONTRIBUTIONS

Boszormenyi-Nagy and Krasner (1986) have proposed that the very birth of a child produces strong family ties, regardless of whether the child is raised with her biological parents. They emphasize the legacy of intimacy that is enacted in the family of the young child. Specifically, the child is obligated by filial loyalty to the parents who gave her the gift of life. This early relationship is shaped by the legacy of intimacy and caring that was received by the parents and is passed along to the child. The relationship is asymmetrical, with parents giving more than they receive. Certainly the child's obligation for filial loyalty is constantly being increased on the parents' side by their acts of caring for the child. We believe, however, that the child's responsiveness repays their acts of caring and encourages further involvement. The infant who is able to be calmed by parents, or who feeds well, or who smiles at his parents, is rewarding parents' nurturing even though in different kind than that which was given.

Boszormenyi-Nagy and Krasner's (1986) theory offers a framework for understanding how intimate relating is recorded and stored, to be passed on to other relationships and future generations. These transactions begin in an atmosphere of trust that there will be adequate care for the infant, and that there will be reciprocity. To the extent that these transactions are successful, trust is built into them. When the transactions are not successful, for whatever reason, trust resources are not built up, and the atmosphere for intimacy is impoverished. When this happens, since intimacy is interpersonal, all members of the relationship system suffer the lack of intimacy and the lack of the opportunity to be involved in intimate relating. This deficit is carried with them into future stages of family life and to future relationships, including future periods in which there are young children.

THREATS TO THE INTIMATE ATMOSPHERE
OF THE YOUNG FAMILY

It has already been suggested that the confusion between intimacy and sexuality may pose a threat to intimacy in the young family. The real confusion between caring feelings and sexual feelings is illustrated by the experience of mothers who report being sexually stimulated by nursing. Is this sexual stimulation, or is it a pull deeper into the intimate relating with the infant which is *like* intimate sexual relating? This is an important question, because, when people are extremely moved they usually

experience physical sensations, often in the genital areas or other erogenous zones. Such feelings are so specifically associated with sex that when
they occur in other than obviously sexually stimulating situations, it is
assumed that they are, nevertheless, sexual.

We treated a 32-year-old schizophrenic woman who encountered
such confusion after the birth of her third child. At times when nursing
the infant, she experienced what she interpreted as sexual excitement, and
she would interrupt feeding and put the infant down. At other times,
when holding her happy, squirming infant in her lap, she again felt
sexually excited and assumed that the child's kicking was stimulating her.
She had no sexual interest in the child, but she repeatedly interrupted
their interactions because she felt that her feelings in response to the child
were "wrong."

The converse of this is that many people believe that the only true
intimacy is sexual intimacy. A father of four daughters tried to teach his
children about intimacy through sexual intimacy. He read them books
about human anatomy and sex, and he fondled them genitally. Whatever
stimulation the father may have experienced for himself through these
activities, he believed that he was providing essential teaching to his
children.

The search for intimacy through sex is also seen in nymphomania
and borderline conditions in which individuals seem to be uncomfortable
with sustained relationships but nonetheless crave physical holding and
may feel that such holding occurs legitimately only in sexual relationships.
It may also be, as we have suggested before, the impetus for teenage
pregnancies, with intimacy and comfort being sought through sex and
then through the relationship with the baby.

Other factors that may interfere with the intimate atmosphere of the
young family are the temperamental characteristics of the child; how the
parents are suited for parenting; the marital relationship of the parents;
and other environmental characteristics such as relationships with extended family, work satisfaction, and economic security.

In describing the atmosphere of the young family, we have assumed
that there are two parents who are married to one another; who are happy
to have a child; and who have supportive families, a certain economic
security, and a healthy, responsive baby. But, of course, some variation of
this is usually the case. If the parents are not married, often other adults
are involved with caring for the child. Kellam, Ensminger, and Turner
(1977), looking at entirely different issues in family structure, did note
that a household headed by two adults, regardless of the adults' relationships to the child, was a stable structure in which children did relatively

better than in a single-parent household without significant access to other adults. It is also clear that, when a child is born, even to an isolated or cut-off individual, other adults are more likely to rally around. But sustained interpersonal bitterness, lack of social resources, and other environmental stress factors, as well as a parent's own discomfort or inexperience with intimacy, can disturb the establishment of an atmosphere of trust and intimacy in the young family.

The child, too, makes a contribution. We have already mentioned how the child's responsiveness stimulates and encourages parental involvement. Imagine the situation of a child who doesn't respond positively. The common example is the infant with colic, who, seen from the point of view of good-enough parenting, is a child who requires better-than-good-enough parenting. Such a child—or one who doesn't sleep well, or one who doesn't feed well, or one who is handicapped so his responsiveness is disturbed—tests parents to the limit, causing them to argue between themselves, making them irritable, and causing them to question their competence. The effect may be to push parents away rather than to draw them in, to promote isolation rather than intimacy within the family.

In many families the marital relationship deteriorates after the birth of a child. Rather than being pulled together, the family seems to fly apart. This most often happens after a first child or a difficult child. Suddenly the father may stay away from home, drink, or have an affair, or become deeply absorbed in his work. What has happened? Is it the difficult child, the preoccupied mother, the anxious father, or something about the revolution in the family system brought about by the presence of this new person?

Kraus and Redman's (1986) interpersonal model for post-partum depression addresses another way of looking at the disturbed young family. The original stimulus for self-doubt may be minor—a sense of being overwhelmed, not equal to the task, or the like. It could also be triggered by an unusually difficult baby. At any rate, the authors describe how the efforts of well-intentioned adults in the mother's system, trying to be of comfort, actually disconfirm her reality and therefore contribute to her deepening depression. Clearly a parent who becomes so emotionally unavailable is not contributing to the atmosphere of intimacy so important for this young family.

Exclusion of one parent is another common hazard. Whitaker* refers to the love affair that arises between mother and child, which essentially excludes the father. He also suggests that the first child is for the mother,

*C. Whitaker (1980), personal communication.

while the second is for the father, so that the father may be brought back upon the arrival of the second child. In many circles fathers are becoming more involved with their young children. The competition that may ensue between parents about who will care for the child can lead to the serious undermining of one parent. For example, a father asked his wife to stop nursing their baby because he felt excluded from this relationship. In another case, a mother whose major sense of competence with her young children was nursing was urged to stop nursing when the children were 3 and 4. She became psychotic, was hospitalized, and was thereafter excluded from the inner circle of the family by husband and children.

We believe that it takes a special mix of contextual and personality factors to interfere thoroughly with the establishment of a culture for intimacy, so strong are the natural forces to create a caring, close environment. Even the stresses of wars, chronic separations, and repeated losses are often compensated for as the needs of young children are addressed.

SENSUALITY AND INTIMACY

We have observed that defining many feelings as sexual and defining the goal of mature relating as mature sexuality may have interfered with the development of healthy intimacy. A certain part of developing strong, differentiated feelings while participating in intimate relationships is a clear, comfortable sense of oneself as a sensual being. Sensuality is often experienced in ways that are taken to be sexual. We may have strong responses to a beautiful piece of art or a landscape, an exquisite line of music, or a magnificently danced movement, and these may be felt in the parts of the body that are most sensitive. Such responses are better identified as sensual than sexual. They also occur when a person is stroked or tickled, or when a person encounters a pleasant tactile experience. Genital areas and other erogenous zones appear to be particularly sensitive to sensuous experience, and this fact undoubtedly contributes to the confusion between sensuality and sexuality.

A case in point is a 5-year-old girl who was routinely tormented by her older and stronger brother. She soon learned that, when tickled, he folded into helpless laughter. Their physical spats took on a new shape as he attempted to beat her up and she strategically aimed for his more ticklish areas. Although both children were fascinated by the differences in their genital equipment, neither experienced the rivalrous physical play as anything but a part of their continuous efforts to establish who they were with respect to each other and, ultimately, a larger world of peers.

The sensuous comfort that a young child gives herself by sucking her thumb and rubbing a familiar object on her cheek while she falls asleep is akin to the comfort discovered by touching a sensuous area, the genitals. Rubbing the genitals gives some children pleasure, and it is something they can do for themselves. Technically, it is masturbation, but it is more constructive to understand the activity as exploring sensuality than as an explicitly sexual act. Developing familiarity with her sensuality prepares an individual for being comfortable with the sensuality that is associated with intimacy and, ultimately, with sexual intimacy.

Children are curious about sex, as they are curious about everything. Relatively speaking, however, feces seem to get a longer focus of attention in the 2- to 5-year-old than sex, and penises are most interesting because they can be urinated from. Both feces and urine are familiar to children, whereas sex is not, even when children may have been fondled. For example, a 4-year-old who had frequently been genitally fondled by her father drew a picture of a dragon having a baby. The baby was coming out of the dragon's stomach. Despite the genital stimulation from her father, quite possibly a pleasing and sensuous experience for her, she had no more sophisticated views of sex and reproduction than many other youngsters her age. A drawing done by her twin sister, also involved in the fondling, expressed considerable apprehension about the danger of strangers, reflecting that, rather than sex, her greater concern was about the intervention of child protective services and the placement of the children in a strange foster home.

ROLE DISTINCTIONS AS A CHARACTERISTIC
OF THE YOUNG FAMILY

The way that roles are differentiated and tasks are carried out in the young family has importance in determining the sex-role functioning of all the family members. An individual's gender assignment is given and imprinted very early in life. Money and Ehrhardt (1972) long ago found that a child with ambiguous genitalia, who was assigned one gender and later found to be of the other, usually retained the personal identity of the earlier assignment. But, while gender identity is fixed, as illustrated by Money's findings, sex-role behavior is plastic and seems to be much more so in the centripetal-period family.

The issue of gender is one of concern in the family systems field, because, as the feminist scholars argue, families are organized around basic assumptions about male and female sex-role differences and the inequalities that are built into them. In the centripetal-period family, sex roles may be open for reworking. Fathers, in particular, have an unusual opportunity for the expression of emotional intimacy with someone other than their wives, which they may accept by assuming certain duties of child care such as night feedings, bathing, and putting the youngster to bed. Evidence of this can be seen in fathers' behavior with their children, such as baby talk and singing, which they would never display at the office or in the company of other adults. Mothers appear to have less of an opportunity for sex-role change in this period of family life, because of the enormous value placed on the mother–infant relationship.*

In our society, forces in the young family currently seem to be more flexible for fathers, while mothers are still usually regarded as primary parents and caretakers. Even in the so-called co-parenting arrangements, or in families in which the mother is the primary breadwinner, it is usually still the mother who plans the meals, arranges for the laundry to be done, sets the standards for the house to be clean, and arranges for child care. We have also observed that even fathers who are primary caretakers of their young children are less likely to stay home with their children and organize their days around either their children's wishes or domestic tasks. They tend to be on the go, and they are more likely to involve their children in activities of their (the fathers') choosing.

Mothers do differ in how willing they are to share intimate parenting with fathers, and in how willing they are to benefit from the fathers' greater involvement with and responsibility for the children, by taking advantage of the opportunities to develop other aspects of their own lives. The most striking example of major sex-role revision in the young family is what Pruett (1983, 1985) has studied at Yale as the "father-mothers." He studied a series of 17 families in which the father assumed the primary nurturing role with the infant, while the mother assumed the primary role of breadwinner for the family. Follow-up on these families until the children reached age 5 demonstrated no obvious deviance in the psychological functioning of any of the family members. While this is not a surprising finding, it could be an important message to mothers about their children's ability to tolerate flexibility in parental roles.

*On the other hand, mothers have a much greater opportunity for sex-role changes in the centrifugal-period family, when their children are grown up. The developmental pressure on the father during that period may not be expressed in sex-role change, but in a more fierce confirmation of a masculine gender identity.

FIRM AND DIFFUSE BOUNDARIES IN INTIMACY
AND SEXUALITY

In describing the close and resonant relationships of the young family, we have characterized the family as naturally highly involved and we believe that this is an essential quality. Infants need to be "read" and responded to, their communications need to be interpreted, many of their needs must be anticipated. As children grow older and begin to speak, the same process of understanding their meaning, in their terms, is required of their parents. Thus, a 4-year-old child who, while walking downstairs to break-fast, cheerfully announced to her mother, "Dennis and I were fucking yesterday" could not be taken literally. The mother said, "You and Dennis were what?" The child said, "Fucking." "What does that mean?" the mother asked. "I don't know," said the child, and they went on to break-fast.

Two things are important in this example. The first is the child's free interaction with her mother—her willingness to experiment with her new word, to try it out, and to learn more about it from her mother's reaction; in short, her confidence in that relationship. The second is the mother's perception of the child as a child. This recognition allowed her to be skeptical about what the child really meant. She saw the child as curious, experimenting, interesting, worth having a relationship with, but not sexual in the adult genital sense. The mother experienced a differentiation between child functioning and adult functioning. Operating within that framework, she was able to accept her daughter's statement as simply trying out an idea, and she was able to sustain the boundary and encourage the child to continue to be curious.

When little boys—or little girls, for that matter—approach their parents of the opposite sex with a proposal of marriage, this is an overt manifestation of the oedipal period. If one places the proposal of marriage in the context of other outlandish proposals made by a 4- or 5-year-old, one sees that Oedipus is only one of the heroic figures whose exploits are enacted by the imaginative youngster. There are conquerors like Agamemnon and travelers like Ulysses, not to mention any number of gods. All of these ancient heroes and gods and their modern equivalents establish an important place in the minds of children and remain as myths throughout their lives. Why has Oedipus been singled out? Is it possible that a proposal of some special relationship to the parent is more interesting to the parent than these many other postures assumed by the child? If this is so, then wouldn't the parent be likely to respond in such a way that lets the child know of this interest? Couldn't such interaction then become a pattern? If that pattern also excluded one parent, couldn't there be real jealousy of the romance between the child and the other parent?

Most people don't grow up to have unresolved Oedipus complexes. This is because, in most families, parents are clear that their children are children and are not capable of marrying or having sex at age 4. Parents can be flattered by the children's attentions and at the same time deal with the proposal in the same way they deal with many other such imaginative inventions. Mothers and fathers don't marry their children, but they may respond to the children's approaches with the closer, deeper relating that the children appear to be requesting. This nurtures the experience of intimacy while maintaining clarity about generations and sexuality. We believe that adults who have the capacity for intimate relating, learned during their own childhoods and practiced through their parenthood, will not be sexually tempted by their children but can be tempted by their children's invitations to experience new depths of intimacy. When this distinction is made, there is no Oedipus complex and no oedipal conflict.

SUMMARY

The family with young children passes through a period in the family-life spiral in which there is an atmosphere of closeness and responsiveness that allows for the learning and practice of intimacy. This natural process is manifested by family members caring for one another and being physically close to one another through holding, caressing, and soothing. It also involves the evaluation of a basic trust in mutual responsiveness.

Sexuality is not a natural part of the intimate behaviors between parents and children. We believe that it is a misperception to describe children as sexual, and to describe the physical arousal in parents in response to their children as sexual. Instead, the feelings are sensual and are a part of a physical response to nurturing and being nurtured, to caring and being cared for. Describing such feelings as sexual interferes with the intimate atmosphere of the family, begets mistrust and self-doubt, and ultimately begets future generations with difficulties with intimacy.

The culture of the young family, dominated by centripetal forces, is ideal for the development and reworking of sensuality and the capacity for intimacy. Doing so will provide a grounding in family relatedness and a basis for healthy intimacy in the future relationships of all family members.

PERSONAL RESPONSES: LEE COMBRINCK-GRAHAM

Influence of Gender and Generational Socialization. It's hard to know what influence my gender has had on the formation of my ideas—I've actually been the same gender my whole life! Possibly being a woman with Ambition (at first, to be as smart and sophisticated as my older brother) in a social setting where I was given modest encouragement of this ambitiousness and virtually no models, has allowed me to go outside the mainstream of theoretical conventions. My brother and I were unique in that our parents were divorced and, when I was 8, we had a stepfather. No one else in either of our school classes was in a situation like this, until we went to high school. This, too, was out of the mainstream. And I watched my mother take her Vassar education [à la McCarthy's Group], worth very little in the wartime job market, leave it behind, and get on with the business of supporting her family. To be successful as a woman has always meant being exceptional (which I have often confused with being eccentric). Although this position does not explain the specific content of my chapter, it does address the fact that I choose to question the logic and usefulness of conventional thinking, rather than accepting it as an explanatory framework.

Influence of Personal Intimacy and Sexual Experiences. As a child and again as a parent, my physically intimate relationships with family members in another generation (first parent, then children) have always been very clear. For this reason, hugging, kissing, sitting on laps, and snuggling have always been important and unambiguous sources and expressions of affection, comfort, and caring. I have found this to be true in relationships with friends, as well. Sexual intimacy is clearly very special, and it is different in form and intensity from that which is shared with most family members. I do not, for example, see sex as a source of comfort or reassurance, but something to be entered into for mutual enjoyment, when both partners are in pretty good form for both giving and receiving.

Implications for Family Therapy Training and Practice. The most important point in my chapter is the distinction between intimacy in general and sexual intimacy in particular, as a specialized form. Families (including parents, grandparents, and children) have a responsibility to communicate the value of intimate relating and to help their members of all generations to become comfortable with intimacy, both in utilizing resources derived in intimate relationships and offering intimacy in return. Boundaries between generations as well as boundaries of conceptual clarity must be recognized and strongly maintained, in order to communicate safety without exploitation.

Practically, in family therapy, these ideas will be useful in assisting families who hold back or maintain too much emotional distance, to come closer, particularly through providing affection and comfort to their young children. These experiences can be enacted in sessions. In families in which there is an exploitative physical interaction—a caricature of intimacy—it can be useful to explore ideas, fantasies, and personal needs in an effort to clarify the distinction between intimacy and sexuality. It means that these families have to be worked with as a whole, rather than in the fragments left by social and legal intervention.

In training, clearly the therapist needs to understand and act on the basis of this distinction, too. Rules of conduct that govern confidentiality and the proscription of sexual involvement with patients or clients are imposed because of the confusion that people experience about intimacy and sexuality. There are many opportunities for intimacy in both individual and family therapy, and there are many intimate moments in which the therapist shares. Some of these moments are accompanied by the physical feelings of sensuality. During these moments it is most important for the therapist to be clear about the distinction between intimacy and sexuality not only to observe the role distinction between therapist and patient, but also to clarify this distinction for the patient.

REFERENCES

Benedek, T. (1959). Parenthood as a developmental phase: A contribution to the libido theory. *Journal of the American Psychoanalytic Association, 7*, 389–417.

Boszormenyi-Nagy, I., & Krasner, B. (1986). *Between give and take: A clinical guide to contextual therapy.* New York: Brunner/Mazel.

Bowlby, J. (1969). *Attachment and loss. Vol. 1: Attachment.* New York: Basic Books.

Bowlby, J. (1982). Attachment and loss, retrospect and prospect. *American Journal of Orthopsychiatry, 52*, 664–678.

Brazelton, T. B., Koslowski, B., & Main, M. (1974). The origins of reciprocity: The early mother–infant interaction. In M. Lewis & L.A. Rosenblum (Eds.), *The effect of the infant on its caregiver* (pp. 39–66). New York: Wiley-Interscience.

Combrinck-Graham, L. (1983). The family life cycle and families with young children. In H. R. Liddle (Ed.), *Clinical implications of the family life cycle* (pp. 35–53). Rockville, MD: Aspen Press.

Combrinck-Graham, L. (1985). A developmental model for family systems. *Family Process, 24*, 139–150.

Erikson, E. H. (1968). *Identity: Youth and crisis.* New York: W. W. Norton.

Kagan, J. (1984). *The nature of the child.* New York: Basic Books.

Kellam, S. G., Ensminger, M. E., & Turner, R. J. (1977). Family structure and the mental health of children: Concurrent and longitudinal community-wide studies. *Archives of General Psychiatry, 43*, 1012–1022.

Klaus, M. H., & Kennell, J. N. (1976). *Maternal-infant bonding.* St. Louis: C. V. Mosby.

Kraus, M. A., & Redman, E. S. (1986). Postpartum depression: An interactional view. *Journal of Marital and Family Therapy, 12,* 63–74.

Mahler, M., Pine, F., & Bergman, A. (1975). *The psychological birth of the human infant.* New York: Basic Books.

Minuchin, P. (1985). Families and individual development: Provocations from the field of family therapy. *Child Development, 56,* 289–302.

Money, J., & Ehrhardt, A. A. (1972) *Man and woman, boy and girl: Differentiation and dimorphism of gender identity from conception to maturity.* Baltimore: Johns Hopkins University Press.

Pruett, K. D. (1983). Infants of primary nurturing fathers. *Psychoanalytic Study of the Child, 38,* 257–277.

Pruett, K. D. (1985). Oedipal configurations in young father-raised children. *Psychoanalytic Study of the Child, 40,* 435–456.

Sander, L. W. (1980). Investigation of the infant and its caregiving environment as a biological system. In S. I. Greenspan & G. H. Pollock (Eds.), *The course of life: Psychoanalytic contributions toward understanding personality development. Vol. 1: Infancy and early childhood* (pp. 177–201). Bethesda, MD: National Institute of Mental Health.

Stern, D. (1985). *The interpersonal life of the infant.* New York: Basic Books.

Winnicott, D. W. (1965). *The maturational process and the facilitating environment: Studies in the theory of emotional development.* New York: International Universities Press.

Wood, B. (1985). Proximity and hierarchy: Orthogonal dimensions of family interconnectedness. *Family Process, 24,* 487–507.

From: Intimate Environments: Sex, Intimacy and Gender in Families, Guilford Press, 1989. Edited by David Kantor and Barbara F. Okun.

5

TRANSFERENCE AND BEYOND

Michael Vincent Miller

In "The Fairy Godfathers," one of his disquieting short stories about our failures at love, John Updike brings together two definitive modern experiences—divorce and psychotherapy. The story concerns a pair of lovers who are in the midst of leaving their marriages in order to be together. In the past they had traveled with their former mates in the same suburban circles: among couples who play tennis and attend early music concerts together; among husbands who borrow each other's tools on weekends and wives who go barefoot in summer, displaying shapely, dancerlike arches. Eventually they had begun an affair. Now, picking their way through the debris of their ruptured families and their own guilt and vacillation, each of them sees a psychotherapist.

They meet regularly at his new fourth-floor walk-up apartment. During these encounters they carry on a rueful courtship, approaching one another with self-deprecating irony which mixes doubt and reassurance, desire and pathos—the emotions of people still haunted by the marriages they have abandoned. But above all, they discuss their latest therapy sessions, which stimulates their desire for each other. Just as being in love can become an obsession, so can being in therapy. Psychotherapy acts upon them like an aphrodisiac; poring over its intricate probings of motive and impulse turns into a sort of spiritual foreplay that overcomes their conflicted feelings. Steered by therapy away from their previous marriages and toward each other, as though this were the passage from neurosis to health, they eventually get married, buy a house, and terminate therapy—whereupon they discover that they have virtually nothing to say to one another! It is as if their romance were little more than an artifact created by the two therapists.

Michael Vincent Miller. Private Practice, Newton, Massachusetts.

As its title suggests, Updike's story is a modernist fairy tale, a kind of grotesque new version of "Cinderella." (In case the title isn't enough to make sure we catch the allusion, Updike nicknames his heroine "Pumpkin.") It also resembles those ancient Greek myths in which gods and goddesses, operating from dubious, all-too-human motives, interfere in the doings of mortals who have managed to arouse their interest or hatred. In "Cinderella" the heroine is delivered by supernatural intervention from poverty and familial oppression to a wonderful fate—marriage to a prince. But in "The Fairy Godfathers," hero and heroine are both delivered to the emptiness of modern marriage. Instead of nineteenth-century fairies or capricious Greek deities, Updike gives us psychotherapists who cast their spells disguised as psychological insights.

"The Fairy Godfathers" reminds us of a danger in the cultural phenomenon that the sociologist Philip Rieff once called "the triumph of the therapeutic" (1966). The avowed purpose of psychotherapy is to help people live better lives. But all too often it manages to insinuate itself so thoroughly into patients' attitudes that it becomes a substitute for the real thing. Has the therapeutic triumphed by defeating life? There is a poignant innocence in our hope that benevolent experts or wizards can purge us of uncertainty and confusion. But as Updike warns, we are not likely to be saved from the pitfalls of love—its illusions, compulsions, and dependencies—by becoming more psychologically sophisticated. Love was probably better off when it was still blind.

THERAPY'S INFLUENCE ON MARRIAGE

In case one is tempted to write off Updike's little fable as poetic exaggeration, let me turn to a research project currently in progress. The Harvard psychologist Carol Gilligan has been interviewing couples with children who are suffering through marital crises, in order to explore how they arrive at decisions to separate or stay together. Gilligan found that a large number of couples in her sample head for therapists' offices before they wind up in those of lawyers.* This is hardly news to me or my colleagues who practice a lot of marital therapy; we depend on this unfortunate turn of events to make a living. Judging from Gilligan's account, the therapeutic results for these couples were not uniformly impressive. Although some of her couples were very satisfied with what they learned from

---

*C. Gilligan (April 12, 1988), personal communication.

therapy that might help them resolve their problems, others were left awash in ambiguity, and some were even plunged into further turmoil over the therapy itself. Gilligan's preliminary findings confirm my own less systematic clinical hunches—namely that all too many patients who turn to therapy desperate for help with marital distress come away feeling that the therapist has somehow maneuvered the rescue or breakup of their marriages, leaving them bewildered and uncertain about their own real wishes.

There are active therapists who move in with a heavy hand, advising, provoking emotions like cheerleaders, criticizing the husband or wife who is unwilling to change, supporting the one who more readily accepts the therapeutic agenda. Such therapists are busy playing the role of saviour or parent and mainly succeed in infantilizing their patients. But therapeutic interference can also be much more subtle; it doesn't take a deliberately active or directive therapist to confuse patients or come between intimate partners. There are plenty of therapists who seem to think that by doing nothing except listening attentively or providing "mirroring feedback," they are assuming postures of neutrality and objectivity, leaving everything else to their patients' imaginations. (Updike's story is all the more convincing because we don't know how much of what the lovers report about their therapists' opinions is real and how much is imagined.) They influence their patients nevertheless. After all, *someone* is there listening, and being heard may be precisely what is missing from a patient's marriage. Even silent therapists can end up caught in triangles as though they were rivals for a husband's or wife's affection.

There are also the therapists in whom love and sex seems to bring out the worst, as psychosis does. These therapists tend to rely on clinical technique and professional formalism, which makes them rigid and abstract. They approach their patients with arrogance instead of tenderness, coldness instead of empathy, and dogmatism instead of open-mindedness. Maybe they manage to avoid the anxiety that their patients evoke in them, but this is a peculiar goal when you consider that sex and madness are the very topics upon which they are consulted as experts.

Of course, there are excellent therapists of every persuasion, and good and bad therapy is conducted along the entire continuum from overt meddling to limp inertness. The point is that therapists have real impact on their patients' lives, whether they behave like psychological athletes or circumspect statues. In either case, they can only be responsible for their intervention to the extent that they both know themselves and are conscious of their effect on others, in addition to recognizing their patients' actual concerns. Passivity may look at first glance like evidence of responsible therapy, but it can turn out to be only a more insidious form of interference. It is no wonder, then, that so many accounts of marriages subjected to therapy are deeply disturbing. Whether or not such therapy serves the best interests of patients in unhappy marriages, whether or not the therapists' roles are accurately perceived, one impression comes through consistently: Psychotherapy is capable of having massive influence on the fate of marriages.

The social implications of this influence are terribly unclear. How are therapeutic decisions about marriages being made, and what values are they based on? Does therapy tend to support or even create a culture in which gratifying oneself is praised and marital ties are disparaged? Are the therapists fighting the last vestiges of Victorian patriarchal tyranny or are they fostering narcissistic self-indulgence? Are they wrecking families through what used to be a civil offense called alienation of affection, or are they helping free men and women from pathological bondage? Has the neighborhood marriage broker of old become a marriage breaker? How much projection occurs, where the therapist's neutral interpretations are distorted by wishful thinking in the case of some patients and by bitterness, fury, or melancholy resignation in the case of others?

That so much is left open to question does not serve this strangely unaccountable profession nor its clients well. It suggests that psychotherapy is not exempt from our general confusion about love, sex, and marriage. More specifically, ambiguities arise from a gap or an incongruity between the theories that psychotherapists espouse and what actually goes on in their practices. The traditional analytic view reduces the intimate, erotic, and other powerful, elemental feelings that arise between therapist and patient to transference and countertransference. This theory implies that the therapist is a neutral bystander, a mere catalyst, the vague object of inflamed regressive feelings on the part of the patient. But at least it does acknowledge the passionate nature of the attachment, akin to falling in love.

Another influential viewpoint, rooted in modern object-relations theory, places more stress on mutuality and empathy, which leads it to suggest that the development of intimacy in therapy may in itself have a curative effect. This theory acknowledges the immediacy and reality of feelings between therapist and patient, although usually in a rather mild and uninspiring way. A third conception, held by many practitioners of family therapy, concentrates on the structure of interaction in therapy and virtually edits out both the therapist as a person and love as a subjective phenomenon. None of these approaches to intimacy in the clinical situation does justice to the demonic complexity that can envelop therapist and patient when powerful emotions, especially erotic ones, are set loose in the close quarters of a therapy session. The impact of the therapist's personality on the patient in particular remains largely unacknowledged and unarticulated. Most of the theories that psychotherapists use to explain their role seem designed to preserve their innocence.

We are not flourishing in our intimacies. My own feeling is that psychotherapy has not yet been very successful in helping men and women grapple with the anxieties of loving one another. Perhaps there is not enough psychotherapy (with the exception of certain existential and phenomenonological approaches such as Gestalt therapy) that focuses on the actual quality of contact between people. Most psychological theories have little to say about how we can surrender to intense feelings for each other and yet keep our differences intact in the struggle to know both ourselves and another man or woman. If anything, a great many couples have found that their bouts with therapy lead them further into self-absorption and away from their marriages. I know of at least three situations where husbands or wives became so steeped in the therapeutic culture that they left their marriages and went into training to become therapists themselves.

Where can a husband and wife turn when their marriage begins to come apart? In the seventeenth-century Puritan village, when it became known that a married couple was helplessly stuck in a severe quarrel, the governor sent in a representative to mediate. This illustrates how important the family's well-being was to the life of the early American community. Since we can no longer depend on much assistance from organized religion, the surrounding community, the extended family, or other traditional bolsters of married life, psychotherapy may be all we have to fall back on.

But the kind of dilemma that Updike portrays with satirical clarity may have been built into the very origins of psychotherapy, and it continues to plague most contemporary therapies. From the beginning, even as it struggled to teach people the liberating power of intimate and sexual speech, psychotherapy developed a peculiar one-sided silence of its own— a technical and methodological silence—to which it gave the name "transference." The concept of transference has proven to be a mixed blessing, because it has been at once a powerful diagnostic instrument for discovering how love can fail and a frustrating obstruction to learning how to love more fully.

SEX AND TRANSFERENCE

Despite Freud's quest for a science that could explain mental and emotional life, his theories remained on more familiar terms with passion than have most subsequent psychologies. He was still only a generation away from the Romantic era, whereas we have tended to bury much of our romantic idealism in an era where sex, marriage, and divorce all verge on becoming technicalities. And perhaps the forbidden sexuality of Freud's times made him more sensitive to the alluring urgencies and tensions of the erotic.

Fin-de-siècle Vienna smoldered with sexual desire and sexual sickness. Based on instinctual repression, the social order of Freud's time seemed about to explode. Its erotic contradictions were "like a dark underground vault over which rose the gorgeous structure of middle-class society with its faultless, radiant facade," wrote the Viennese novelist and critic Stefan Zweig (1953, p. 82). When Freud looked underneath the ornate scaffolding of Viennese life, he discovered lustful fantasies and yearnings, including grotesque ones, lurking everywhere—among both children and their parents, psychotics, mobs, dreamers, mystics and priests, artists and poets, aristocrats as well as laborers. This was certainly a cultural setting that would tend to produce ripe specimens of eros in neurotic disguise.

Freud became occupied, even preoccupied, with the sexual issues that led him to develop the concept of transference before the turn of the century. During the 1880s he collaborated with Breuer on experiments using hypnotic suggestion to treat hysterical symptoms. Not only did it become apparent to them that repressed sexual urges and related emotions might produce these symtpoms, but there was increasing evidence, bewildering but unmistakeable, that their work itself awakened strong erotic longings in their patients, most of whom were women.

One evening Breuer received an urgent call to go to the home of his patient Anna O. Upon arriving he found her suffering from phantom labor pains. Writhing in her bed, she announced that she was about to give birth to his baby. Breuer, a married man, fled in panic and abruptly ended her treatment. His colleague Freud had a less exotic but equally unsettling experience: As Ernest Jones describes the incident, when Freud leaned close to hypnotize a certain hysterical patient, she suddenly flung her arms around his neck "in a transport of affection" (1953, p. 250).

These were among the more blatant incidents. A few years later Freud concluded that the feelings stirred by analysis could also appear in much more subtle and subterranean forms, which included hostility toward the therapist as well as desire for closeness to him. Much to his dismay, Dora, the sexually pent-up and suffering adolescent of his most famous case history, quit therapy at the point where he thought that they were on the brink of success. Not until it was too late did Freud realize that she might have been prompted by a blend of secret love and vindictiveness.

If Freud's scientific curiosity was provoked by these events, one can imagine that he must have felt anxious and defensive as well, given the dim official view of sex that dominated his times. He decided to step back (rather than flee like Breuer) and observe his patient's erotic overtures with detached vigilance. The resulting turn-of-the-century Viennese tableau—an attentive but objective bearded man of science and medicine who appears lost in thought and a female patient on a couch, inflamed with symptoms—was to have wide influence on the subsequent evolution of psychotherapy. It became the standard psychoanalytic stance for dealing with emotions such as sexual desire and feelings of love and hate, whatever the patient's personality, background, or gender.

The following is one of my favorite recent examples of this approach, because it displays such impeccable psychoanalytic decorum: An eminent analyst received a phone call one night from a female patient in a state of panic. He immediately scheduled an emergency session, and she arrived at his office in a low-cut evening gown with a fur wrap around her neck and shoulders, explaining that she had been on her way to a social engagement when she called. At the end of the hour, she rose from the couch, considerably calmed; picked up her fur from a chair; and gave it to the analyst. Turning her back, she indicated that he was to drape it around her shoulders. The analyst, a worldly man, realizing that she was assigning him the role of her escort, handed her back the wrap without a word.

One can guess that her hurt and angry feelings about the analyst's rejection might be included among the material of the next session. But this analyst, known to be a man of considerable composure, would betray nothing of his emotional response to the episode nor her reaction to it, though he might decide to remind her of its resemblance to incidents in her early life when her father had also frustrated her expectations.

Freud coined the name "transference"—it first appears in the book he published with Breuer (1957)—to describe those feelings and behaviors, overt or disguised, that kept surfacing to trouble his therapy sessions. He explained them as libidinal attachments and frustrations that patients imported from childhood and pinned on the therapist as a way to repeat the past in the present. At first he considered them to be resistances, neurotic obstacles threatening the course of treatment, but then he found that they could be extremely useful in unraveling the early history of neurotic illness. Later Freud saw another benefit for analysis in the desires awakened through transference. Only something like passionate love for the therapist, he concluded, could sustain the patient through the anxious and painful self-scrutiny necessary to achieve a cure.

There is no question that transference was one of Freud's most significant clinical discoveries or, perhaps more accurately, inventions. By linking sexual desire and infantile dependence, Freud built an entire theory of human development and behavior on the ancient Greek intuition that Cupid is a child. He added that the sexual roots of our conduct are hidden from consciousness as well. Transference lent support to the theories of infantile sexuality and the unconscious and provided the clinician with a concrete means to implement them in therapy. It would not be an overstatment to say that transference made psychoanalysis feasible.

In its initial formulation psychoanalysis emphasized the regressive and pathological facets of love, rather like those ancient cultures which considered falling in love akin to madness or spirit-possession. It ignored the possibility that strong emotions between a therapist and patient, especially those aroused in the therapist by the patient, could in any constructive way be regarded as an end in themselves. In psychoanalysis, such feelings are allowed to flow only in one direction—from patient to therapist. Transference theory is, as John Shlien put it, "the analyst's proclamation of innocence" (1987, p. 28).

Is the analyst somehow invulnerable to arousal? It is said that Freud was obliged to conceal an erection at the end of a therapy hour spent with an attractive female patient. If this were true and had become generally known, the theory of transference as a regressive sexual attachment of the patient to a neutral therapist might have been amended. Freud's erection is not easily reconciled with the canon of analytic objectivity. Its exposure would have weakened the authority of those patriarchs of analysis— medical doctors explicating in "dry and direct" tones (Freud's characterization of his manner of talking frankly about sexual acts to innocent young girls) the unconscious, forbidden desires of their patients (Freud, 1963, p. 65). Transference, among others things, was a brilliant tactic which enabled Freud to avoid Breuer's terror, so that he could stay with the patient when sexual feelings started to heat up the therapy office. It wasn't that Freud was blind to the therapist's own longings and fears, but he regarded them as dangerous to the course of treatment. Subjugating the "counter-transference," as he called it, became a crucial part of every analyist's training.

If we hold the psychotherapist more responsible for the effects of his feelings on the patient, we soon begin to burst the confines of transference. From this perspective we can discover in transference theory a thinly cloaked politics, a therapeutic ideology or myth in which the therapist figures as absent hero, and we find ourselves increasingly uneasy about the psychotherapist's cultural role.

SEX AS POWER: THE POLITICS OF TRANSFERENCE

The question is not whether transference exists or whether it is useful, but whether psychotherapists mistake it for the whole of intimacy in therapy. To the extent that they do, they offer a reductive vision of love—one that leaves out both its complex, terrifying politics and its almost religious yearning for transcendence.

Even at their best, intimate relations exist in a precarious balance. They are always on the verge of being pulled in two directions at once— toward union and toward conflict—because they are continually buffeted by the competing claims of love and power. The contradictoriness makes intimacy vulnerable to anxiety-ridden, even violent turbulence. As though it were not hard enough, love and power have a way of disguising themselves in each other's clothes. For instance, "surrender" can describe an ecstatic loosening of the self or a capitulation to another's will. "Bonds" can refer to a freely chosen close and persistent attachment or to the bondage of enslavement or imprisonment. "Commitment" can mean a voluntary, enduring loyalty or a miniature version of what society does to people it defines as criminals or insane. Our language for describing erotic experience reflects the mixture of freedom and determinism that makes love difficult and ambiguous. Updike's story plays on such difficulties: It dramatizes how confusion of love and power can occur between patients and therapists as well as between lovers. Therapists presumably ought to help us disentangle the sexual from the political when the confusion damages our intimacies. We hardly need them to add more complications.

Insofar as therapists veil themselves and their procedures in mystification, they promote further confusions of love and power. I don't think that this is a satisfactory way to help people deal better with their intimate lives outside of therapy. For example, the classical transference model reduces the therapist to a silhouette, a projection screen dispensing occasional insights. One could argue that the shape of love and power in the transference situation—the yearning sexiness of the needy patient and the detached neutrality of the distant therapist—parodies a patriarchal social order with its emotionally unavailable, power-wielding fathers. Freudian analysis may have succeeded in freeing people's sexuality from neurotic symptoms by clarifying their origins in childhood, but it left them in the grip of patriarchal authority. It is not surprising that so many analyses ended in so-called transference cures, where patients gave up symptoms to please or spite the therapist and then returned to their lives eventually to develop new ones. The political structure of transference has as much to do with the maintenance of patriarchal authority as with the protection of patient and therapist from each other. This is probably why psychoanalyses, which began as a radical enterprise containing an implicit critique of the established order, gradually became a therapy of adjustment to that same order.

Psychoanalysis returned its patients to the danger of further illness because it returned them to a social order built on a foundation of sexual repression and male domination. Feminist historians have shown how the Victorian era's severe, inhibiting attitude toward sexual desire was tied to the oppression of women as a class. For all its usefulness in gaining insight into the patient's history, transference can also be viewed as an ideological instrument of male domination in psychotherapy. Recent developmental theorists, such as Nancy Chodorow and Carol Gilligan, have explained why women seek interdependent intimacy, whereas men tend to detach themselves from it. Transference denies the mutuality of intimate feelings between the therapist and the patient.

The dismantling and revision of classical psychoanalysis has been underway for some time. Nevertheless that part of its legacy involving a powerful, inaccessible therapist has been inherited by many of its successors, as though the invisible God of the bible still reigns in psychotherapy. New therapies have produced new reductionisms. There are behavioral therapies that rob the patient of his subjective experience and give the therapist the paternalistic task of distributing rewards and punishments. Strategic family therapy, the school founded by Jay Haley and his coworkers, scrutinizes intimacy, including that between therapist and patient, for signs of hidden power struggles with as much fervor as the Freudians searched for signs of hidden sexual desire.

Strategic therapy has been valuable in showing us how underground battles for domination figure in marital and family life, but it has let eros slip away in the meantime. According to this school, all love is power, symptoms are tactics to gain control over others, and therapy is like a chess match in which the therapist is the superior player. Haley (1969) wrote a long essay in which he argued that Jesus Christ, the archetype of spiritual love in western religion, was a brilliant political tactician who rose to power by organizing a mass movement of the wounded and dispossessed. As far as I can recall, Haley never mentions love in this essay.

As strange as it may seem, family therapists, with a few exceptions such as Nathan Ackerman, Carl Whitaker, and R. D. Laing, have simply ignored love and sex as serious subject matter. They interest themselves in the forms of intimacy—patterns, structures, systems, and cybernetic loops—and hardly at all in its content. Their tendency is to equate the therapist with his technique for altering dysfunctional patterns of behavior in individuals, marriages, and families. As a result, the person of the therapist is not just neutralized, as in psychoanalysis, but virtually eliminated. These therapies are perfectly in tune with the era of technology and information processing. So austere is their perception of intimacy that they make transference and countertransference seem in comparison like an operatic duet.

SEX AS LANGUAGE

"There is no sex without talk," wrote the psychiatrist Leslie Farber (1976, p. 167). Erotic love always contains the option of revelatory conversation, even though it may choose to be silent. But sex without self-disclosure is no more than lust. Neither the silences nor the conversations of lust are eloquent; they echo down the stark corridors that reflect the participants' absence from each other. At least such encounters are often mercifully brief. But what about the hopelessness that afflicts unions like that of Updike's adulterous lovers after they marry? These marriages may resound with superficial chatter or interminable complaints or violent quarrels to disguise the deeper silences. Modern marriages too often recall Ford Maddox Ford's description of a troubled marriage in *The Good Soldier* as "a long, silent duel with invisible weapons" (1951, p. 123).

It is perhaps worth reminding ourselves that self-expressive talk is also the primary medium of psychotherapy. Through its work with hysteria, classical psychoanalysis stumbled on the deep, inevitable connection between desire and speech. The repressive sexual morality of the Victorian era tried to make sexuality nearly mute, so that it remained almost unknown and incommunicable. Perhaps this speechlessness was the true meaning of the unconscious. Hysterical symptoms, so widespread during those times, were themselves a kind of language—a distorted, wordless language of sexuality, especially the sexuality of women painfully confined to the wrong parts of the body. Psychoanalysis made an important contribution to the relief of human suffering when it learned to use the give-and take of free association and interpretation as a method for transforming the unconscious language of symptoms into explicit sexual speech.

The failure of modern psychology to do justice to love and sex is in part a failure of language. Our problem is not that we labor, like the Victorians, under the tyranny of secrecy—certainly not in this age of overflowing information. If the nineteenth century suffered from too much sexual repression, it may be that the twentieth century suffers from too much random sexual expression—which may yet accomplish what repression failed to do: Kill off sex as a passionate and transcendent experience. The formula that has dominated our times—sexual freedom plus social science used as a basis for moral values—however liberating at first, has ended up playing a part in draining the erotic of vitality and mystery. In trying to be scientific, our current psychologies and psychotherapies have contributed almost as much as pornography and narcissism to the waning of sexual love.

Contemporary psychiatrists and psychologists writing about love have produced a pretty uninspiring reading list and, if anything, could improve things by introducing more pornography. Neither the language of object-relations theory, nor the stimulus-response accounts of behaviorism, nor the cybernetic categories of systems theory contain any passionate utterance or imagery. In general, the social sciences have not provided us with a rich vocabulary for understanding intimacy. For example, one of the most flattening (and most inescapable) words we use in talking about intimacy is the word "relationship." In a college math course, I learned that a relationship is something that exists between two variables that affect one another, which can therefore be described in an equation. Lovers affect one another, but variables do not make love (or go through struggles at failing to make love) nor is the act an equation.

What would a behaviorist or a systems therapist make of the scene in *The Magic Mountain* where Hans Castorp passionately celebrates Madame Chauchat's x-ray? For Castorp, her x-ray is a metaphor, a blueprint of his beloved's soul; it's as if he can still see her radiance through it. Sexual love is the poetry of contact. It involves the discipline of connoisseurship, an aesthetic appreciation of another's being. As long as psychotherapeutic theory and practice continues to be dominated by mechanistic thinking, all we are left with is the x-ray.

The best writing on love and marriage comes not from social scientists but philosophers such as Plato, Kierkegaard, and Ortega y Gasset and novelists such as Thomas Hardy, D. H. Lawrence, and Virginia Woolf. Freud admired poets and novelists and thought of them as his precursors.

He came as close as any psychological theorist has to understanding the complexity of erotic life, yet he seems to have had a sense of his own limitations. He backed off from portraying the subjective experience of love and sex in his writings, just as he backed off in therapy through the use of transference. Instead, he presented a theory of the preconditions in mental life which cause love to succeed or fail. When psychological writers come up with "empathetic communication" and other such empty abstractions in their quest for operational definitions of intimacy, one wishes they would back off too.

Psychological theory does not have to be mechanistic. In his book *Thalassa* (1968), Sandor Ferenczi described sexual intercourse as though it were a mixture of paradise and catastrophe. He went on to link sexual desire with a primitive instinctual urge to return to the sea-life from which we came. This may be more imaginative than scientifically accurate, but at least it gives eros the kind of cosmic scope that D. H. Lawrence always reached for. At times Ferenczi almost managed to adapt the ideas of biological science and psychoanalysis to the unruliness and unpredictability of human passion.

Not all the signs of our times are discouraging. There is a shift away from mechanistic conceptions in modern psychoanalytic practice as well as in other modern schools—Rogerian therapy and Gestalt therapy, for example. Some practitioners insist that therapists can make valid use of their feelings—that it is not enough to view the patient's emotions through a one-way mirror; that awareness or insight heals mostly when the patient feels supported by not only close but affectionate attention. And what is love but close, appreciative attention?

I am not saying that the intimacy of psychotherapy is the same as the other intimacies in our lives nor that it represents any substitute for them. The therapist's job is to pay attention to the patient's needs and not the other way around, whereas husbands and wives or lovers ought to be aware of each other's needs. The asymmetry of therapy is part of what patients pay for. You could say that psychotherapy is to life what a painting of a landscape is to an actual landscape—a carefully edited and condensed version of the real thing. Like a painting, the therapy session exists within a frame that lifts it out of the everyday flow and sets it apart, making it more simplified and finite than life. The idea is that when spectators leave the museum or patients the consulting room, they will walk outside and see the world (and themselves in it) differently.

What intimacy and psychotherapy have in common is that both are emotionally charged, difficult enterprises, demanding persistence, courage, discipline, and self-knowledge. William Carlos Williams wrote that

"The business of love is cruelty *which*, by our wills we transform to live together" (Williams, 1962). There's always pain in therapy, as there usually is in love. But the outcome of contending with the painfulness can be a more satisfying human existence.

In many cases, the psychotherapist is the only person that the patient is free to love. That sad truth is among the reasons why people come to therapy in the first place. Maybe only the therapist sees the patient truly naked. Even lovers do not really see each other naked; they are usually still clothed in self-protection. We don't know how to show our souls to each other, and we try to learn in psychotherapy. How can therapists not help but feel intimate when they are being given something close to the total knowledge of another that most of us only dream of? How could they not feel a poignant affection wash over them at such revelations of the human condition?

Freud pointed out that love for the analyst enables the patient to tolerate the anxiety of therapy. We might add that only love for the patient enables the therapist to tolerate therapy without taking refuge in mechanistic theory and technique. Whatever relief it provided from Victorian neurotic symptoms, the formal, studied neutrality of analytic transference is out of date in our day. Yet many influential attempts to go beyond the transference model in psychotherapy seem at least as unsatisfactory. We need to develop a psychology that is more lyrical and ironic, richer in the phenomenology of erotic experience, one that can make the psychotherapist a more daring, compassionate explorer and teacher amid the tragicomedies of love and sex in the modern world. Such a theory might help bring the therapist to life in the therapy session. If it is to speak with real conviction to our anguished, faltering, still persistent willingness to risk loving one another, psychotherapy may well demand more emotional communion between therapist and patient than anything psychological theory has yet suggested.

REFERENCES

Breuer, J., & Freud, S. (1957). *Studies on hysteria*. New York: Basic Books

Farber, Leslie H. (1976). *Lying, despair, jealousy, envy, sex, suicide, drugs, and the good life*. New York: Basic Books.

Ferenczi, S. (1968). *Thalassa: a theory of genitality*. New York: W. W. Norton.

Ford, F. M. (1951). *The good soldier: a tale of passion*. New York: Vintage Books.

Freud, S. (1963). *Dora: an analysis of a case of hysteria*. New York: Collier Books.

Haley, J. (1971). *The power tactics of Jesus Christ and other essays*. New York: Avon Books.

Jones, E. (1953). *The life and work of Sigmund Freud*. New York: Basic Books.

Rieff, P. (1966). *The triumph of the therapeutic: Uses of faith after Freud*. New York: Harper and Row.

Shlien, J. M. (1987). A countertheory of transference. *Person-Centered Review*, 2, 15-49.

Williams, W. C. (1962). *Pictures from Brueghel and other poems*. New York: New Directions.

Zweig, S. (1953). *The world of yesterday*. London: Cassell.

6

THOUGHTS ABOUT SEX, LOVE, AND INTIMACY

Carl Whitaker

WHO AM I?

First I must define the setting for my participation in this book, beginning with the fact that I was born in 1912 and therefore am at least two generations out of phase with our cultural movements. The reader should take that into account in reading what I extrapolate from my belief system.

WHAT IS A FAMILY?

I guess we should begin by defining what, in general, a family is. It is really a combination of two families, his and hers, and the term has been so variously used that we need to define the kinds of families. I discern three types of families.

The most prevalent type of family is the *biopsychosocial family*, whose members are biologically related because of the genetic fact of inheritance; psychologically involved, whether the affect is negative or positive, low or high voltage; and, finally, socially combined, since they live in the same territory. In this kind of family, the parents are biologically reincarnated in their children so that the father sees in the face of each child his own face and the mother's face and the mother sees in the face of each child her face and the father's face. This produces a kind of unique identity or identification, which, although frequently below the

Carl Whitaker, Department of Psychiatry, University of Wisconsin Medical School, Milwaukee, Wisconsin.

level of awareness, is very profound and expresses itself either positively or negatively to the degree or intensity that the individuals can tolerate, in spite of or because of their life experience and their investment in each other. The investment is irrevocable and profound, whatever the degree of recognition.

Second, there is the *psychosocial family*. This is a family whose members have "fallen in love" or are invested more and more in each other by virtue of their psychological closeness and by the degree of their investment in each other and their social life. This irrevocable love is based on psychological investment rather than the biological identification characteristic of the biopsychosocial family. Again, the investment may be positive or negative. Usually it is a combination of both, and there are, of course, multiple variations of this. The psychological investment may be momentary but results in pregnancy and continued family development. On the other hand, it may be long continued and fairly independent of sexuality—the so-called platonic psychological involvement which I think of as whole person to whole person but with an agreed-upon dissociation from a sexual relationship.

The psychosocial family would include blended families. Of course, you also have his, hers, and their families, in which there would be a biological subfamily within the two psychological and psychosocial families living together. Both the biopsychosocial and psychosocial families are typical patient families.

A third kind of family is the *social family*. Ordinarily, I use this term to talk about a football team or a tennis duo, a sorority or a fraternity, or a political group. This type of family is often time limited and resembles a friendship-based (chosen rather than inherited) intimacy or closeness in which there are team investment, team objectives, and organizational and psychological social investment, in addition to individual investment. Although this kind of family takes multiple forms, it frequently evolves into a "family-set" (family type of organization) with important generation gaps between the older and the younger members. Along with these generation gaps come role responsibilities, which are assumed or assigned in a manner and way similiar to a family pattern. Examples of this type of social family would be the therapist and patient dyad or the network of colleagues. This concept of social family as sharing family-type roles and rules but differing in terms of time limits and its voluntary team objectives provides a context for my comments about intimacy and sexuality in family therapy.

I would also describe modern sexual games as social-family experiments. And, of course, the social family, if it includes sexual intercourse, can produce a sudden new biological investment, which may indeed be fairly low or very high voltage as time goes along. This could lead to a new or different type of family or could remain time and investment limited.

The fact that the biopsychosocial and psychosocial families consist of a combination of two families produces a conflict in the usual problems of integrating the two cultural backgrounds. The rules, mythology, and organizational patterns of one family are different from those of the other family and comprise the foundation for stress in families. In blended families, the combination is more complex, as it includes several families of origin as well as previous spouses and their families. In social families, there are influences from several or many families, but the time limitations and team objectives may soften the necessity for integration.

DIFFERENCE BETWEEN THE SEXES

We usually think of the family as originating from the dyadic relationship between two persons, usually of different sexes. One of the classic philosophers—which one, I don't remember—said there is no such thing as a dyad. It is merely the remnant of an extruded third. So, when I talk about families, I am really talking about my family, the result of my excluding my mother and my wife excluding her mother. Part of my belief system is that fathers are, as Margaret Mead says, a social accident and are, for most of their lives, unable to be humanistic and merely in love with things. This gets us into the issue of differences between the sexes, which I first learned about from my mother, who was always right. The differences between the sexes powerfully influence how families form, develop, and function.

If in my fantasy I go back 100 million generations, I can assume that the men who produced the next generation were the ones who were the most powerful in killing for food and protection and most turned on by the lure of sexual experience. If we carry that process through 100 million generations, it becomes more and more clear that the selection process is very specific and has happened inexorably. One can also define the sexual evolution of the female. If I go back in my imagination 100 million generations, the women who produced the next generation were the ones who not only were seductive but who cared for and protected their children. This process itself went on for 100 million generations. It produced the evolution of the kind of maternal investment evident in 93% of the "single-parent families" that now make up an increasingly large population. The mother is the person who cares, and the father is her chosen teammate who, of course, has a psychological investment in the mother. But this investment is relative and easy to disguise by combining it with feelings about his mother or some other woman. He will, of course, maintain some affect, usually having to do with his pride at possession or his effort to protect his turf.

So it is the "natural selection" differences between the sexes that lead to the current notion of family where the father's role is peripheral and executive compared to the mother's role.

EVOLUTION OF A NEW FAMILY

What I am getting at is the differentiation of sexual investment and psychological investment in the evolution of a new family. One of the obvious sources of a new family is the symbiosis between two families. But in our culture the usual process involves two separate families, many times unknown to each other, each sending out a scapegoat to reproduce their family. Once these two parents have produced offspring, the critical question is, Whose family are they reproducing, his or hers? And, of course, this is never settled and never readily resolved on the deeper level.

Critical to the dynamics of the family's origin is the obvious fact that, although the attraction between these two parents-to-be may be vibes, also known as electrical excitement about some cue stimulus (sexual investment), there is also some complementary or supplementary interlocking dynamic (psychological investment). There is usually also a contract for bilateral psychotherapy: He is sure she will be the ideal wife as soon as he gets her over being compulsive, and she is sure he will be the ideal husband as soon as she gets him over his drinking problem. As we know, this marital contract is open to the usual impasse in pseudopsychotherapy!

Marriages also can be originated on the basis of the panic about being 16 years old and the belief that, if you combine with another 16-year-old, you become one 32-year-old and a member of the powerful adult world, overnight. This is also one way to escape from one's parents.

Thus, the biopsychosocial family includes many generations—certainly the parents and children, but also the two sets of grandparents and the siblings of each of the parents. It consists basically of a series of subgroups: all the males, all the females, the males in one family and the females in the other, the cross-generational groupings, and the infinite numbers of triangles. Simultaneously, there are many stress-inducing triads: husband–wife–child; husband–wife–his mother; husband–wife–

golf; husband–his son–his son's mother (previous wife of husband); husband–wife–his sister; husband–wife–her father; husband–wife–her mother.

INTERPLAY OF SEX, INTIMACY, AND LOVE

The definition of sex is based on the sexual games of the lovers. Frequently, the sexual game consists of a penis and a vagina going off on a trip together. But there are *no people* along. The issue is whether or not the people will ever arrive in order to have a love relationship.

One of the problems with the territory of sexuality as experienced or struggled with in psychotherapy is the fact that, in our present cultural orientation, sex has become a substitute for developing a loving relationship. Unfortunately, most times the sexual experience is one of the most successful ways of short-circuiting any whole-person-to-whole-person relationship. This means that love never arrives. It is short-circuited each time by the sexual separation process.

Malone* said many years ago that sex is not a way of getting together; it is a way of getting the other person out from under your skin. Sex is a way to become independent or noncaptured, to escape from the togetherness, to escape from the we-ness that mother nature is thrusting upon us. Sex, then, can be a diversion from love.

The struggle to adapt to or tolerate family living is involved with two general territories—the commitment to closeness and the ebb and flow of intimacy. Closeness consists of more and more investment in each other. Intimacy, upon which I will elaborate further, consists of a temporary state of sacrificing one's personhood for the privilege (momentary or episodic) of belonging to a larger system. Intimacy is, then, the psychological interpenetration of two persons, symbolically represented or metaphorically described in the process of sexual intercourse. It also occurs in the moment of excitement and the we-ness that leaves one temporarily free from the boundaries and interfaces between individuals and families.

Closeness, of course is algebraic. It can be positive or negative. Many times it is more powerful when it is negative than when it is positive. Closeness is like the stock market. The investment will grow, but it can also slump on its own or from inside trading.

The sexual experience itself can be one of the moments of interpenetration, either increasing the current of intimacy and lovingness or short-

---

*P. Malone (1953), personal communication.

circuiting and avoiding lovingness or closeness by diverting the person-to-person relationship into a body-to-body game. Whereas the biological family consists of a quality of identification which is visually and nonverbally present, though usually unrecognized, the sexual experience can provide an infrastructure that makes life operate as a form of we-ness, of belonging to a bigger system in which one is willing to invest part of one's personhoood. In the biopsychosocial and psychosocial families, the relationship involves a relative sense of belonging to a bigger system, mostly operated on the basis of cue stimuli with an open-market freedom to invest or withdraw. The social family, of course, is a casual acquaintanceship around a common purpose. In a social family, one can avoid the stress of more intimate relationships. Thus, sexual experiences can take a different form and meaning in different types of families.

A decade ago, I wrote that love, sex, and the committed relationship covary with each other through the life span (Whitaker, 1976). At some periods, all three variables seem to summate into a marvelous suprasystem, while at other times they seem to fragment, occasionally resummating. The continual reciprocal balance of I-ness and we-ness seems to underlie and enhance the flourishing of these variables on the biopsychosocial and psychosocial families. Time-limitedness affects the balance of love and commitment in social families. Different types of intimacy will be present in different types of families at differing times of the family life-span.

INTIMACY MODELS

As I have continued to think about the interrelationship of love, sex, and the committed relationship, I've been able to describe three types of intimacy and some of the variables that disrupt or activate these types of intimacy. This elaboration will enable us to consider the formation and development of intimacy in families and in the process of psychotherapy.

The first type of intimacy is what I call *cultivated intimacy*, a bilateral process. This occurs typically as a predominant form in the social family. The most obvious example is the therapist and patient. Others include a singer and accompanist, a husband and wife, business partners, and teams (football or baseball). Cultivated intimacy may also apply to opponents, such as boxers, business competitors, and labor union associates, who are intensely bound by common objectives or processes. This type of intimacy is usually voluntary and time limited around a common objective. It may develop into a longer-range relationship and a different type of intimacy.

A second type of intimacy is *forced intimacy*, usually situational. This type appears in cellmates, persons in a prison camp or adrift in a lifeboat, a couple who have been pushed into a shotgun marriage, and siblings in a blended family. This also is usually time-limited but may or may not develop into a different type of intimacy.

A third type of intimacy is *natural intimacy*. This arises out of constructive sources in the relationship between persons, for example, the greater intimacy among the citizens of a country where there is a common enemy. We saw this after Pearl Harbor or during the post–World War II fear of the communists, and it is present when siblings bond in fear of their father. We see this with persons who live in the far North and share in their common fight to stay alive in the face of Mother Nature. Another natural intimacy may develop out of situational pressures, such as in the therapeutic impasse or among schoolmates in their struggle to pass a course or exam.

We may see each of these types of intimacy in a family at different times of development. One is not necessarily exclusive of another, and they may coexist or evolve in varying combinations.

DISRUPTION OF INTIMACY

The disruption of intimacy can come about as a result of many different forces, including the following:

1. Presence of a third person. Although we ordinarily think of the third person as disrupting a one-to-one intimacy, it is possible, paradoxically, for this to take place in reverse. The third person can *increase* the intimacy, because, with the arrival of the third person, the one-to-one relationship, in which there was a certain degree of togetherness and a certain degree of againstness, is altered in the fact that the triangle now forces the separation into two sides. If the one-to-one relationship pushes the third person into being the antagonist, then the one-to-one is an increasingly intimate relationship, whether negative or positive. As therapists, we often depend on this paradoxical triangulation to increase couple intimacy.

2. A time and space separation. This happens when soldiers go overseas and leave their mates at home or when illness or occupation require long physical separations.

3. A competing intimacy. An obvious example of this would be a sexual affair. Others include the intrusion into the husband–wife relation-

ship by the competition of one or both mothers-in-law or by a child or professional/work absorption.

4. Accumulating roles and role responsibilities. These may result in a loss of spontaneity and restriction of the resources that provide for intimacy development. Examples are the 10-year syndrome in marriage or the gradual neurotic interlocking in a partnership or a clinic group. This accumulation of role responsibility may be around a single role, such as the responsible older brother, or around multiple roles, such as the mother in her relationship to the various children, her husband, her job, and the community.

5. Long-term denial of self. The person who represses her hostility in a marriage and gradually builds up a degree of denial of herself will find intimacy with the other person lessening and becoming disrupted.

6. The break of an implicit contract. In the husband–wife therapeutic marriage, the implicit arrangement that each shall be patient to the other is gradually or suddenly broken by one or the other, and this is seen as a rejection resulting in the intimacy being badly disrupted and distorted. In the Edward Albee play *Who's Afraid of Virginia Woolf* this happens when the husband stops playing along with his wife's fantasy that they have a child.

It seems pertinent to note parenthetically that there is NO LOSS OF INTIMACY, BUT MERELY A DISTORTION OF IT. INTIMACY CANNOT BE DESTROYED. IT CAN ONLY BE DISRUPTED AND DISTORTED.

ACTIVATION OF INTIMACY

Assuming that intimacy is a quality, it seems that it should be possible to activate it, or that it could become activated, by certain situational sets or certain types of experience. I have identified the following:

1. Isolation. Intimacy in a couple is activated in the isolation of the honeymoon, and the intimacy an individual has with himself may be activated in a similar way during a religious retreat. The increasing intimacy with the significant other on the honeymoon is somewhat different from the increasing intimacy of Christ's 40 days in the desert, but there are many similarities.

2. A team product. The arrival of a child marks the reincarnation of both the the self and the other. When the husband sees himself in the

child's face, he also sees his wife's face. This leads to a "weness," in that he sees the "we," not just the "I" or "you," in the child's face. This identification increases intimacy.

3. An ending that people anticipate. This structure has long been recognized in the pattern of the summer romance, a time-limited psychotherapeutic relationship, or the intimacy people experience on airplane and train trips.

4. Expression of negative affect. This is most conspicuous by the aftereffects of a fight between boyfriend and girlfriend or between husband and wife, when there is intimate lovemaking that ameliorates the pain after the expression of negative affect.

5. Variables of time. Intimacy undoubtedly has a quality of ebb and flow, a quality of with-ness and without-ness. The time for intimacy may be spontaneous or planned, predictable or unpredictable.

6. Significant experiences. Peak mystical or meditational experiences such as the Zen state of satori, or another significant type of moment, can increase the move toward intimacy, due to the anticipation of such an experience occurring again.

7. Denial of self. It is possible that the deliberate denial of self can also bring about an increasing intimacy. This means diverting self-preoccupation to concern for the other.

8. Denial of purpose. It is possible that denial of one's own desire, impulses, or gratification in order to please the spouse can, like denial of self, activate intimacy. For example, if I want to go fishing, but my wife doesn't like to fish and I deny that desire in order to be with her, our intimacy will grow.

9. Denial of pseudo-intimacy. Conscious denial of pseudo-intimacy (superficiality) can activate intimacy.

PSYCHOTHERAPY AND ISSUES
OF LOVE AND INTIMACY

All psychotherapy, by its nature, is parenting. That is, one person is dependent and trying to be more of his whole self, and the respondent, called the therapist, is an actor. A therapist is enacting a role, just as any parent is enacting a role. A parent, rather than being a whole person, is deliberately denying some of her responses and activating others. Both parenthood and therapist are roles. And the patient is a whole person, not a role, in the sense that the child is a whole person. This difference—

therapist as a role and patient as a whole person—is critical to an effective therapeutic relationship.

The patient can become confused by this because he is deluded into thinking that this therapeutic relationship is as profound as a parent's love for a child, when, in fact, it is not. The role of the therapist is conditional upon a bilateral agreement that the imitation intimacy that occurs in psychotherapy shall be maintained by the twosome—or, if it is the family, by the therapist and the family. Now, if the therapist has not had therapy herself, she may assume that the therapist–patient setting is one of whole person to whole person or of role to role. In other words, she may not recognize the necessary difference between the therapist's genuine role and the patient's genuine whole investment of self needs and demands. Assuming, as I do, that everyone's need for intimacy is greater than her tolerance of it, there may develop a co-transference setting such that the therapist allows herself to get out of the therapist role and become a whole person, with the natural whole-person demands for intimacy. The therapist's demands for such delusional intimacy should have been satisfied by her own therapy. Co-transference thus makes the therapist vulnerable to the complex and powerful intimacy experience of the patient.

Probably this co-transference is best stated by the covert contract that is made between therapist and patient(s): *I will be your mother if you will be my mother.* If this process is not broken up by the other family members, the family as a whole, or a consultant or a co-therapist, it can rapidly evolve without the awareness of either one into a profound bilateral delusional intimacy. Such intimacy can be extremely frightening and may well lead to the kind of short-circuit characteristic of falling in love. This kind of falling in love includes the discovery that sexuality is one way of preventing the danger of being victimized by the paranoia that goes with bilateral intimacy on this infrastructural level of every therapeutic relationship. The therapist's professional role disappears. The crucial contract that the therapist will be an imitation or foster mother and the patient will have the freedom to be his whole self is broken. The social roles lose their power, and the dynamics of the twosome are profoundly pathologized without any awareness that the initial contract has been broken. The covert co-transference delusion makes the therapist and patient each victims of the process that supposedly entailed the therapist staying in the role as a foster parent rather than as a whole person. In actuality, the therapeutic relationship becomes a psychological affair, or, if you will, cross-generational incest. Such pathologizing of the therapeutic relationship can lead to sexualizing the therapeutic relationship.

The danger of cross-generational incest is minimized if a co-therapist or consultant is used, so that it becomes clear to the patient, whether an individual, a couple, or a family, that the relationship between the two "parent" therapists is more important than the relationship of either to the patient. Then the generation gap is intact and the psychological connection between the patient and the therapist is an "AS IF" relationship. The responsibility for maintaining the generation gap within the therapeutic process is clearly and completely with the therapist. The therapist is hired to maintain a role and NOT to be a whole person.

The process of psychological love that takes place between the foster parent (therapist) and the family or individual patient only becomes sexualized if there evolves a sense of peership and the parent role is disguised by this illusion or delusion of peership. That is, it happens if the generation gap is not intact. Remember, the therapist is hired to maintain a role, not to be a whole person. The therapist is hired to belong to an older generation. The process of therapy is most simply described as that of foster parenting. The psychological love that goes on between the foster parent and patient(s) is indeed significant, powerful, and valuable. But there is a difference between the biological identification of self with offspring that takes place in a real biopsychosocial family and the psychological love characteristic of the therapeutic relationship. The therapist's responsibility is to maintain the generation gap, to maintain the role structure of his participation, and to protect the family—both the individuals and subgroups within the family—so that they become more whole as individuals, as subgroups, and as a family.

In the infrastructure of every therapeutic interview and, more specifically, in the ongoing psychotherapy, the therapist, if he is male, is reliving his own mother–son relationship, but without the benefit of the taboo they were protected by. Moreover, this reliving is concealed by the kaleidoscope of the pornographic word games that constitute psychotherapy. The whole psychotherapeutic relationship is highlighted by the bilateral recall of childhood memories and childish enthusiasm and the voltage on the part of each of them of the "what-if" extra thoughts. Overlaying all of these fantasies is the counterculture paranoia and the freedom of their isolated time–space setting, as well as the standard "I'm for hire" contract. Is it any wonder that in the one-to-one psychotherapeutic relationship this cross-generational psychological incest between the therapist as a foster mother (although he's male) and the patient as a love-hungry child may be suddenly precipitated into an acting-out pattern completely intolerable to either one of them, outside of that setting? The impulse is often reinforced by the frustration of everyday living and the reality of social adaptation and real-world demands. These impulses are inevitable, and we need to counter them in order to prevent pathologizing the therapeutic process.

The pathologizing of the therapy process is essentially losing the necessary generation gap. The problem then becomes how to prevent the therapist from becoming a peer with one or more members of the patient family. Acting against pathology rests with what the therapist has done in preparation for becoming a professional.

The most obvious method for prevention of pathologizing the therapy process is to develop the maturity of the therapist as a person. The therapist must become enough aware of herself that she is endlessly suspicious of her own participation and endlessly concerned with self-critique. A very important method for preventing pathology in the therapeutic process is for the therapist herself to have had psychotherapy. This not only helps make her more tolerant of the role restrictions inherent in being a professional therapist but also provides a more thorough understanding of the process of transference.

TRANSFERENCE

Unilateral Transference

The power of transference is not really experienced when one is the therapist. This is very similar to the experience of being a mother. Any one of us knows the power of the mother over the children, but I have never seen a mother who really *sensed the power* she has over her children.

Mothers see their offspring as the children they used to be, regardless of the age or stature of the offspring. Likewise, children see their mother as she was when they were young. This explains why so many adults still react to the omnipotent mother they have kept in their head from their childhood. A patient will often transfer this idealized, omnipotent parent from childhood onto the therapist.

Transference is only experienced from the side of the victim, and that is true in the process of therapy as well as in the process of child rearing. The victim—that is, the people who are patients—are rarely able to understand and critique their own participation. They really should not need to, as that is the therapist's responsibility. *The victim of transference is not able to understand the power* that transference exerts and is only reveling in the return to childhood, the regression that takes place in the process of therapy. Since patients are not aware of it, they very frequently do not express it, so the therapist may not really be given the opportunity to critique it or become aware of it on a conscious level. The therapist is seduced by the the devotion of the victimized patient and the seductive temptation of his own humanness. The transference phenomenon, from the patient's experience in this relationship, becomes distorted only if the therapist also develops a delusional system transferred from his own life. This occurs when the therapist uses this patient as his own reincarnation, as a parent would in the case of biological or adopted children.

One needs to know transference as a process of investing, in the therapist, the affect one has had toward one's primary caretakers, usually mother and father. It is an intrapsychic phenomenon. This does not happen behaviorally, although it may express itself behaviorally. It happens in the inner world of fantasy and may be taking place and expressing itself in behavior or in the living process without the patient knowing about it or having any sense that something is going on below the level of awareness that affects the interrelationships among people.

Bilateral Transference

It is equally true, but little mentioned, that this process of transference may take place bilaterally. For me, love by its very definition is a process of looking at the other and seeing onself. This bilateral relationship involves the readiness to reinvest oneself in another. Thus, the transference that the patient has is often matched by the process taking place within the therapist. The therapist also may not know what is involved or what result it is producing in the relationship being established with the patient on a deliberate role-defined basis. Once this transference and co-transference have developed, however, the therapeutic relationship becomes an interpersonal experience. That is, there is an action–reaction and interaction or synthesis, if you will, of the two transference components.

Projection

Behind the transference, or interlocking with it, is a process called projection. It is the means by which the transference experience inside may make a victim of the other person. For example, if the transference is toward a punitive father, the projection of that may make the patient see the therapist as a punitive person, even though that may not be true in any outsider's view or in the therapist's own character structure or perception of her participation in the interaction. But the intrapersonal transference has then become an interpersonal projection. Not only is there projection, but it is quite standard for the person who is being projected upon, the therapist, to react in response to the projection. So the therapist, sensing the patient's infantile dependent state, responds to it as though she were the nurturant mother or the punitive father. This is what Ronnie Laing (1965) calls *praxis*: The projection is accepted and lived up to by the person who is receiving the projection. *dreaming up*

The setup between therapist and patient is much easier for the patient to tolerate if it is a peer relationship, not a cross-generational relationship. But, as previously discussed, the patient's illusion of being a peer can be a very profound complication in the whole process of therapy. Actually, this illusion can become more and more prominent until it becomes a transference psychosis, an actual belief rather than just a misperception. The individual patient or the family itself can develop the delusion that this is not a therapist, this is just another individual who has been incorporated and coopted for the individual patient or family's own purposes, or without any purpose, just for their own strength.

A bilateral delusion of role fixation can produce problems in family therapy. The therapist can be convinced that he is carrying out his role as anticipated and trained for, and the patient can pick this up and respond to it, resulting in a bilateral delusion that each one is carrying out the role the other one projects, with neither one of them being open to change.

Family therapy can become further complicated by the fact that the therapist, or even the therapeutic team, can be triangulated by the family, within its own structure. This can be subtle and out of all awareness. For example, the father can project his protective role onto the therapist, and the mother can project her nurturant role. The therapist can become triangulated between the two of them. So the therapist, in order to break through this triangulation process, must free himself of the mother–father transference he has accepted. The therapist must also break away from the dependencies and role fixations assigned by the culture. The culture actually demands he adopt the patient. The therapist may even need to break out of his previous role fixation to his own spouse or parents. In other words, therapists need to understand their own bilateral transferences, in order to free themselves from limiting role fixations.

If the structure of the family interactional system is successful, however, there are several things that take place. Probably the most critical is the loss of the time anchor. It is possible for the family to move back or ahead in time within the fantasy of the interview microcosm. Then the loss of a role and the arrival of a freedom to be their whole selves and to even evolve a bipolar craziness can occur. There can develop an irrational relationship between the family and the therapeutic team so that there is new freedom on each side of the polarity.

I think one of the big things that family therapy does is to make the available intimacy in a family more usable and more openly present, because of the freedom to flip back and forth in the transference set. The therapist is free to be intimate, free to bond, to love, and even cuddle the little children in the family, as a way of physically cuddling the adults, since that is not permitted in our social structure. This freedom to play and symbolically express the lovingness and the emotional coupling with children, this freedom to flirt—emotionally, nonverbally, or even verbally—comes from the security of the family's presence. The therapist can move rapidly from person to person, expressing intimacy with the father and then with the mother, or with one child or another, or with the male subgroups or the female subgroups. One of the most difficult things about family therapy, on the other hand, is to develop intimacy with the family as a whole, rather than playing competing games with one or another family member or creating intimacy turn-ons with one or another family member. So, the playing with an individual member needs to be in the context of developing and maintaining a relationship with the family as an organism.

Commitment and Intimacy

The therapist who commits herself to a patient risks the danger of uncontrolled involvement. Commitment usually implies a future time and is not merely a present state. The committed therapist presumes that there will be an end point that will be tolerable to him. Like family life, psychotherapy is an endless crisis, a rhythmic crisis involving surges of intimacy and ebbs of loneliness. Will I look at the patient and see an insignificant other, or will I look at her and see my very self? Will I manage to be more and more naked with this other of my selves? Will she hurt me? Of course. Will I hurt her? I hope so. Can she take it when I hurt her? Yes, if I enjoy it. Can I expose my aloneness?

If I can commit myself to greater intimacy with myself, the patient will, in her reciprocal aloneness, be pressured to commit herself to a self-intimacy that is, in itself, authentic. The therapist must force the patient to be herself and not merely act the patient role. This can only be done if the therapist insists on being himself in his most intimate way, but within the therapist role. Is my inner self being or waiting? Being or doing? Can I dare to share my inner self with me? Can I dare to be more full of myself?

Each crisis is the effort to force myself to a greater commitment to intimacy with myself. From that, and only from that, can the patient be encouraged to be, that is, to commit herself further to intimacy with her person.

One of the problems of being a therapist is the problem of the recurrent empty nest. The foster child comes and stays for a while, and, often without any decision made by the participants, the relationship ends. This is very painful because the foster parent—the therapist—is stuck with an empty nest. And the problem is how to rebuild the empty nest or how to keep from resting in it. Resting equals decay.

Thus it is important to learn to be interdependent with the patient family and not independent of them. It is critical to learn to foster democracy and not be tempted or seduced by the offer of monarchy. Accepting the offer of being the king is one of the ways of destroying the kingdom. It is critical that the therapist concern himself with the *process* of therapy, not the progress of the family or even his own. Progress thinking is double thinking and, as such, is a way of destroying the creativity that makes therapy operate. It is important that the therapist learn to tolerate anxiety rather than try to relieve it. It is important that the therapist struggle for strength in himself and not seek relief and strength in or for the patient family.

The critical movement is toward an integration process, not knowledge. Unification makes for strength, whereas knowledge makes for an observation distance, which means relative nonparticipation. It is critical that the therapist be alert and waiting for a chance to surprise himself, not struggle for cognitive awareness of what is happening or should, could, or might happen. Cognitive awareness is distance from emotional experiences and should be a by-product or fringe benefit of participation. It is important that the therapist have increasing flexibility, not increasing stability, for stability is decay. It is more important that a therapist struggle for fullness in himself than direction, for a global living process rather than a focused life, for joy rather than for success. The therapist should, therefore, strive for the adventure of the therapeutic experience, not the security of it; for teaming up with the family, not for adequacy in himself.

TRAINING FOR THE PREVENTION OF SEXUALIZATION OF FAMILY THERAPY

As mentioned earlier, the maturity of the therapist as a person and the development of her self awareness through personal psychotherapy are important methods for preventing the process of sexualizing family therapy. Prevention of pathological sexualizing is also possible during the training period. Good training to become a professional psychotherapist moves from the stage of learning about therapy to the stage of learning how to do therapy and finally to the stage of being a therapist. This is very similar to learning how to be any other kind of actor, where one learns about acting and then how to act, finally becoming, in essence, an actor. One thus becomes a person who is invested in the role of therapist in much the same manner that a parent learns to put more and more of herself into the role of parenthood. It is interesting to recognize how tempting and alluring this role is, because of its power. For many people, the powerful role of parenthood is, unfortunately, never ended. For therapists, training can help one learn to understand and be in charge of this powerful allure and to anticipate and prepare for termination of treatment, for the pain of the empty nest.

Training itself necessitates both experience and being responsibly related to the experience. To be doing therapy with somebody directing it from behind a one-way mirror always seems to me like the problem of raising children under the careful guidance of the grandmother. It takes the real power as well as the level of participation out of the experience itself. The trainee, I think, should have to carry the responsibility for what is happening and critique it afterward, rather than have it supervised during the experience or imaged beforehand. A series of simulated experiences, of course, may make it possible to relieve some of the trainee's anxiety and make the postinterview critique more tolerable. It is very important for the trainee to be able to maintain the therapist role in the face of the power of the family. The family members are not really in a role but are coming with their full selves, much the same as children are their full selves and not in a role with their parents.

It seems critical that the therapist should initiate her parental role, the foster-parent set, by leading, by being in control. The nurturance offered by the therapist, then, should be secondary to the establishment of control of the therapeutic situation. The therapist must be clear that this space is her home space and that she has certain ways of operating that are important to her. The patient family should know these ways before they get started, so that they may understand the limitations and the routine of this setting. While this is automatically done in the process of setting a time schedule, it should also be deliberate. The therapist should decide before the first interview starts who shall be there, when, and where. Such control is necessary to avoid patient maneuvers to establish a peership, as this would destroy the generation gap and hence the success of the therapy. Through control, the generation gap is established. Then the therapist/parent can comfortably support and nurture her foster child, the patient family.

The use of a consultant in the therapeutic process is also important in the prevention of pathology. It is my belief that there is no such thing as a family therapy process in which one individual can effectively handle the therapeutic experience. I am convinced that there should be a second therapist in on the second interview, no matter how simple and routine the situation. The pathology in any individual erupts from a disordered functioning in the family as a whole, and the power of the family as a whole is exerted to maintain this, their latest effort to cure themselves. They may seem dependent in the same way that a foster child seems dependent, but they really are not. They are powerful, and they are coming for therapy as a result of having tried a long series of therapeutic maneuvers that have not worked. They are much more frightened—and therefore manipulative—than we give them credit for!

If, during the second interview, another therapist reviews the first interview in front of the family, the strength of the therapist taking control both before and during the first interview is augmented. This sets up a pattern of one system trying to help another system take control of itself more effectively. It decreases the amount of humiliation that the family is enduring. Even if the consultant never participates in another session, the therapist represents a therapeutic system and, as such, is much more comfortable being herself.

Being able to tolerate the empty nest syndrome helps prevent the pathologizing of the therapeutic process. The therapist must discuss with the family very early in the process their taking control of themselves, implementing new understanding and their new energy organization. One way of teaching the therapist to tolerate the empty nest is for her to write up the termination interview after it has taken place. Or, she can share her loneliness with the family before and during the last interview. She can review with consultants or with other members of the training group those factors that remain alive and within her as a person. It is very difficult to learn how to disconnect from the therapist role, just as it is hard for actors to avoid carrying their role over into real life. Of course, this is just another way of talking about the importance of the trainee's personal maturity before the beginning of training. The trainee has a real life and must not be tempted to make her professional work role a substitute for living.

When it comes to preventing the sexualization of the therapeutic relationship, being an unmarried therapist is almost as bad as being an unmarried Marine and guarding the American Embassy in Moscow. Without adequate training and protections, the therapist can be very vulnerable to alluring temptation. Because the patient is the full, whole person and the therapist is enacting a role, the therapist is much weaker than the patient. It should be remembered that plays fail because of actors, not because of audiences.

Every psychotherapist has a secret agenda. Most of this is nonformulated and below the level of awareness. Yet the power of this secret agenda, whether or not we are aware of it, is constant and pervasive and sometimes painfully destructive. Rules should be made that set up protection from one's own pathology, and this involves defining a series of settings or attitudes for one's own participation in the role of therapist.

The first one of these may be the most critical: *Being* as opposed to *doing* is what counts. Doing is usually a way to avoid being who one is, what one is in the role. This is similar to the notion that sex can be a way of doing rather than loving, which is more like being. The freedom to be opening oneself and not penetrating others is another way of helping to clarify the fact that the therapist is in a foster-parent role and the patient/family is a dependent who is a whole person and not in a role. I believe that the freedom to hypnotize oneself is one of the ways of not being or staying hypnotized by another, whether that other is family of origin, nuclear family, personal therapist, supervisor, or, most painfully, the patient family in treatment.

One of the important things for therapists to learn is the joy of triangles. Most therapists learn to fear and avoid triangles, but triangles are inevitable. Better they should be enjoyed and reveled in and thus flexibly rearranged. Otherwise they become fixated and therefore destructive.

Obviously, I am advocating creativity and freedom to be oneself and flow with the process of therapy. Acknowledging and understanding the ebbs and flows of the intimate therapeutic process and the essential generation gap in the therapeutic relationship allows family therapists to experience and foster therapeutically the intimacy and sexual fantasies inherent in bilateral transferences and projection. This enables them to take full responsibility for preventing the sexual pathologizing of the therapeutic relationship and process.

PERSONAL RESPONSES

Influence of Gender and Generational Socialization. It is clear to me that early life forms the basis for most of the significant components in any individual's belief system. I grew up on an isolated farm, a quarter mile from the nearest farm and one mile away from a little village of 400 people. This isolation for my first 13 years included, however, my father's father and mother. They lived in our big house as part of our family. Father's father was my basic playmate until my brother, 3 years younger, became a peer. This occurred when I was 7 or 8, at which time my three grandparents and my step-grandmother died. We then became a nuclear family of four.

These losses certainly affected the intimacy in my family. My mother failed to resolve her grief over losing her mother when I was 11, and I suspect that contributed to the concealment from me of intimacy between my parents. Farm life had a natural effect on family intimacy. The intimacy between my mother and me and my father and me was typically New England, satisfying but limited.

Influence of Personal Intimacy and Sexual Experiences. Fifty years of marriage and the raising of six children create by necessity the massive evolution of a two-person intimacy endlessly activated by babies and growing children. During college, I experienced intimacy from several profound episodes of nonprofessional psychotherapy with a two-person peer group. Studying the body as an organism during my 4 years of medical school and my 2-year residency in obstetrics and gynecology were symbolic influences on my understanding of myself, others, and relationships.

My experiences of personal professional psychotherapy—including 10 interviews in a one-to-one relationship, several sessions of individual therapy with a two-person therapist team, and marital therapy and later family therapy with one or more children with two therapists—were powerful stimuli to intimacy and the freedom to break some of our culture-bound influences.

I know that I was strongly influenced by the necessity of adapting to a new and very different social structure when my family moved from the farm to the city during my freshman year in high school. I later learned to live by myself at medical school when my family left the city to move back to the country.

It is important to note that my very extensive experience with animal sexuality during my first 13 years on the farm seemed to have very little conscious input in my later discovery of human sexuality.

Implications for Family Therapy Training and Practice. Learning about psychotherapy is like learning about painting. One of the best ways to keep from becoming a painter is to study painting. Likewise, I'm wondering about the dangers of supervision and how it may impede one's evolving into a psychotherapist. Frequently, the process of supervision leads only to the evolution of a better and better imitation of the supervisor. This can rob therapists of the support needed to prevent the suppression of their individual personhood.

As I've written in my chapter, becoming a professional demands the capacity to involve onself in the foster-parent role that psychotherapy demands. As you can see from my own psychotherapy experiences, I'm intrigued with the possibility that a peer twosome of learners would be the ideal way to learn how to be a psychotherapist, because it would provide not support for but protection from the transference dangers of supervision and/or the suppressive dangers of learning alone. I hope that we will develop methods for cultivating the therapist's creativity and personhood. It seems to me that that is the only way to protect the therapist from the fatal disease of mechanical pseudo-intimacy. I believe that creativity needs to be taught from the very beginning, protected from public evaluation and criticism so that it does not become a process of shedding creative efforts or impeding evolving theoretical belief systems.

As learning increases, the need for ongoing evaluation and criticism increases. I hope that psychotherapists will be like Wanda Landowski, a world-famous harpsichordist, who was still taking lessons and being criticized when she was 85. I'm only 76. Know a good therapist?

I'm emboldened to raise a more politically controversial issue by suggesting that the struggle between the man and his unresolved hypnosis by his mother is a much more critical issue than whether the man can get over the booby prize of running the material world or the woman can get over the dangers of being in charge of the world of intimacy.

REFERENCES

Albee, E. (1962). *Who's afraid of Virginia Woolf?* New York: Atheneum.
Laing, R. D. (1965). Mystification, confusion and conflict. In I. Boszormenyi-Nagy & J. K. Framo (Eds.), *Intensive family therapy*. New York: Harper & Row.
Whitaker, C. A. (1976). Sex, love and the committed relationship. *Journal of Sex and Marital Therapy*, 2(4), 263-264.

7

THERAPISTS' BLIND SPOTS RELATED TO GENDER SOCIALIZATION

Barbara F. Okun

How does a therapist's gender help or hinder her dealing with intimacy, sex, and sexuality in family therapy? Do male and female therapists define intimacy and sexuality differently? Why do some therapists avoid sexuality and intimacy concerns, even when they are presented openly by client couples and families? Does gender affect therapists' attraction to a particular approach over other ones? Why do some routinely verify or check their effectiveness while others express absolute certainty about their perceptions of and work with clients? Why do some feel the need to work on teams while others will not do so? Does gender influence therapists' effectiveness with couples or families who have not been helped by other therapists? Do male and female therapists evaluate the same data differently? Do they interact differently with male and female family members? Do they acknowledge and/or treat the power aspects of sex roles differently? Are there gender-linked differences in their focus? Their assessment? Questions such as these constitute the basis for this chapter.

The therapist's personal characteristics, comprised of gender, personality, culture, class, race, and generation, influence her decision to become a therapist, her choice of route to implement this occupational decision, her later theoretical allegiance, and her consequent selection and use of treatment approaches. Gender socialization is a primary determinant of our personality and a major contributor to our capacity for relationships. Dominant (male) or subordinate (female) gender socialization, more powerful than innate biological gender variables, results in pervasive

Barbara F. Okun. Department of Counseling Psychology, Special Education & Rehabilitation, Northeastern University, Boston, Massachusetts.

gender-linked cognitions and behaviors. Gender-linked feelings, thoughts, and behaviors underlie therapists' anxieties, leading to their hesitation to acknowledge and address intimacy and sexuality in both their personal and professional relationships. There may even be some truth to the common folklore that therapists become therapists in order to experience intimacy with control, or without activation of their own dependency needs, and that family therapists in general choose their specialty in order to gain leverage over controlling parents, particularly engulfing, overwhelming mothers!

The effects of gender conditioning on us as individuals and as therapists are deeper and more widespread than most of us can readily grasp. Yet, while the authors of family therapy literature devote increasing attention to exploration of how gender differences affect client families' health and functioning and to the dangers of therapists promulgating and perpetuating stereotypical and unequal male-dominant family structures and roles, there is little discussion about the impact of gender socialization on the therapist herself. We are concerned with the context of our clients, but we ignore the context of ourselves as therapists.

In addition, most of the writing about gender ignores other variables, such as age/generation, ethnicities, religion, and socioeconomic class. Whereas gender is clearly the predominant variable, due consideration must be given to the reciprocal influences of these other characteristics. They shape the development of both the personal and professional identities of the therapist. Likewise the therapist's professional acculturation influences her adult personal and professional development, both of which in turn affect the attention paid to intimacy and sex in personal and professional relationships. There are indeed reciprocal influences of the therapist's personal and professional relationship experiences over the life-span.

LITERATURE

There is little if any discussion in the family therapy literature about the person of the family therapist, although increased attention is being paid to gender in families, feminism, and family therapy (Goldner, 1985, 1988; Hare-Mustin, 1978, 1987; Hare-Mustin & Marecek, 1986, 1988). What reference there is to the gender of the therapist is based on clinical experience and the implications of family systems theory, rather than on actual research. Family therapy writers do consider, however, the findings of the research about the effects of individual therapists on the therapy process and outcome.

These findings, as summarized by Kaplan (1985) and Howard and Orlinsky (1986), point out that, although there is no clear, replicable evidence of a strong and specific gender effect, therapists' level of professional experience and therapist–client relational bonds are more clearly related to client improvement than any particular theoretical view or treatment technique. The therapist's capacity for relationships involves his ability to form attachments—that is, to engage and invest, to be empathically attuned and expressive, to be warm and accepting—and to endure separations.

This capacity is elaborated by Kantor and Neal (1985) in their thought-provoking article on the therapist's distance–engagement stance with clients. The authors suggest that therapists should learn about their "boundary profile" in order to understand the types of relationship distance they establish and maintain with clients. This boundary profile includes one's preferred system type (closed, open, or random), one's preferred psychopolitical style of interacting (mover, follower, bystander, or opposer), one's preferred theme for interacting (affect, power, or meaning), and one's most preferred and least preferred bystander stance (distracting, passive, or aggressive). The therapist's boundary profile will determine the therapeutic stance—disengaged/detached, professional, or engaged/informed. This concept is, perhaps, the most thorough systemic consideration of the interactional styles of family therapists in the literature. Kantor and Neal suggest that different therapeutic styles will be effective with different types of families. Obviously, therapists' levels of personal comfort with closeness and distance in relationships will affect their acknowledgment and responsiveness to intimacy issues.

SOCIALIZED DOMINANCE

The thesis of this chapter is that gender, because of socialized dominance in our society, does affect therapists' and clients' capacities for and ease with intimate relationships. By socialized dominance, I mean that we are born into a dominant or a subordinate position that is based primarily on gender (male being dominant and female subordinate) but is also affected by class, ethnicity, and the structure of our family of origin. Our gender determines our psychic structure and the meaning of our experiences of attachment and separation from birth onward. These experiences, in turn, determine our capacities for intimacy, for sustaining and tolerating the ebbs and flows of closeness and distance within long-term relationships. There are obvious biological differences between men and women, but these are far overshadowed by the primacy of social, political, and economic variables which construct not only a dominant, power-based context for men and a subordinate, devalued context for women, but also a belief system that reinforces the dominant notion and, in fact, defines lifespan experiences and relationships according to a male model.

On a broader scale, our affiliation and experience with male-dominant or female-subordinate cultures or subsystems shape our cognitive schema (Bem, 1981), which are comprised of the content, form, and process of all our perceptions and thinking. Cognitive schema determine our beliefs (views of self and the world) and our blind spots (things on the edge of our line of vision that we cannot see). These beliefs and blind spots influence our willingness to be exposed and sensitized to or integrated into differing cultures and systems, such as other gender, race, ethnicity, generation, professional, or family systems. Once we open ourselves up to differing views and perspectives, we become vulnerable to the anxieties that accompany the doubts and uncertainties of questioning our premises and assumptions.

Acculturation refers to the process by which two distinct cultures or subcultures (i.e., male and female genders) share space and process information—that is, assimilate from each other—and which results in changes in each culture. Acculturation, therefore, depends on an open-system flow of information allowing the transformation—change, movement, and growth of all parties.

Our experience in a dominant or subordinate culture based on our gender shapes our beliefs, values, and attitudes about gender identity, relationships, intimacy, and sexuality, which naturally affect our relationship opportunities and experiences. If we are open to the acculturation process, we can learn to be empathically attuned to others, and this fosters intimacy in both personal and professional relationships. Therapists' effectiveness with clients from different cultures (based on gender, age, class, ethnic, and professional groupings) depends on their capacity for acculturation, for empathically learning to understand and appreciate differing perspectives and belief systems. This acculturation is necessary in order to form and develop both intimate personal relationships as well as helpful therapeutic relationships with client family members of different genders and ages, as well as client families of different ethnicities, classes, and religions. The process is reciprocal and includes the capacity to learn from others just as we expect them to learn from us and also enables us to change our theories and the fittingness of our beliefs.

Socialized dominance more than biology accounts for gender uniquenesses. As a powerfully pervasive variable, gender influences the effects of other dominant or subordinate variables, such as class, age, ethnicity, and family structure. Ignoring the impact of any one variable, however, results in a skewed assessment of clients. Regardless of how weighted the variable is, each is necessary to understand the whole person. A therapist's natural or chosen membership and experiences (both dominant and subordinate) in all subsystems shapes his person and his personal and professional characteristics. These shapings affect his views of client couples and families, as well as of family therapy theory and practice. More specifically, his views of himself and the world may limit or expand his capacity and willingness for empathic understanding of similar and different subsystems.

The concept of socialized dominance suggests that relationships based on hierarchy are likely to foster the dominant person's development at the expense of the subordinate's development. Hierarchy—if movement is at all possible—naturally promotes a climate of competition and adversity, and we see this in our couple and family clients' presenting problems and struggles. An example is a couple who come in because the wife is unhappy and the couple's fighting has escalated to the point of becoming unbearable to both. The husband is angry because the wife refuses to have sex. Underlying their lack of sex is their struggle for control, to determine whose needs will be met at what costs. Our patriarchal society fosters male dominance and female compliance, and it has only been in the past 20 years that we have begun to acknowledge the ramifications of this assumed dominance in all types of relationships, for both males and females. There are consequences for everyone when we acknowledge and challenge the socialized dominance in our personal and therapeutic relationships. The issue is if and how intimacy can survive in a power-based relationship. We may believe that relationships based on equal power can develop, over time, a context of mutual commitment, trust, and security in which authentic mutual sharing and mutual empathy can occur. Moreover, we may hold that such equality leads to mutual enhancement, which is the goal of an intimate relationship. If we do believe these things, our therapeutic objectives will focus on confronting power and meaning imbalances and abuses within couple systems, in order to heighten intimate functioning.

Intimacy may or may not involve sex. Sex may be intimate, based on commitment to the relationship and mutual enhancement, or it may be recreational, based on maximal pleasure from performance rather than from interaction with the person. There are many different styles and levels of intimate and sexual relationships. Many writers today also cite gender differences with intimacy issues (Miller, 1976; Rubin, 1983; Scarf,

1987), suggesting that men are more likely than women to eroticize intimacy, to assume power dominance, and to value performance over relationship.

With regard to the therapeutic relationship, Howard and Orlinsky's (1986) exhaustive review of process and outcome research in psychotherapy stresses the importance of collaboration—the therapist's encouragement of client initiative and active participation—over the therapist's hierarchical directiveness. The critical issue becomes whether male and female therapists have different capacities for collaborative, egalitarian relationships with clients and others. Do males by nature or by training feel more comfortable with an action orientation and females more comfortable with relational aspects of the therapy process? Do male and female therapists equally avoid dealing directly with intimacy and sexuality issues?

When we do acknowledge and treat intimacy and sexual problems of clients, our own personal and sexual concerns cannot help but be affected. Recently, one of my female therapist clients commented on how jealous she is of her clients' "more exciting sex lives," and I've heard many other therapist colleagues compare their own relationship experiences to those of clients. In fact, therapists who speak critically and disparagingly about their clients are often reacting to personal anxieties that have been triggered by their clients' concerns.

The remainder of this chapter is devoted to a review of some of the recent work regarding gender differences and how these differences affect us both personally and professionally.

GENDER EFFECTS IN PERSONAL AND PROFESSIONAL SPHERES

The works of Dinnerstein (1976), Chodorow (1978), Gilligan (1982), and Miller (1976) have alerted us to the reality of different male and female socialization. The essence of these differences lies in the female's attached, relational self compared to the male's separate, autonomous self. Females have been seen as expressive, capable of intimacy, in touch with dependency needs, and concerned with others' needs and development at the expense of their own. Males have been viewed as success oriented, competitive, independent, and more concerned with their own needs and development than others'. Because the traditional goal of psychotherapy for both males and females has been "individuation," "self-differentiation," and "autonomy," and since the capacities of females to form, develop, and sustain relationships have been given low value and pathologized, these feminine and masculine polarizations have resulted in a traditional rigid classification of gender stereotypes and the further continuation of patriarchal social and family structures. Sex roles obviously apply to therapists' personal roles in their own families as well as to client families.

How do therapists' own sex-role socialization and experiences affect their assumptions about and views of sex roles within client families? Do therapists, for example, strive toward the traditional goal of autonomy as the sign of psychological maturity and health for both males and females? Are female family members expected to comply with more powerful males? Are female therapists more skilled than male therapists in forming empathic therapeutic relationships?

Object relations theorists, who have stressed the need for individuation (development of a self) in order for mature attachment relationships to occur, have provided a framework for writers such as Dinnerstein (1976), Eichenbaum and Orbach (1983), and Chodorow (1978) to formulate the different ways males and females experience relatedness and separateness in their psychic development. Males are taught to separate from mother, the opposite-sex parent, whereas females are taught to remain attached to mother, the same-sex parent. Same- and opposite-sex parenting relationships with the primary parent have significant influence on the development of self-concept and relationship behaviors. Later work by Gilligan (1982) developed those essential differences between the genders based on dualistic poles of female relational and male logical modes in moral development.

These works paved the way for separate-but-equal tracks for the genders. This dualism, however, has furthered polarization by stressing differences and minimizing similarities between females and males. The elucidation of the differences is probably necessary before we can consider similarities and even areas of overlap. While it seems clear that gender differences do have a profound effect on how men and women value relationships and how they are able to develop and maintain them, these theories do not address the different capacities for both autonomy and relationships that exist within each gender and to what these differences may be attributed. Based on what we do know about gendered socialization, female and male therapists might be expected to have different views and values about intimacy and sexuality in relationships. However, because their experiences have been different does not mean that their capacities for intimate relating are different. Gendered styles and values of attachment and separation stem from early infant and childhood relationship experiences with primary caregivers, not from innate biological capacity.

Miller (1976, 1987), for example, focuses on the self-in-relation and on mutually enhancing relationships as the goals of psychic maturity for women, rather than the traditional male-formulated "illusions" of autonomy and independence. It is unclear, however, whether goals of relation and autonomy are *appropriately* gender-differentiated. Perhaps we therapists should lean more toward an androgyny model, helping women to become more adept at autonomy and men to become more adept with mutually interdependent relationships. While androgyny perhaps makes ideological sense, it does not always work in actual therapy. Over and over again in our clinical practices we find that autonomy as a goal for women may be resisted by the women themselves, both because of their adherence to traditional values and because the family system cannot toleate more equity of power. We simply cannot ignore the significance of economic, social, and political power in family and larger social structures.

In my work with female clients who are therapists, I continually find women who appear to behave autonomously and powerfully in their professional roles but who behave in traditionally stereotypical subordinate roles within their own families. When I point out this discrepancy, they are confused and uncomfortable. The power of the dominant cultural views cannot be underestimated or easily resisted. It is possible that clients wonder whether therapists practice in their own lives and relationships what they advocate for clients, just as youngsters often wonder about the inconsistencies between what their parents practice and preach. Like children, clients are sensitive to a therapist's cues and often sense more of the therapist's true person than the therapist realizes. It may be, as recent research (Petry & Thomas, 1986) suggests, that androgynous therapists, regardless of gender, produce more favorable therapeutic relationships with both men and women. Therapists who live according to androgynous values and sex roles should be more effective than those who merely give lip service to androgyny.

What do these gender issues mean to us as family therapists? It is obvious that female and male therapists perceive things from different vantage points because of their different socializations, opportunities, and experiences. It may be, however, that gendered relationship values are less prevalent among therapists than in other professional groups, given that both females and males may choose to become therapists because of their desire and capacity for valuing and working with relationships. Despite consciousness raising, however, the effects of socialized dominance are hard to overcome. Therapists' ongoing professional development may help to enhance their personal relationship capacities, just as their personal relationship opportunities and experiences may influence their professional opportunities and experiences.

Differences with Regard to Gender: Blind Spots

Perhaps women therapists have a subtle advantage over men with regard to gender-type blind spots. Women therapists have been acculturated in two systems, (1) the male-dominant system in which they were raised and in which they have, by necessity, learned to achieve some separation in order to live and work as therapists and (2) the female subsystem where they have naturally and empathically identified with other females and shared the effects of attachment and lifelong subordinate experiences. This experience may enable them to relate more naturally than men to both genders within client families, since they have, by necessity, learned the "language" of their own group as well as that of the dominant group. (This situation is parallel to the French in Alsace-Lorraine learning German when occupied by the Germans, whereas the Germans, as a dominant culture, did not have to learn French.) Male therapists, on the other hand, may not have had the opportunities to experience and learn about nonthreatening, gratifying, egalitarian attachments that lead to intimacy. They may need to work harder to develop and enhance their relationship skills.

Therapists' messages and actions about sex roles are sometimes incongruent. We sometimes see both male and female therapists give contradictory messages to their female clients: "Go home and be more assertive with him, don't let him do this to you," is offered simultaneously with, "Be dependent on me and don't argue or disagree with my interpretations and directives." Therapists, both male and female, are in a position of authority over clients and often fail to recognize and appreciate the ramifications of their power and dominance. Clients, too, may respond differently to same- and opposite-sex therapists, indirectly reinforcing hierarchical relationships. For example, female clients may overcomply in order to please male therapists, and male clients may resist the therapeutic process and insist on more symmetrical buddy-buddy relationships with male therapists or "little boy" or flirtatious, seductive relationships with female therapists. Therapists may unintentionally or intentionally play into these sex roles.

Recently, the wife/mother in a family I had worked with the prior year came to see me after I had been away for several weeks. Originally this family had been referred by a school psychologist, due to a child's difficulties. While working with the family on parenting issues, I had the youngster evaluated at a children's hospital and he turned out to have severe attentional deficit disorder, which certainly explained some of the behavioral problems at school and home. The family and I had worked hard together to change their views and strategies with this child, while engaging the school system in developing an appropriate educational program. When this had been accomplished, serious marital issues had surfaced around intimacy and sexuality. I had begun to work with the couple on these issues, and the youngster and family were seen by a male psychiatrist to evaluate the possibility of medication for the youngster. Several joint sessions were held, and the psychiatrist and I had collabo-rated on our treatment plans. The father was most resistant to couples therapy, so we had ceased those sessions, and I had worked with the wife/ mother to provide support and help her to differentiate from both her husband and son.

When the wife/mother returned to see me, she was very depressed and reexperiencing the agoraphobic symptoms of 8 years earlier, when her marriage had been in acute distress. In discussing her feelings and symptoms and why they resumed at this time, she reported her rage at her husand for refusing to work on the marriage and for resisting her at-tempts to "become closer." She then reported that the psychiatrist had told them that I was wrong to work on couple issues, that is, because the husband only wanted help in parenting, that should have been the only treatment focus. He advised her that she would have to accept her family situation as is and not press for closeness. In fact, she claimed that the psychiatrist told her to cease withholding sex from her husband and to adapt to his needs. Although this psychiatrist had been trained in family systems therapy and considered himself to be aware of gender issues, when he and I met to discuss this situation, it became clear to me that our differences were based more on our gendered experiences than our different professional experience levels. He learned from this case that intimacy and sexual issues in a marriage can underlie larger family problems and need to be addressed. The fact that the wife/mother had such a strong symptomatic reaction to his evasion of her needs was a powerful lesson.

This anecdote reveals the gap between men's intellectual awareness and their deeply ingrained socialization, which may be a blind spot even though they may believe that they are enlightened or feminized. They may be totally unaware of the impact of their inherent dominance by gender, as well as by their professional role. Women therapists, on the other hand, may have been so strongly acculturated into the dominant power system of their profession that it may override their subordinate gender affiliation. In fact, some women's professional acculturation detracts from their more natural tendency toward empathy, resulting in the "Queen Bee" syndrome in which they exhibit less empathy for women's issues than do men. They become stronger examples of male power models than many males. We cannot, therefore, assume that all female therapists are more attuned to intimacy and relational concerns than male therapists are. Gendered attributions to male and female roles, to husband/father and mother/wife roles, stem from multifaceted socialization processes.

Power

Power is the underlying force of these gender socialization differences. There are two types of power that predominate: publicly attributed status power and privately attributed relational power. The former is masculinist and the latter feminist. Most women therapists' power is manifest in their ability to form and to maintain nurturing relationships and in their capacities for and experiences with empathic and intuitive relating. This relational strength has been expressed both overtly and covertly in their own family systems and more covertly with client families.

The use of public power is praised in men and castigated in women. The use of power by typical men therapists has been more overt and directive than the use of power by women. Men's power is pervasive and cuts across many social subsystems, including family, local community, professional, economic, religious, and political groups. Traditionally in our society, men have been willing to give women relational power within family systems while retaining economic, social, and political power in all their social systems. Their power comes from perceived *birthright* and is readily available to them, whether or not they choose to share it with women. Women, on the other hand, have had to struggle to gain and retain power outside of their families. Thus men are more comfortable with their power, taking it for granted, whereas women are more anxious about using power, fearing "punishment" for such behavior and lacking skill and practical experience with male models of power.

For example, in the field of family therapy, Virginia Satir, the lone female pioneer, was known for her incredible ability to relate empathically and was referred to more as a gifted therapist than as a major theorist. The development of theory is viewed as more powerful and of a higher status than therapeutic skill. The language and theoretical contexts of family therapy have been formulated and promulgated by men whose birthright provided them with an overriding innate power dominance.

Until recently, most of the training and supervision of both female and male family therapists was predominantly conducted by men, another form of power. Many men, while willing to have women trainees and co-therapists, assume that they will automatically retain authority and leadership. Thus, women have been supported and encouraged as long as they have not challenged this assumption. When women have insisted on acknowledgment of their own power and status, they have typically either had to leave the male-dominated organization and form their own or had to take their power needs "underground," playing it "both ways." This is similar to the "Oreo" attitude that many blacks have to assume in white-dominated organizations, where their black concerns are undercut by the necessity of giving in to white hegemony. Kanter (1976) has documented the costs of tokenism in organizations, for all subordinate tokens. It is interesting to note that, even though a small but increasing number of men at national conferences are talking about gender inequities, there are few men who attend the sessions and meetings presented by women regarding gender issues. More women than men seem to attend the few sessions on gender issues presented by men. This supports the higher value placed on males by both males and females. It also suggests that gender may be an issue women perceive and struggle with more than men.

Working for Change

The underlying current of struggle between male and female family therapists does not negate the fact that an increasing number of male therapists are "feminist" or "androgynous" in their perspective. It is their very openness and sensitivity to relationships that, as mentioned earlier, may have influenced their occupational choice. However, to learn the "language" of the subordinate female culture in both their personal relationships and within the male-oriented field of psychotherapy requires intense energy and effort on their part, as they must seek entrance into a cultural subsystem that will not easily admit them and with which they are not naturally affiliated. Acculturation requires motivation and effort, along with desire and willingness. Furthermore, in so doing, men risk alienation from their own dominant male culture as well as messages that "it is not enough" from the subordinate female culture.

When gender roles are discussed, many male therapists become exasperated and throw up their hands, saying, "What more can I do; what more do you want?" We end up with frustrated clashes between women and men therapists, with both sides being angry and defensive, and these clashes only serve to polarize us further. This polarization is maintained

by men therapists' blind spots about the impact of their natural dominance and power and by women therapists' blind spots about the equal
importance of self-differentiation and attachment. Women project onto
men the anger they justifiably feel about their social subordination and
mens' contribution to it; and men project onto women their fears of
closeness, dependency, and ultimate rejection reminiscent of their separation from their mothers. These projections, while providing temporary
psychic relief through ventilation, divert energy away from the improvement of social conditions. They also, according to social learning theory,
reinforce the status quo.

Some of the defensive resistance to feminist challenges can be explained by the natural reluctance of dominant cultures to change and give
up power. Just as women have been reluctant to relinquish their power
over relationships within their families, men have been reluctant to
relinquish their political, social, and economic power within society. It is
necessary for women and men to work together to learn about themselves
and each other—their similarities as well as their differences. As individuals, we do share the same aspirations for love, achievement, interdependence, and freedom. The differences lie in the opportunities for realizing
these aspirations. Women's opportunities are systematically obstructed by
our society. This reality must be acknowledged by both men and women,
in order to develop theories and treatment interventions that are equitable
and effective for both genders, that attend to social as well as individual
change and to the collective as well as individual struggle necessary to
achieve such change. We need to value equally relationships *and* performance, thinking *and* feeling.

There is no evidence to suggest that women therapists do not have
the capacity to wield economic, political, and social power in their lives
and professions; to deal powerfully with clients; and to assume effective
leadership roles in clinics, universities, and institutes. Nor is there evidence that men do not have the capacity for intimacy and nurturing
relationships with family, colleagues, and clients. It is true that both
genders have had to strive to develop those capacities deemed appropriate
to the other gender. Gender socialization is restrictive and imprisons us by
emphasizing stereotypical feelings, attitudes, and behaviors. When we
feel, desire, or behave in what is commonly perceived to be opposite-
gender fashion, we are likely to experience anxiety, which leads to defen-
siveness.

For example, women who exercise power directly are referred to as
"bitchy," "castrating," and "angry" by both men and women. Men who
relate empathically and considerately are referred to as "soft," "wimpy,"

"ineffective," also by both men and women. The language we use is gendered and value laden. It restricts us in that we think of gender differences as either/or constructs, rather than both/and, the former ascribing the larger Cartesian quality. An example might be the use of the term *gender differences* rather than *gender uniqueness*.

No wonder people feel uneasy and uncertain about expressing agreement or support for subordinate gender behaviors. Defensive anger covers up this discomfort, and projection can result in feelings of victimization that lead to further self-defeating behaviors, rather than to growth and change. Because male behavior is of dominant value and power, both males and females strive to agree with and support that type of behavior. There is a cost attached to supporting devalued, subordinate positions. For example, the cost to the therapist may be loss of clients, because male clients are usually the financial providers for the family and the therapy. This explains why women feel anxious and confused when faced with the conflicts between their own needs and values and those of the dominant society.

Most women have had to struggle, without benefit of female mentors or role models, for entry into male-dominated professional power systems in all fields. Socialized dominance exists in all professional systems, even though it is rarely acknowledged. Whereas female deferment may be more subtle than it used to be, it is still rampant. In many organizations, women find that opportunities for advancement to leadership positions do not exist for them, regardless of their competence. Both female and male therapists are influenced by their formal education and training experiences, identification with theoretical and mentor role models, information, knowledge, and skills, which develop and become refined over time. Since the family therapy professional system has been formulated, developed, and managed by males, just as psychological and family theory has been formulated and developed by males based on male criteria, female therapists are automatically subordinate in their professional systems, too.

Now that women have entered these professional systems, however, they are struggling to exercise significant influence and to transcend their subordinate status. Many women have had to overfunction, overachieve, and repress some of their feminine characteristics and relational and affiliative needs in order to achieve dominant status. Women typically have difficulty learning comfortable, appropriate ways of experiencing and expressing power, both within their organizations and as therapists with families. An example is that some female family therapy trainees are uncomfortable with powerful, active techniques and are initially resistant to structural and strategic approaches (Okun, 1983). As more women supervisors become available, role modeling can alleviate this discomfort.

As women are becoming more articulate about their achievement needs and concerns, so are many men getting in touch with the female, relational parts that were repressed and frozen in early childhood when they first became aware of their differentness from their mother and sisters. The women's movement has liberated men, too, who are now able to acknowledge their yearning for intimate relationships. Both women and men feel more open to alternative interpretations of stereotypical roles. Many male family therapy trainees are initially uncomfortable dealing with affect and intimacy and are more comfortable with active, directive strategies. With supportive supervision, they can learn to develop this part of their self as therapist. Likewise, today we are seeing more client couples where the man is verbalizing his desire for closeness and intimacy and the woman is desiring more separation, in order to have time and space for her career. This phenomenon applies to therapists' personal relationships, too. Balancing relational and achievement needs are human concerns for both men and women.

Awareness of Overlapping Characteristics

We must also acknowledge that, just as there are many men and women in our society who are choosing to retain the status quo and maintain their gendered views and behaviors, there are also family therapists who choose not to question traditional family roles and rules. This fact is often reflected in the types of theory and therapy that a therapist is attracted to. Purely strategic and structural approaches may be more likely to reinforce the status quo than a more eclectic, integrated approach. Just as there is a continuum in our general population of gender variations and gender overlapping, so is there a similar continuum among therapists, with both feminine and masculine ends of the spectrum being unequally populated by females and males, respectively.

So there may very well be a male–female difference in terms of which therapists continue to expose families to the symptomatic and problematic consequences of accepting the current male-dominated society and family structure, which therapists suggest alternative models, and which therapists help clients seek equitable solutions to their dilemmas. Even if women are more "naturally" attuned to these issues, more and more men today are becoming acculturated and sensitized to them. There is a growing awareness of gender overlap as we find more male and female family therapists acknowledging the existence and influence of gender differences.

With experience, I have learned that stereotypes do not apply across the board. Some of the male members of the families with whom I work and some of my male supervisees, supervisors, and professional colleagues possess more empathic relationship capacities and skills than some of the females. There are many variables other than gender that influence the absence or existence of these relationship behaviors, and I can only suggest that autonomy and relatedness are not clearly opposite poles.

Gender Advantages

When I consider the variety of families with whom I work, I can see that my femaleness is an advantage in some cases and a disadvantage in others. My experience and acculturation in both the dominant groups to which I belong (therapist, life stage, class, current family structure, employer organization) and the subordinate ones (gender, family of origin, religion, profession) can facilitate my client assessments and my ability to join, design, and implement treatment plans. My blind spots, however, can impede these processes. Clients know that I am female when they are referred to me, so they have already made that choice and come into my office with a set of expectations. The wife or mother, who is often, but not always, the initiator of treatment, may expect an ally; the husband or father may expect an adversary. I work hard to join with both, usually first by empathizing with all members of the system and then by reframing their presenting problem (changing it to a nonblaming, nongender-biased, systemic perspective). I feel at an advantage here in that I have been acculturated in both the male and female systems as an adult for several decades and can draw upon an experiential base that very few males can utilize.

My blind spots are signaled by my anger and impatience. What can get me into trouble is when the family's view of the world and their sex roles are at direct odds with my own views. If their views underlie their presenting problem, and if this problem provides enough leverage for me to engage the family in questioning their views and becoming willing to change in order to resolve the problem, then we can explore what kinds of changes the family system can tolerate. This process must involve consideration of larger social systems: What types of options and supports exist for clients within their own realities.

For example, in one stereotypically gendered family referred to me because of the teenage son's truancy and drug involvement, the father, a prominent psychiatrist, continually berated his nonworking wife for failing to be a "proper mother." The wife was intimidated by both her husband and son. She was emotionally and financially dependent on her husband and refused to speak up for fear that he would leave her. She had no desire whatsoever to change her family structure or lifestyle or to become more independent. However, the son's difficulties provided leverage in that this couple was very concerned about their status and position in their community. With therapeutic assistance, this woman learned to seek support from female friends and make some minimal moves to change the balance of power in her marriage. She did achieve some economic independence by insisting on a separate bank account and a weekly deposit by her husband. In return, she was more agreeable about attending his professional social functions. This slight shift in the couple relationship took the focus off of the son, who was able to return to school. To the parents' surprise, this allowed them to make some tradeoffs so as to work more collaboratively than they ever had. In fact, they resumed sexual relations after 4 years of abstinence due to warfare. I could not help wondering how this psychiatrist acknowledged or dealt with his own clients' sexual issues, given his reticence to acknowledge his own lack of sexual activity.

If the family does not wish to change their gendered structure, it is best to work within their value system as best as possible, to help them achieve symptom relief and change. Therapists do not know what is best for others, but they do have educated thoughts and opinions. One can *expose* one's views to others but not *impose* them on others.

It is important to acknowledge the economic, political, and social realities as well as the consequences we and our clients may experience both as a result of changing and of not changing. As eloquently argued by Hare-Mustin (1987), the process of change is continuous, arduous, and complex. We can advocate and support change, but we must help clients to understand the power of dominant cultures and what the risks are for resisting or defying this power.

Clearly, gender will affect how therapists deal with sex and intimacy within families. Their definitions of intimacy may differ. Because of gender socialization, female therapists may be more comfortable with closeness and with talking about feelings, while male therapists may feel more at ease with activities and talking about things. Discussing sex and intimacy with members of the same or opposite gender may be uncomfortable for some therapists. Both men and women therapists often report feeling like voyeurs or intruders. Their own anxieties may lead them to avoid more than cursory attention to sexual issues, even when clients introduce these issues. More important, gender stereotypes may influence therapists' views about sexual relationships. For example, some males may focus more on performance aspects and some females may give more attention to affection and the intimate relationship conditions of the sexual relationship. Certainly, therapists' values, attitudes, and experiences with their own intimate and sexual relationships cannot help but influence their acknowledging and handling of these issues with clients. Their comfort with active and passive participation, frequency, initiation, and sexual variety in their own relationships will affect their comfort dealing with clients' sex lives. Therapists who have led restricted sex lives are probably more likely to avoid sexual issues, whereas therapists who are engrossed in their sex lives may inappropriately or voyeuristically overemphasize these issues with clients.

Therapists' experience of gender socialization in their family of origin is certainly the most powerful influence on their adult personal and professional capacities to acknowledge and address intimacy and sexuality. As family therapists, they will continuously be pulled by client families— both consciously and unconsciously—to experience the residual gendered feelings, beliefs, and behaviors derived from their own upbringing. How open they are to these stirrings will affect their approach to or avoidance of learning more about themselves and their clients.

Effects of Age, Class, Family, and Profession

Other variables contribute to the personal characteristics that influence therapists' occupational choice, relationships, and lifestyle throughout adult life. These other variables may be viewed as aspects of overall gender socialization. They are areas of potential difficulty for us. In order to be effective therapists, we have to recognize our biases and look for our blind spots. There is a danger, however, of leaning too far in an opposite direction, in an attempt to overcompensate for our biases and blind spots. We need to let people and families be themselves and not try to make them over into our model. There is no one correct model or degree of intimacy or sexual functioning; each family needs to expand their possibilities and choose what is comfortable and best for them. As we think about the variables of age, class, family, and profession, as well as gender, we can view them as positive, expansive resources rather than as causes of deviance. We can assume what Katz (1981) refers to as a "synergistic paradigm" where differences become valued and supported rather than devalued and discouraged.

Age/Generation

Although cultural and ethnic issues have been explored in the family therapy literature (see McGoldrick, Pearce, & Giordano, 1982), little attention has been paid to the age or generation of the therapist. It is difficult for therapists truly to appreciate and relate to the developmental tasks and issues of adults in an older life phase. We tend to project onto clients those attitudes and expectations derived from our experiences with our own family members of those age stages. It is usually easier for us to relate to people younger than we are, as we can identify more readily with their struggles.

Furthermore, there are socialization differences affecting each generation. For example, the generation raised during World War II has very different perspectives and experiences on just about everything than the generation that grew up during the 1960s. Generational empathy, as reflected in language, thinking, and shared experiences, can certainly help therapists understand the type and meaning of issues presented. Therapists need to be sensitive to changing sexual mores and norms. Gender as well as generation differences prevail for both therapists and clients, both in terms of sexual attitudes and sexual experiences. These differences can underlie discomfort in acknowledging sexual issues, especially if therapists are not secure in their own sexuality or comfortable with others' different values and orientations.

Dealing with intimacy and sex with older people can also create discomfort that is reminiscent of old boundary issues with their parents and older close relatives. Talking about sex with an older couple may make us feel like we are intruding upon our parents' sex life (which we may have denied existed). Often we do not have enough current close relationships with people in older life stages to allow us to feel familiar and comfortable with their intimacy and sexual concerns. For example, a young therapist may not realize that older people have strong sexual needs and desires. Their capacities may differ from earlier in life, but sex still provides vigorous gratification. In fact, many older couples report more enjoyment sexually as they focus more on intimacy and less on performance. It is as if gender stereotypes merge into more androgynous attitudes and behaviors. Older couples sometimes need help with adapting to changes in their bodies, such as helping older women achieve adequate lubrication, helping older men understand that a longer time is required for erection, or helping couples learn new ways of lovemaking when illness or aging has affected their usual formats.

Just as family therapists need to understand issues of childhood and adolescence, they also need to learn about the issues of adulthood at different life phases, in order to differentiate developmental, medical, and psychological problems. When parenting and/or careers are no longer the primary functions, couple relationships change and intimacy and sexual issues that have been successfully ignored tend to emerge. The qualitative aspects of the couple relationship become more important than the earlier functional imperatives of raising a family and developing a career.

More important, as therapists grow and learn themselves, their world views and perspectives change. They become aware of their own "pathological certainties."* They can recognize and acknowledge how little they know, how little certainty there is, and how few answers there are. Many therapists who have attained considerable success and achievement have written and talked in their later years about their increased sensitivity to their own relationships and, therefore, to the relationship aspects of client families. This tendency to reprioritize achievement and relationship strivings is discussed in adult development literature (Okun, 1984). It becomes clear to therapists in both their professional and personal spheres of life that as one ages, the quality of relationships becomes more highly valued than performance and achievement.

There is more power associated with midlife attainment and stability than in the establishment processes of early adulthood. In our culture, established middle-aged therapists are in positions of power over younger, struggling entry-level therapists. This is similar to the natural dominance of parents over youngsters in family systems. In fact, as in family systems, the middle-aged group is dominant also over the older age group, which is either clinging to power and status or eagerly relinquishing it to enjoy the challenges of retirement or semiretirement.

Socioeconomic Class

Socioeconomic class differences can also create blind spots in therapists. Most psychological and family theories have been formulated by middle-class professionals and do not take into consideration class differences any more than they do gender differences. As with ethnicity and gender, class functions as a determining force in how individuals and families relate to their environments. There is a tendency for middle and upper classes to

*"Pathological certainties" is a term that was introduced by Dr. Edward R. Shapiro (1982) to describe the pathological development of certainty individuals acquire about the experiences of others.

devalue lower classes, just as males may devalue females in our hierarchical society. The white middle-class in this country has always dominated the blue-collar working classes. The struggle involves mobility: Attainment of respected professional status is one way of achieving upward mobility, and therapists who have done so may always find themselves struggling with the remnants of their original socialization in another class. This struggle may be reflected in their comfort in working with clients from the same class or from other classes.

Intimacy and sexuality issues may be far removed from the presenting issues of those lower-socioeconomic-class families struggling with survival. However, this generalization must always be challenged to be sure that we are not imposing an unchecked stereotype. More likely, lower-class families do not have the economic resources to engage in anything but concrete, short-term, problem-solving therapy. This situation does not mean that they lack intimacy and sexuality issues, but that their priorities may be different from middle-class clients who have the luxury of resources with which to explore and contemplate the qualitative nature of their relationships. The point is to focus on perceiving and hearing *what* clients themselves present and value and *how* they do so, and to keep in check our own class assumptions so that we do not automatically presume that they apply to others.

Family

Much reference is made in the literature to the therapist's family of origin, and many trainees are actively encouraged to reconnect with extended family in order to understand their own multigenerational family themes and patterns. Little mention is made, however, of our current family system—our intimate relationships and marital and parental status and experience.

While it is true that our relationships in our family of origin influence our later family dynamics, current family relationships also powerfully influence professional and other interpersonal interactions. This is particularly true for therapists whose professional work focuses on interpersonal relationships. Are male family therapists more involved with their wives and children than other men? Are family therapists better able to parent because of what they learn from clients?

We have not discussed how therapists deal with couples and families when they themselves are undergoing crises in their own marriages and families. Does a divorcing therapist subtly influence struggling couples to separate? How does the family therapist whose teenage daughter just had an abortion deal with a family whose teenage daughter is acting out sexually? How do the heterosexual presumptions of many family therapists impact on homosexual families?

We seem to presume that we are always in control of the boundary between our personal (private) and professional (public) functioning. We can acknowledge that our work can impact our mood, energy, and behaviors at home, but we do not seem to want to acknowledge the possibility of our home increasing our vulnerability to blind spots at work. Therapists believe that their training has given them permanent protection from contamination resulting from the dangerous confusion of personal and professional concerns. This obviously is not true, given the known existence of inappropriate overt and covert sexual acting out in therapy.

It is not unusual for therapists to identify most with the members of the family or couple closest to their own age and status. For example, younger, unmarried therapists tend to identify with offspring, and therapists who are parents of adolescents tend to identify with the parents, and so forth. What is astonishing is how often our blind spots prevent us from recognizing this identification and its impact on therapy. If we identify with a subordinate culture, we are more likely to identify with the subordinate member(s) of the family; if we identify with a dominant culture, we may identify more readily with the dominant member(s) of the family. Or, because of our dominant or subordinate roles and experiences, we may deliberately identify with the opposite.

In families, the system can dominate the individual. The family therapy literature reflects this dominance by diminishing the existence and impact of the individual on the family system and the family–therapist system. Likewise, the family therapy literature has ignored or played down the impact of larger sociocultural systems on family systems and on the individual. The fact is that an individual can affect a larger system, even if this effect is less powerful than that of the system on the individual. And family systems are powerfully affected by the larger sociocultural, political, and economic systems within which they reside.

Nowhere is this "conspiracy of silence" about individual power better illustrated than in the literature on abusive families. Our collusion with these systems in avoiding attributing responsibility for abuse to the individual perpetrator has led to our stance of claiming, just as the abuser does, that "the victim is as much to blame" (Bograd, 1985; Hare-Mustin, 1978; Okun, 1986, 1987). Furthermore, there is a tendency for therapists to blame resistant family systems for treatment failures, thus emphasizing the power of systems over any individual, including the therapist. Perhaps this is why teams and co-therapists are so highly valued in family therapy,

particularly with highly resistant families: Therapy teams are more dominant and powerful than a solo therapist. While acknowledging the powerful effects of a family system over the solo therapist, family therapy
training is more likely than individual therapy training to minimize the
effects of the therapist's personal responsibilities, since the very nature of
family therapy and family therapy training does not allow for the careful
scrutiny of an intense, personal, intimate relationship between the therapist and the client. The individual system within the larger family system
is devalued. Unless we attend in training to the importance of individuals
and of intimate relationships between individuals, it is unlikely that family
therapists will be attuned to intimacy and sexuality in their practices.

The underlying point is that our experiences in dominant and subordinate or nondominant systems of both our family of origin and our
current relationship systems will affect how we perceive and relate to
clients. This will be reinforced by our experiences in subordinate training
systems and our entry and assimilation into the dominant establishment
of the family therapy profession.

In the preceding chapter of this book, Whitaker suggests that "being
an unmarried therapist is almost as bad as being an unmarried Marine and
guarding the American Embassy in Moscow." This refers to the possibility
of an individual being seduced by and into foreign territory. Blind spots
are foreign places. Although it is unpopular, heterosexist, and perhaps
discomforting to suggest that one must be married and a parent in order
to be an effective family therapist, it is ludicrous to ignore the impact of
that experience on therapists. It is not necessary for all couples therapists
to have been or be married, but they do all need to have experienced a
long-term, committed, intimate relationship in order to deal effectively
and affectively with the intimacy and sexuality of families and couples.

Applying Our Experience

Our understanding of the vicissitudes of intimacy and sexuality over the
course of marriage and parenthood can be strengthened by our personal
experiences. Professional training and experience can provide only partial
appreciation of the complex and intricate relationship issues inherent in
family systems over the family life cycle. As a supervisor, I am continuously struck by therapists' assumptions about the way people should relate
or parent. When this is processed and discussed, these assumptions are
revealed to be based on the therapist's own personal issues and biased
expectations. Our blind spots are at work, whether or not we are aware of
them. Inevitably, they are primarily traceable to our experiences in subor-

dinate child subsystems in our family of origin as well as our dominant and nondominant experiences in other ecosystems of childhood and youth.

Just as the research by Howard and Orlinsky (1986) clearly points to therapists' professional experience level as a major variable in the outcome of individual therapy, so is it likely that therapists' family relationship experiences affect the outcome of both individual and family therapy. For example, I certainly am more sensitively attuned to career womens' complaints about being (1) overloaded and overburdened with career and family responsibilities and (2) less available for intimate and sexual relating to their husbands, than I might be if I did not also experience the realities of these pulls. By legitimizing these issues, I can help couples to reassess and rejuggle their competing demands and pressures so they can include a cushion of space, time, and energy for nurturing their intimate relationship. I can help them learn how important as well as how episodic this intimacy is and how necessary it is to learn to balance the pressures of family and work life. When I am experiencing an intimacy drain in my own relationships and am overinvolved in my work, my blind spots about this are apt to be activated and I may be less sensitive to the importance of this balance issue with clients. It is important to use our experiences positively and openly, rather than in a biased, restricting manner. In order to do this, we need to become aware of the biases inherent in our own experiences.

We learn how to love and be—or not to be—intimate from our families, first from our family of origin and then from our current family. These experiences set the stage for our own capacities for relating to clients and helping them develop their abilities for intimate relating. The realities with which we live in all aspects of our lives can impair our opportunities and capacities for intimate relating. Many people today are so busy performing and achieving in order to obtain pleasure and gratification that they simply do not allow the time necessary for deepening the qualitative nature of both their personal and professional relationships. Therapists who have successfully recognized the importance of intimacy and sexuality in their own relationships are more likely to foster and value these relationships in their client families.

Likewise, therapists who have personally experienced parenting are likely to feel more confident and relaxed when dealing with families struggling with parenting issues. They are less likely to be intimidated and confused and more likely to be sensitive to the fluctuations in and varieties of parenting styles and processes. They are therefore more likely to comprehend that the eroding impact of a difficult youngster on the couple relationship is just as significant as the impact of a disturbed couple relationship on the youngster. The dynamics are cybernetic and do not always lead to a "chicken or egg" understanding. Intimacy and sexuality issues underlie many of the problems that bring families into therapy. We need to bring them to the surface in order to understand what is really going on in any family system. This is more likely to occur if the therapist has a strong basis of personal family experiences with intimacy and sexuality. This does not mean that we have to be parents to work effectively with children and adolescents, but that we need to acculturate ourselves to a variety of parent systems and issues in order to "learn the language" and comprehend what we are seeing and hearing.

An example of my own blind spot in this regard occurred recently when I accepted a referral of a female client from a male colleague. I perceived his intention to be that I should support the client in coping with her husband's suicidal depression. In my first session with this woman (her husband refused to come and would see his therapist only during suicidal periods), I was upset by the type of psychological abuse she was experiencing in her marriage and by her passive, dependent acceptance of this abuse. This couple, in their mid-forties, had not engaged in sex for 3 years. I also learned from her presenting commentary that we both had a child in the same social group and we both knew socially many people in common. I suggested that these relationships might interfere with our working together. She, however, perceived this as a plus. I told her that I would need to think about it before contracting for therapy.

I discussed this "conflict" with several colleagues, expressing concern about personal and professional boundaries. One perceptive male colleague gently suggested to me that boundaries were not the real issue; rather, I was using this to cover up my anger at my male colleague for what I perceived to be his request that I help this woman accommodate to her husband's needs. As soon as he said this, it resonated and a subsequent conversation with the referring therapist confirmed my suspicion that I had projected onto him one of my issues—women accommodating to men's needs at their own personal expense. In fact, he had no intention of my helping this woman to accommodate; he had referred her to me so that I might help her gain self-esteem and decide from a more individuated position of strength what she wanted to do. He was also hoping that I could help her to get her husband in for couples work.

This example illustrates how therapists need to check out their own feelings and assumptions, as well as the client's, in order not to project their own issues onto others. It also is a reminder to me that rules are made to be modified; in this case, our having mutual friends and sharing gender, ethnicity, life stage, and class enhanced the therapeutic relationship and provided an encouraging context for this woman to explore her participation in this unhappy marriage, despite vociferous resistance from her husband. Whenever possible, therapists need to communicate verbally with other professionals within clients' relational systems (e.g., medical, legal, and school), in order to check out their perceptions, thoughts, and feelings. Obviously, permission from clients must be obtained in order not to breach confidentiality.

Profession

There are varied routes to becoming a family therapist, including psychiatry, psychology, social work, nursing, the ministry, and family therapy training institutes. Whereas there is no evidence that one route is better than another, it is important to acknowledge the different attitudes, values, beliefs, and expectations inherent in each route.

All of the variables previously discussed affect our experience in professional training. Our gender, age, class, ethnicity, family relationships influence how we perceive, experience, and interpret our training. Our education affects how we think and how we perceive the world. The varying fields from which we come to family therapy are all male created and controlled. Our gender also affects how we are accepted and dealt with within these fields.

Professional systems are like our family systems in that we enter them as dependent neophytes in a subordinate role and go through the processes of attachment, individuation, and separation. As in families, males and females experience these processes differently, and this affects their identity and functioning. As we adapt to the system and it adapts to us, we learn the rules and develop characteristic roles. Our "boundary profiles" as therapists include both our professional and family systems experience. The latter influence our occupational choices as well as the types of professional systems we seek, enter, and remain affiliated with. For each individual, then, there is a particular ongoing reciprocal influence of professional and family systems.

Acculturation to a professional system occurs gradually. Our mental set begins to be shaped from the first day of training. As pointed out by Kingsbury (1987), however, rivalries and friction between mental health professions are not based solely on economic and power concerns but are also significantly engendered by different training experiences, other disciplines, and the hierarchical nature of training organizations. Each profession has a unique definition of professionalism, professional distance, and objectivity. The medical model, for example, teaches objective diagnosis in a hierarchical, impersonal context; whereas doctoral programs in psychology foster a research orientation and moderate distance between clinician and client. Social workers and nurses, meanwhile, are socialized in a relationship orientation. Each profession has different values and attitudes about therapeutic relationships; however, they all view sexual seduction by therapist or client as destructive and unethical. Sexual seduction aborts the process of therapy and denies clients the opportunity to learn about intimate relationships and better, more effective ways to function in relationships.

Many family therapists have allegiances to more than one professional system, considering themselves psychiatrists, psychologists, or social workers who specialize in family therapy. Others consider themselves family therapists and do not continue affiliation with other professional subsystems. Current identification is strongly influenced by initial training and professional acculturation, but it may change over the professional life-span. Often therapists are surprisingly oblivious to the pervasive influence of their professional acculturation, especially that of early adulthood. Whether or not we subsequently modify our training, our early acculturation is as powerful on our current life functioning as is our family-of-origin system on our current family relationships.

Our reasons for choosing to enter a profession and for selecting a particular route underlie our expectations and attitudes. In today's uncertainty regarding credentialing and practice opportunities, these expectations and attitudes are often sorely challenged. A natural result is that some therapists are resentful if they are required to find alternative routes.

Within the mental health professions as a whole, there are hierarchies that result in dominant and subordinate cultures. These pecking orders are perpetuated by third-party payers, credentialing structures, fee structures, training institutions, and societal values. Psychoanalysts dominate the psychiatry profession. Psychiatrists are dominant over psychologists, who in turn are dominant over social workers, who are dominant over psychiatric nurses. Individual therapists dominate over family therapists, just as psychodynamic theory dominates family systems theory. The bottom line is economics—the ability to practice and make a living. During this current era of human service and health care cutbacks and restrictions, competitive rivalries between groups flourish. Which of our professional affiliations prevail depends on social, political, and economic considerations.

Furthermore, as we develop and age, our needs, dependencies, and attitudes about our work and profession change. Levinson (1978) points out how in middle age one is able to let go of earlier mentors and "become one's own person." We mature and develop the interest and opportunities to become a mentor ourselves, to grow up and to assume an adult rather than a trainee role, and to function within our profession. In other words, in midlife, we reassess our professional values, beliefs, expectations, and practices, based more on actual development and experiences than on what was learned from teachers and supervisors. We can challenge and reformulate, where advisable, many of our initial academic assumptions and premises about families and family therapy. How much leeway there is to change our thinking and practice depends on the larger context of professional opportunities, which is affected by social, political, and economic issues.

CONCLUSIONS

Issues of gender, age, class, family, and professional socialization are broad and complex and typically overlap. They have many varied effects upon behavior and relationships and upon the ways individuals view themselves and their world. As therapists, we need to understand how these issues have affected us, how they affect our clients, and how these effects impact our work. Dominance and subordination issues must be addressed in terms of gender, power, and relationships, in order to consider sex, sexuality, and intimacy.

As we become more confident and independent, we are freer to take risks and to learn from our clients. We can be less defensive about limitations and blind spots and learn to trust our hunches and intuitions. It is at this time of reassessment and values clarification that we can become most aware of the subtle and pervasive influence of our professional acculturation. It is also at this time that we can look back and see how we have been shaped by our experiences in dominant and/or subordinate social subsystems. We can choose whether to become actively acculturated into other systems, that is, whether to "learn other languages." This entails risks, challenge, discomfort, and all of the other processes of change that occur when we question our assumptions, premises, and certainties. We need to acknowledge and become more aware of our blind spots. In effect, we need to reassess continuously our personal and professional philosophies and to recognize how deeply sociocultural factors influence them.

Beavers (1977) proposes that "growth-oriented treatment always strives to equalize the overt power between therapist and client since the major weapons used to alter behavior and attitudes are the empathic relationship and problem-solving with the patient" (p. 295). In hierarchical systems such as those of the family, the therapist–client and the professional how can we foster intimacy? The very nature of a hierarchy excludes attending to intimacy or intimate sexuality because such a system is run on dominant–subordinate power, while true intimacy is egalitarian. One solution is to focus on concrete behaviors and performance and on immediate gratifications, and skip the anxieties that accompany grappling with less clear, more elusive relational aspects.

Or, as stressed by Kohut (1977), Miller (1976), and Paul (1970), we can attempt to develop and foster empathic and egalitarian, or twinship, relationships (collaborations) within family systems and between therapists and clients by modeling, experiencing, and developing intimate therapeutic relationships. This requires open systems and mutual respect. It also requires restoration of the importance and primacy of relationship formation and development in our professional training programs, as well as involving trainees in the study of their personal, professional, and client relationships.

Intimacy, sexuality, and relationship issues are not "feminine" issues. They are human issues, and they need attention from both males and females. Family systems, object relations, feminist, and self psychology theories have much to contribute to our understanding and treatment of relationships.

Intimacy and sexuality issues have been ignored in mainstream family therapy training. Perhaps it has been assumed that trainees were exposed to these issues in previous types of training, which may not be true. We might speculate that therapists who have originally been trained "traditionally" and who have, for example, received medical training, may be more knowledgeable and comfortable dealing with sex. Therapists who have experienced supervision in long-term individual therapy may be more comfortable talking about intimacy and sexuality on a one-to-one basis but may feel strained talking to couples and families about such issues. When and where and how narrowly or broadly in our professional development we have received what type of training and how effective our role models and supervisors have been will influence our views of ourselves, of client families and their intimacy and sexual issues, of family therapy, and of the entire mental health profession.

Therapists, like anyone else, have human yearnings for intimacy, for playfulness, for mastery and achievement, and for approval and acceptance. We need to experience membership in different systems, both dominant and subordinate, to remain humble and sensitive to the vulnerability and fragility of the human condition. Our sensitivity to our own issues and needs as well as to those of clients, friends, relatives, and colleagues will help us to keep intimacy and sexuality in our line of vision, which is likely to enhance greatly our effectiveness with clients. When we draw our blind spots into our line of vision, they are no longer blind spots and can be dealt with consciously. Open-system collaboration with others within our own personal and professional systems enables growth and change as a result of the availability and accessibility of feedback. Continued self-questioning and exposure to differing cultures provide opportunities for growth and learning. Isolation and self-absorption preclude this growth and learning and will result in stasis rather than evolution.

Like other aspects of life, intimacy and sexuality ebb and flow. As core components underlying family-system formation and development, we need to understand that there are phases in a family's development when distance may be more appealing and functional than closeness, when separateness is more important than togetherness. It is when this ebb and flow gets stuck or blocked that we often see family problems emerge. Our client families have much to teach us about the differing rhythms and modes of this ebb and flow.

Depending on our gender, we are born into a dominant or subordinate culture, as well as into family and social hierarchies. Our condition of birth determines many of the attachment and separation proceses we will undergo. These influence our experiences of and capacities for intimacy and sexuality in adulthood, as well as our attention to these issues when dealing with client families. As the basic tenet of therapy expounds, we are not rigidly confined to earlier patterns of relationship. We are capable of changing them, once we learn to recognize them. Becoming aware of our own blind spots is the first step toward recognizing their influence on us in our professional and personal spheres.

PERSONAL RESPONSES

Influence of Gender and Generational Socialization. I grew up in a very disturbed upper-middle-class German Jewish family. We lived in a New York suburb except for two separate and confusing years in the Deep South. Males certainly had more privilege in my family. Concurrently, children were expected to be totally deferential and compliant, following the family rules of parental absolute certainty and of upholding the importance of outward perfect appearances and agreement. There was little, if any, genuine affection or verbal relating, and sexual abuse was denied and ignored.

It has only been in the past decade that I've really been able to fathom the enormous impact on me of the rigid doctrines of not just my family, but the women's college I attended and the southern city in which I lived during the latter part of adolescence, where achieving females were considered deviant. Rather than capitulate, I chose consciously at the incredibly early age of 10 to comply outwardly in order to get an education (my ticket to independence and freedom) but to go my own way inwardly.

While my route to independence was indeed lonely and painful, I was fortunate to find real, literary, and fantasied supporters along the way. They provided encouragement and, at the same time, fulfilled some of my yearnings for both giving and receiving emotional responsiveness. The therapist I selected at the age of 19 offered me my first opportunity to experience an intimate, trusting relationship and launched me into adulthood. The 3 years I lived in New York as a single career woman after college—against my parents' wishes—enabled me to experience freedom and independence as a female. Therefore I felt strong and confident when I married at the age of 24. For me, dutiful but emotional distance from my parents and siblings has been both releasing and relieving. This distance has freed me for other gratifying intimate relationships.

The upheaval of the 1960s brought me tremendous relief in that I finally realized I was not alone in my inner questioning and desire to relinquish the shackles of doctrinairism. This resulted in many years of learning about myself as both an achieving and relational woman. My strongest ally was and is my husband, who has a similar need to question conventional thinking and lifestyles and who provides supportive companionship along the way.

Influence of Personal Intimacy and Sexual Experiences. I think the people who contributed most to my increasing capacity for intimacy are two extraordinarily warm, competent male therapists (one I saw in late adolescence and the other in midlife), my husband, my daughter, and my two sons, as well as two long-term women friends. What strikes me is how I've learned about myself as a loving woman from both males and females, and how my capacity for personal and professional relationships has subsequently deepened. My relationships have become more affectionate and cherished each year since I left college, when I insisted on physical, emotional, and financial independence from my family of origin.

The primary relationship in my life is my marriage. It has offered an enriching opportunity for love, intimacy, and sexuality, as well as for growth and awareness. Although this has not been without struggle and regressions, my expectation was and is that struggle and progress are intertwined in any close relationship.

Implications for Family Therapy Training and Practice. Since I've written about the person of the therapist, it is pretty obvious that I believe that "who" we are affects how we conceptualize and practice therapy. Whatever model we espouse is filtered through our own experiences and belief systems. I'm aware that my decision to become a therapist was strongly influenced by a need to be emotionally responsive, and by apprecation of my first therapist as a nurturing "psychological father." The therapy I undertook in midlife (with a superbly skilled, empathic, flexible male) after years of clinical practice not only helped me to grow as a woman but has had more impact on deepening my effectiveness as a therapist than any other trainng or supervisory experience.

Certainly I was attracted to family systems theory and therapy to help me understand my own family of origin and to help me raise my current family. It's what we are not aware of that can get us into difficulty.

Just as I am appalled by parental abuse of children, I am deeply pained by the abuses therapists wittingly or unwittingly heap on clients. I think I have particular abhorrence for therapists who abuse their power and their boundaries, as I cannot help but feel that, with their training, they should know better. These abuses are sometimes overt, more often insidious; but they are always deplorable. It seems to me that our only safeguard as therapists is to look continuously at ourselves, open ourselves up to feedback and evaluation, check out our assumptions, and acknowledge the reciprocal influences of our personal and professional experiences. If I could, I'd insure that all therapists be required to engage in personal therapy and/or supervision with both males and females throughout their professional life-spans.

REFERENCES

Beavers, W. R. (1977). *Psychotherapy and growth: A family systems perspective.* New York: Brunner/Mazel.

Bem, S. (1981). Gender schema theory: A cognitive account of sex-typing. *Psychological Review,* 88(4), 354–364.

Bograd, M. (1985). A feminist examination of family systems models of violence against women in the family. In M. Ault-Riche (Ed.), *Women and family therapy* (pp. 34–50). Rockville, MD: Aspen.

Chodorow, N. (1978). *The reproduction of mothering.* Berkeley: University of California Press.

Dinnerstein, D. (1976). *The mermaid and the minotaur: Sexual arrangements and the human malaise.* New York: Harper & Row.

Eichenbaum, L., & Orbach, S. (1983). *Understanding women: A feminist psychoanalytic approach.* New York: Basic Books.

Gilligan, C. (1982). *In a different voice.* Cambridge, MA: Harvard University Press.

Goldner, V. (1985). Feminism and family therapy. *Family Process, 24*(1), 31–47.

Goldner, V. (1988). Generation and gender: Normative and covert hierarchies. *Family Process, 27*(1), 17–32.

Hare-Mustin, R. T. (1978). A feminist approach in family therapy. *Family Process, 17,* 181–194.

Hare-Mustin, R. T. (1987). The problem of gender in family therapy theory. *Family Process, 26*(1), 15–28.

Hare-Mustin, R. T., & Marecek, J. (1978). The meaning of difference: Gender theory, postmodernism, and psychology. *American Psychologist, 43*(6), 455–465.

Hare-Mustin, R. T., & Marecek, J. (1986). Autonomy and gender: Some questions for therapists. *Psychotherapy, 23*(2), 205–212.

Howard, K., & Orlinsky, D. (1986). Process and outcome in psychotherapy. In S. L. Garfield & R. E. Bergin (Eds.), *Handbook of psychotherapy and behavior change* (3rd ed., pp. 311–381). New York: Wiley.

Kanter, R. M. (1976). Women and organizations. Englewood Cliffs, NJ: Prentice-Hall.

Kantor, D., & Neal, J. (1985). Integrative shifts for the theory and practice of family systems theory. *Family Process, 24,* 13–30.

Kaplan, A. G. (1985). Female or male therapists for women patients: New formulations. *Psychiatry, 28,* 111–121.

Katz, R. (1981). Education as transformation: Becoming a healer among the Kung and the Fijans. *Harvard Educational Review, 51*(1), 57–78.

Kingsbury, S. J. (1987). Cognitive differences between clinical psychologists and psychiatrists. *American Psychologist, 42,* 152–157.

Kohut, H. (1977). *The restoration of the self.* New York: International Universities Press.

Levinson, D. (1978). *The seasons of a man's life.* New York: Knopf.

McGoldrick, M., Pearce, J. K., & Giordano, J. (1982). *Ethnicity and family therapy.* New York: Guilford Press.

Miller, J. B. (1976). *Toward a new psychology of women.* Boston: Beacon Press.

Miller, J. B. (1987, March). *The power of women in families: Fictions and realities.* Panel Presentation at American Orthopsychiatric Association Conference, Washington, DC.

Okun, B. F. (1983). Gender issues of family systems therapists. In B. F. Okun and S. Gladding (Eds.), *Issues in training marriage and family counselors* (pp. 43–59). Ann Arbor, MI: ERIC.

Okun, B. F. (1984). *Working with adults, individual, family, & career development.* Monterey, CA: Brooks/Cole.

Okun, B. F. (1986). Incest in family systems. *Journal of Counseling and Human Service Professions, 1*(1), 67–78.

Okun, B. F. (1987). The family systems perspective of child abuse. *Topics in Acute Care and Trauma Rehabilitation, 2*(1), 27–42.

Paul, N. L. (1970). Parental empathy. In E. T. Anthony & T. Benedek (Eds.), *Parenthood: Its psychology and psychopathology* (pp. 337–352). Boston: Little, Brown.

Petry, R. A., & Thomas, J. R. (1986). The effect of androgyny on the duality of psychotherapeutic relationships. *Psychotherapy, 23*, 249–251.

Rubin, L. (1983). *Intimate strangers: Men and women together.* New York: Harper & Row.

Scarf, M. (1987). *Intimate partners.* New York: Random House.

Shapiro, E. R. (1982). On curiosity: Intrapsychic and interpersonal boundary formation in family life. *International Journal of Family Psychiatry, 3*(1), 69–89.

8

PASSIONS OF THERAPY: HIDDEN SEXUAL DIMENSIONS

Michele Bograd

The practice of family therapy is a passionate enterprise. Although family therapists speak easily of how families struggle for intimacy, absorb or act out rageful disappointments, search to fulfill deep longings, or wither from frozen missed connections, we seldom acknowledge how we as very human therapists experience and grapple with these same yearnings and feelings in every therapy hour. Given that family therapists of a variety of theoretical persuasions share a common focus on the context of current interpersonal relationships, it is particularly ironic that silence shrouds the phenomenological experience of the therapist. Even those family systems approaches that pay special attention to the therapist–family interface tend to describe its technical or systemic aspects, rather than its very human realities and dilemmas. And, although intimacy is the goal of many family therapy approaches, our theories seem to take for granted the complex nature of intimacy in the therapist–client system.

A comprehensive description of the passions of therapy encompasses strong feelings ranging from love to hatred, from boredom to fascination, from helplessness to potency. In this chapter, I focus primarily on clinicians' experiences of sexuality as a hidden dimension of the therapeutic relationship. Sexuality in therapy, as in our culture at large, is a delicate and verboten topic. Yet it is my belief that intimacy and sexuality are interrelated in complex and sometimes quirky ways, and, as in any other relationship, sexuality can profoundly color and influence the connection between therapist and client. Scheflen (1965) some time ago got to the heart of the

Michele Bograd. Kantor Family Institute, Cambridge, Massachusetts.

matter by characterizing the therapist–client relationship as a dance of "quasi-courtship."

Yet, nearly 25 years later, silence shrouds this relational dimension in family therapy: A relatively thorough review of the family therapy literature turns up almost nothing of direct relevance. A rich and vivid description of the variety of ways that family therapists may experience sexual dimensions in therapy is lacking. This chapter provides a forum for the detailed accounts of family therapists who risked sharing their vulnerabilities by revealing this side of their work. To set a context for the accounts, I will briefly define key terms, state the organizing premises of this chapter, summarize recent research on prevalence of therapist–client sexual activity, and analyze the professional and theoretical constraints that contribute to the fact that family therapy as a field has almost totally ignored sexual dimensions in the therapy relationship. Then I will describe the characteristics of the groups of therapists who contributed their perspectives to this chapter, as well as how they came to do so. Following the therapists' actual narratives, I will present some perspectives on ethical and theoretical issues, in the hope of orienting future discussion and analysis toward collaborative dialogue.

BACKGROUND

Definition of Terms

Drawing on the comments of family therapists who described experiences of sexuality with clients, it is obvious that conventional definitions of *sexuality* do not adequately capture the multilayered texture of these experiences. Language seems to limit, if not thwart, the enterprise by dividing up intimacy and sexuality, commitment and sensuality, feeling and sensation, as if they were totally separate domains. No single term easily describes what remains an unnamed dimension in therapy, as the phenomenon at hand is comprised of the overlapping components of caring, intimacy, attraction, sexuality, and sensuality. Each of these terms has physical, emotional, psychological, and interpersonal aspects.

Stiver (1986) distinguishes between caretaking and caring in psychotherapy. *Caretaking* rests on a hierarchical relationship between therapist and client that allows the therapist to guard an objective, impersonal stance in the delivery of care. In contrast, *caring* derives from a more egalitarian relationship and implies deep emotional investment in the other's well-being. Even as Stiver cautions against burdening the client with the therapist's personal data, she challenges the conventional clinical notion that defines caring as interfering with therapy rather than as a healing therapeutic response.

Intimacy connotes closeness, familiarity, thorough knowledge of another, and access to another's most private personal details. Although intimacy often involves mutual exchange, it also refers to the experience of connection resulting when one is the trusted recipient of highly personal information from another. Intimacy exists in complex relationship with *sensuality* or our physical experience of bodies, arousal, titillation, and longing for physical closeness. Sensuality is closely related to *sexuality*, which includes simple genital arousal of erotic interest but also encompasses the kinesthetic–emotional experience linked to how we fundamentally experience ourselves as men or women—gay, straight, or bisexual; asexual or full of desire. Cross-cutting these components is that of *attraction*, which may or may not be specifically sexual. Extrapolating from its definition in physics, attraction is the force exerted by component parts of a system that holds them together through affinity, appeal, or fascination.

In practice, some of these terms carry negative connotations. For example, the dictionary offers *lustful, self-indulgent,* or *lecherous* as synonyms of sensuality. In contrast, I use sensuality (and the other four terms) descriptively, with no implied judgment about the moral acceptability of these feelings. For ease of discussion, I will employ the term *sexuality* throughout this chapter to refer to this textured constellation of emotions and sensations.

Guiding Premises

Conventional approaches to sexuality and the therapeutic relationship commonly assume that the very presence of sexual feelings needs to be explained, as if they were anomalous, unanticipated, or inappropriate. I begin from a very different set of premises:

- Intimacy is at the heart of most psychotherapeutic relationships.
- Most intimate relationships include sexual dimensions.
- Sexuality takes many forms.
- Feelings between therapists and clients are real.
- Such feelings potentially enhance the therapy and are not by definition countertherapeutic.

To flesh out these premises somewhat more formally. I am taking as a given that the psychotherapeutic relationship is a *relationship*. Therapists and clients alike need and create a connection that is mutually enhancing, affirming, and healing. Although this relationship is professional, it is also intimate, as feelings of care, attention, investment, and interest grow from shared intensely private information, constancy of connection, and patterned physical proximity. Since intimacy of this sort is often associated with sexuality in our culture, sexuality may be a natural (and possibly inevitable) by-product of the special bond between therapists and clients (Edelwich & Brodsky, 1982).

This hidden sexual dimension is complex and variable. It can develop on first meeting, over the evolution of treatment, or not at all. It may be the predominant feeling or a fleeting fancy. It may be mutual or one-sided, and it may change over time in nature and intensity. It may carry positive charges of attraction, excitement, and interest or negative charges of boredom, repulsion, or emptiness. But the feelings cannot *not* exist (Edelwich & Brodsky, 1982). Although these feelings derive in part from unconscious needs, current longings, and images from family relationships, they exist as real emotions that understandably develop in a context of nurturance, care, profound sharing, and connection. As such, it is not necessary to explain them away as unusual, irrational, or dangerous. Although they can be misused, and although acting on them severely compromises or destroys the safety of the therapy relationship, they also are forces of profound growth and constructive change.

Prevalence of Sexual Activity in Therapy

Only recently have systematic studies revealed that between 7% and 10% of therapists, primarily men, have had sexual contact with clients (Gartrell, Herman, Olarte, Feldstein, & Localio, 1987; Kardener, Fuller, & Mensh, 1973). Few studies address the question of other forms of physical contact (such as hugging), and almost none examine the emotional facets of a sexual dimension. A survey study of 456 primarily psychodynamic psychologists found that 87% had been attracted to clients, although 82% never seriously considered acting on it (Pope, Tabachnick, & Keith-Spiegel, 1987). Men acknowledged having sexual fantasies more often than women. About 25% of the respondents reported kissing their clients rarely or more often, 44.5% hugged them rarely and an additional 41.7% hugged them more frequently, and 2% reported engaging in sexual contact with a client (a number significantly lower than the rates revealed in most studies). There are no available studies of family therapists' sexual feelings or actions toward clients.

Why the Silence?

How can we explain why family therapists have barely addressed this dimension of the therapeutic relationship? Reference to individual resistance or discomfort seems too facile an answer, since most family therapists are sensitive, self-questioning, and thoughtful clinicians. Several theoretical and contextual constraints shift attention away from therapists' experiences, minimize interest in the dimensions of intimacy and sexuality, or create conditions of shame and exposure that significantly limit clinicians' willingness to address these issues openly.

Irrelevance of the Construct of Countertransference

In psychodynamic theory, the construct of countertransference facilitates examination of the internal experiences of the therapist and legitimizes (while it interprets) therapists' strong feelings toward clients. But early family systems models developed in strong opposition to traditional psychodynamic approaches. Family therapists directed attention to current interactional sequences between family members, minimizing the importance of understanding the emotional nature of the therapist–client relationship.

Theoretical interest in countertransference also prescribes the form of the therapist–client relationship, which subsequently influences the visibility of intimacy and sexuality. The paradigmatic psychoanalytic stance of relatively opaque, responsive neutrality elicits feelings and fantasies of clients and therapists alike. In contrast, many family therapy models permit (if not prescribe) an active, directive therapeutic stance, which includes humor, self-disclosure, and authority. Many family therapists seem to assume that becoming more "real" or three-dimensional lessens, rather than heightens, the presence of intense feelings of longing, interest, or connection for all involved. Furthermore, since family therapists often work with two or more family members, most clinicians presume that the intensity of the therapist–client relationship is "diluted" and of relative insignificance, or that intrafamilial dynamics take theoretical or practical precedence over therapist–family interactions.

Therapist as Technician

To somewhat oversimplify the matter, family therapists tend to view themselves either as outside the family system and acting upon it or as a constitutive part of an interactional system. These relatively mechanistic models of family therapy can depersonalize or take the heart out of the therapy relationship, as they guide us to describe our proactive and reactive sequential moves behaviorally or to think strategically about shifting, confusing, or directing a system toward positive change. At its extreme, this leads family therapists to focus on the consequences of our actions on systems in relatively pragmatic or measurable ways, rather than on the more ephemeral texture of the emotional currents between therapist and family members.

Constraints of the Professional Context

Factors contributing to the silence about sexuality and intimacy also derive from the professional milieu. Particularly important are cultural images of caretaking relationships and their integration into clinical ideologies, and the threat of strong professional sanctions against therapists who acknowledge experiencing sexual feelings.

Culture provides powerful images of the "appropriate" relationship of heart and body in various social contexts. One archetype is that of the caretaker and the dependent: A parent, doctor, priest, or therapist supposedly has no sexual feelings for the recipient of care. But we must question whether this archetype reflects reality. If there is a discrepancy between the social image and the human experience, complex situations emerge. A loving mother experiences sexual feelings toward her small son. Because this experience deviates from the social image of maternity, she struggles with guilt and shame. A committed therapist experiences a strong attraction to a client, deviating from the social image of the asexual caretaker, so he berates himself for the feelings themselves and doubts his capacity to be protective and nurturant.

Cultural images of caretaking relationships are often integrated into clinical belief systems, without critical analysis. If it is taken for granted that caregivers are asexual or neutered, then any sexual feelings are, by definition, inappropriate, unprofessional, countertherapeutic, and evidence of therapeutic error or weakness (Edelwich & Brodsky, 1982). In the face of this professional belief system, therapists experiencing deep personal feelings toward clients often struggle with feelings of shame, self-doubt, and professional insecurity.

A significant number of therapists have abused their power by in-itiating sexual contact with clients, resulting in devastating psychological and interpersonal consequences for clients. This has legitimately led to the creation and enforcement of strong prohibitions and legal sanctions. Although this is absolutely necessary to protect the rights and psycho-logical safety of clients, fear of malpractice suits and personal exposure contribute to many therapists' unwillingness to acknowledge, discuss, and examine openly their feelings of deep connection and attraction to clients.

Description of Therapists

In this context of silence, a final step entails frank exploration of the sexual dimensions of the therapeutic relationship. Toward that end, I began to broach this topic with trusted colleagues. They ranged in age from 28 to 62; had at least a master's degree in counseling, psychology, or social work; and had practiced family therapy for at least 5 years. The majority described their primary theoretical orientation as "eclectic sys-tems," blending primarily structural family therapy with transgenera-tional approaches. Strategic and systemic therapists were underrepre-sented in this nonrandom sample. To my knowledge, most were heterosexual and 75% were currently married. The resulting dialogues were relatively unstructured, often taking place over dinner or away from the workplace. I knew the nine men and seven women very well, having worked closely with all of them in training and clinical settings. I shared warm and long friendships with some of them and felt safe with all of them, given the many professional dilemmas we'd discussed over the years.

Concurrently with these in-depth conversations, I led a series of workshops, at national family therapy conferences, on the topic of sexual-ity and family therapy. I was moved by the intensity of these workshops, as participants eagerly welcomed the opportunity to explore dimensions of our work that are usually ignored or harshly judged.

From these experiences, I collected numerous anecdotes, which are but an initial foray into how family therapists perceive, experience, and evaluate sexuality within the intimate caregiving relationship. These ac-counts were tape recorded, noted in writing, or reconstructed from mem-ory. Essential details have been preserved and all but minimal identifying data removed. Given the preliminary nature of this exploration, I selected vignettes highlighting some of the major dimensions emerging from the accounts. All conclusions are tentative, as only qualitative content analysis was employed.

Invitation and Caveat

One way to gain safer distance on sexuality is by employing detached professional language that is neither self-revealing nor evocative. In this chapter, family therapists reveal and document *in their own terms* the variety of ways they experience sexual dimensions in therapy. Naming is necessary before formal analysis; understanding is necessary before the development of models on how to manage or utilize sexual feelings. This first task of witnessing requires suspending judgment, in order that the tales may be told. It invites a potentially disturbing awareness of our own reactions, needs, and longings. Such a stance may threaten or relieve, or it may do both. Most important, it requires an immediacy, a presence, an openness.

The fear and vulnerability we feel in acknowledging our sexuality as therapists is deep and profound—so profound that people fear the naming itself. This fear sometimes takes the form of accusations against those who begin the dialogue, that they are supporting, if not promoting, active sexual contact between clients and therapists. Thus, the following clarification is in order: Uncovering the hidden sexual dimensions of therapists' relationships with clients is not equivalent to supporting the gross abuse of power manifested in overt sexual contact. Nor should the open examination of such complex feelings be confused with idealizing or justifying them. Although some fear that danger lies in uncovering these feelings, I believe the greater harm rests in hiding and suppressing them, such that their influence remains unexamined and perhaps uncontrolled. Rather than question frank discussion of this dimension, we should question and challenge the silence and pervasive discomfort that surrounds its existence. This can only clarify our ethical mandates of care, not compromise them.

THE ACCOUNTS

What follows are the words of family therapists, organized around eight themes that emerged from the hours of conversation: (1) therapists' reactions to inquiry about sexuality; (2) sexual dimensions and therapists' awareness of them; (3) objects of desire; (4) the treatment unit; (5) personal vulnerability: the example of marital status; (6) therapist as voyeur or caregiver: treating family sexual issues; (7) family-of-origin issues; and (8) gender and power: women as sexual objects.

Therapists' Reactions to Inquiry about Sexuality

The beginning conversations were tense and anxious. My colleagues were very willing and eager to share but concerned about the risk of professional exposure. Talk about sexuality left us giggly, vulnerable, and—as some honestly confessed—aroused. The boundary between descriptions of therapy experiences and intensely personal revelations felt tenuous and blurred. In spite of our professional air and sometimes detached clinical assessments, there was no easy way to talk about our work or respond to the statements of the other without revealing a great deal about our sexual selves—in and out of the office.

> I don't feel that uncomfortable talking about this (*laughs*). Or maybe the way I know I *am* uncomfortable is that nothing comes up for me right away. But I don't just think it's repression. You're asking me to think about something I just don't think about that consciously. It's like something is out there but it's out of focus. [woman]

> It's hard to begin, even though we've known each other for years. How can I talk about something so personal about myself and my work? This is different from tales of the latest man I'm tracking or yet another piece of work on my own family. It's too intimate, and I feel exposed. [woman]

> I'm worried about how you'll see my work. I feel embarrassed talking about having these feelings because *good* therapists don't have these feelings, do they? I feel I should have this all under control. And, by definition, I think I'm doing a poor job if my own needs are getting met in therapy. [man]

> I'm afraid of making this public because I know I'm not part of the mainstream dogma. We can't talk about this easily in our culture in general, and not in the therapy culture, either. I think caring and the sexual energy that sometimes generates are major curative factors. I can say that to you, but a part of me fears being different when I'm not observing the traditional rules. It is really risky. [man]

Sexual Dimensions and Therapists' Awareness of Them

For these family therapists, sexuality within treatment was not a unidimensional experience. It ranged from a relatively simple physical rush to a more complex experience of attraction, care, investment, and commitment. Upon initial inquiry, male therapists more quickly described experiences of physical arousal or "lust," while women discussed the more gradual development of sexual dimensions contingent upon a deepening relational connection. It is unclear, however, whether these suggestive gender differences reflect distinct sexual experiences or whether each gender follows socially prescribed rules for talking about sexuality. For example, some of the female therapists reported feeling uncomfortable experiencing sexual arousal without an intimate connection. In addition, most of the men, upon direct questioning, revealed a qualitative shift in the nature of their attraction as a function of the increased trust and intimacy of the therapy relationship.

> I've never felt sexual with my clients. I just work off of a different part of myself. [man]

> You know, when we first talked (several weeks ago), I said that I wasn't aware of feeling much attraction or sexuality with my clients, ever. I've been thinking about it since then, and I realized I steer clear of dealing with it in any way. Like, I don't talk about sex with my clients—and I do a lot of couples work—unless they bring it up. Even then, I'll do some behavioral stuff around their sexuality, but I feel more comfortable shifting the focus to talking about intimacy and family-of-origin stuff. The other thing is that, since we talked, I have felt more with my clients. It's like I'm allowing myself to feel something new, or maybe to feel what was always there anyway. [woman]

> It's sometimes just physical. I botched one family case because I couldn't stop looking at the daughter's legs. It was a difficult case anyway, and my energy just got focused on the wrong thing. [man]

> Yes, I've felt something for clients, but I didn't even know what to call it. Outside of therapy, when I'm attracted to someone, I feel out of control, too emotional, anxious, elated—like a teenager. But those feelings don't belong in the therapy room. Or, as we talk about it, they don't belong with my image of what a good therapist feels like with clients. [man]

> There's sexuality that is just a rush because something is in the air, and then there is the attraction that comes out of having worked hard with someone or seen them through a real vulnerable time. The attraction grows out of loving the family. And I think the family's awareness of that love and that attraction makes the work more powerful. The question is how to keep your balance. [woman]

> I see the world as filled with sex. And I don't just mean genitals, I mean a whole dimension of energy. I feel comfortable with it, it's exciting and

sometimes anxiety provoking. [I know you well enough to know there's almost nothing that's not sexual for you.] And I know you well enough to know you don't always like it. So our therapies probably look real different. You have a lot to teach me about protection and constraint, and I can teach you not to be so reactive to a more assertive vital energy. [man]

Objects of Desire

Although most of the therapists easily admitted sexual attraction to clients, hesitation or discomfort became evident when I inquired about whether they were attracted to men, women, or both. In general, men more emphatically stated they were attracted only to the opposite sex. (To my knowledge, no gay men were in my sample.) Men who acknowledged attraction to both sexes explained they experienced sexuality as a global life energy; hence, attraction to other men in no way reflected a desire for sexual contact. In contrast, women were less reactive to my inquiries and tended to acknowledge attraction to both sexes. This attraction, however, grew out of feelings of intimacy or connection and was not primarily sexual. Women also described distinctly different sexual experiences, contingent on whether they were treating heterosexual or lesbian couples.

I notice women's bodies a lot, but I never feel attracted to men in my practice. I don't outside of my office, and I don't inside it. [man]

I think of sexual feelings as positive, so it's never disturbing to me. And by sexuality I mean an energy. I have sexual feelings about men and women. I find that comforting. It's a good check against abuse, because I'm more likely to treat men and women the same, rather than different—rather than investing my attraction to women with more meaning. And there's no question in my mind that I'm straight. [man]

As a lesbian, I have to deal with the misconceptions of my clients. Some straight women get worried that I'm interested in them. I've never understood that. You don't assume that your straight therapist is going to be interested in you necessarily, but our culture really scares people about women loving women. Men sometimes seem confused. I'll sometimes be playful with them or flirtatious—and it's like they can't make sense of it. [woman]

I don't quite know how to explain it, but I can feel a real change in my sexual energy. With a straight couple, if I'm kind of turned on by them, I have a more flirtatious edge. I know that dance and am pretty good at it. I relate to how the couple is together, and it reminds me of the way I am with my

husband and other men who've been in my life. With two women, there
sometimes is this very sweet, warm, physical sense between us. I just feel
different sexually and emotionally. Part of it is that it's so familiar to be with
women. [woman]

The Treatment Unit

Common sense suggests that individual therapy enables the development
of highly charged sexual feelings. It is often assumed that family therapists
treat primarily couples or larger social systems, but the majority of family
therapists interviewed practiced a significant amount of individual treatment—albeit from a systems perspective. In individual psychotherapy,
these therapists reported a greater awareness of sexual energy or tension,
and greater ease in addressing its presence with the client. However, there
is no simple correlation between cognizance of sexual dimensions and the
size of the treatment unit. Some therapists experienced a reduction of
sexual energy while working with couples or families because the presence
of others served to constrain or inhibit sexual interest. In contrast, other
therapists reported greater personal comfort with feelings of sexuality or
intimacy when working with more than one client. For these therapists,
the larger client system somewhat lessened the intensity of the treatment
relationship and so provided the proverbial safety in numbers situation.
Interesting data emerged as therapists described the phenomenological
experience of shifting from one treatment modality to another.

I sometimes see partners individually, along with conjoint meetings. Somehow working with the couple distracts me from my own interest. I am more
aware of my attraction in individual meetings. I'm thinking of one case where
I worked with the man for several weeks while his wife was out of town on
business. He did a beautiful, intense piece of work on his family. There was a
lot of warmth between us. It's strange to admit, but I felt the loss of that
special connection when his wife returned. [woman]

I'd been working with a couple for about 6 months. One day, the husband
called to say he'd be late, so I started the meeting without him. I don't even
remember what we were talking about, but when the husband arrived, he
came into the office without knocking. Really, it felt to me like he burst into
the office. And I had the strangest reaction. I felt like I'd been caught with his
wife. I still haven't figured out whether there was something going on
between me and her on some deep level, whether I'd somehow played a brief
role in some dance of theirs, or what. [man]

There's something to the saying "safety in numbers." When I'm working with a whole family, I'm less aware of myself altogether. There is more to attend to, to keep an eye on, to orchestrate. It really is less intimate than one-on-one contact. But sometimes I find I notice my sexual feelings more, the more people there are in the room—as if it's safer to feel that then. [Can you give me an example?] I work with this man who gets very animated when he's talking to his girlfriend. I'm touched by his earnestness and energy. It's like a quick flash of interest, but when his partner is there I feel the limit, and somehow it allows me to have the attraction and worry less about it. Alone with him, I'd feel more anxious or aware of it or wondering whether he was feeling the same. [woman]

When I work with couples, I'm aware that I complete the triangle. I expect certain things to happen, and I expect the sexual energy. In other words, I assume its presence. So I expect certain things to happen. For example, the wife feels a strong attraction to me. After all, for an hour a week, she sees me as a caring man, attuned to feelings and relationships. Whether it's conscious or not, I expect her to compare her husband to me. And sometimes it's not subtle at all, like when a woman directly states she wishes he'd be more like me. And I expect the man to have feelings about that or about my interest in his wife. He may be angry, threatened, insecure, jealous, or indifferent. Depending on the case, I sometimes bring that out explicitly. But I always keep in mind that I'm in a triangle, hopefully a helpful one, and that it's charged—sometimes lusty, sometimes poignant, sometimes competitive, sometimes playful. [man]

Personal Vulnerability: The Example of Marital Status

Two factors promoting the intimacy of the therapeutic relationship are continuity of contact and intensity of connection. Proximity and constancy, coupled with my premise that psychotherapy is a relationship that serves both therapist and client needs, mean that clients are often valued parts of therapists' lives. Some therapists acknowledged having more regular contact with clients than with friends. When a therapist is experiencing increased vulnerability, clients can become the focus of therapists' wishes, fantasies, or longings. Personal vulnerability takes many forms, ranging from traumatic loss (the death of a parent or the end of a marriage) to more sustained stress (studying for licensing exams or nursing an ailing child). Notable in these therapists' accounts was vulnerability around life-stage issues. Perhaps because of the developmental stages of the therapists, marriage and singlehood were often mentioned as critical factors influencing the presence of sexual attraction and/or the perceived safety of experiencing the attraction. But the relationship between marital status and sexual attraction is not a simple one.

It is also important to note that traditional clinical literature defines personal vulnerability as professional liability. Yet these family therapists also described how periods of loneliness, stress, dislocation, or confusion in their own lives enhanced a more responsive sensitivity to the needs and feelings of clients. Awareness and conscious regulation of one's fragility are key elements in protecting the therapeutic relationship.

> I come from a family where there were no boundaries. There was a time when all my clients were game when I was hurting, horny, needing. It was a mess. But with the work that I've been doing on my sexuality and with my marriage, I can work better because I'm not leaking as much. My sexuality is still being worked; it's always being worked—that will never be over. But what's crucial, I think, is what the therapist in his own personal life is or is not getting and what is working off of clients. Because if I'm frustrated in my primary relationship, I'm more susceptible to getting healing from clients where I'm "in power." How could I do this work and not go home and get my needs met? It would be intolerable. [man]

> My marriage ended several years ago. And it was clear to me all along that my work—the structure it provided, the intense connections with my clients— gave me something I needed during the months that I was so lonely and desolate. During that time, it was taking care of my clients and getting back from them that I was doing something good and caring that was important. I didn't feel sexual in my real life, and I didn't feel sexual with my clients. Then, as I began to think about beginning another relationship, I found myself strongly attracted to several men in my practice. I'd be aware of what I was wearing on the days I was seeing them and sometimes would be distracted in the sessions, acutely aware of how they were sitting. On a vacation, I fantasized about one of them. Now I can come up with a lot of explanations for it—but the feelings felt quite real. Sometimes I couldn't concentrate; sometimes I'd wonder whether they found me attractive, too; sometimes I'd find myself flirting with them. I was excited, embarrassed, and worried about what the hell I was doing as a therapist. Though I talked about this in supervision, I focused more on them and what role I was playing for them— as if it was simply a question of their dynamics or some family-of-origin pattern. But I wondered a lot about how my own loneliness and neediness fueled the attraction. [woman]

> I feel attracted to women in my practice. But it's totally safe because I'm happy in my marriage and I know the boundaries are there. [man]

> I don't believe all this about marriage as contraception. I know married therapists who have been inappropriate with clients, or had affairs. You

could make the case that married therapists are more vulnerable because it sometimes happens that the only contact they have with people outside of their husband or wife are their clients. My single friends have a lot of intense, close connections. I'm happy in my marriage, but the demands of family life mean that it's only with my clients that I get to explore other parts of myself. I've never acted on anything and don't plan to. [man]

Therapist as Voyeur or Caregiver: Treating Family Sexual Issues

Family therapy has just begun to address healthy sexuality and sexual dysfunction as crucial dimensions of family life (Simon, 1988; Weeks & Hof, 1987). But, outside of prescribing professional empathy, few articles address what family therapists might feel as they initiate and promote delicate, painful, and detailed discussion about sexual issues among family members. Although most family therapists have formal training in how to broach sensitive topics, sexuality and sexual practices are not on that list. But for the therapists interviewed here, frank discussion of clients' sexual practices or difficulties often resulted in disturbing—though not always unpleasant—feelings for the therapist.

It's almost embarrasing to say this, but I sometimes find myself getting aroused as I get detailed sexual histories. I feel it's purely a professional inquiry, but I sometimes wonder whether my own titillation isn't behind some of my questions. Voyeuristic—you know what I mean? I was taught about objectivity and professional detachment, and my training dealt with the anxiety I might feel. But no one suggested that I might have sexual feelings of my own. [man]

I was treating a young unmarried couple for sexual dysfunction. I dealt with family-of-origin issues for weeks until I realized it was my own discomfort that kept me from exploring the obvious. And then, it turned out this couple was into mild bondage and domination and the woman relished the submissive position. I felt angry with her and more humiliated than she did. It was hard for me to stay neutral about how they made love. So my feelings weren't of attraction or interest, but bordered on repulsion and criticism. [woman]

I was working with this sweet couple who'd experienced incredible deprivation in each of their families of origin. They'd been married for 16 years and had had little sexual contact. Very carefully, I found myself using myself as a model of a different kind of sexual experience. I talked familiarly with them about sex and dropped a more formal didactic tone that I feel more comfortable using with clients. I was kind of flirtatious with the husband, who was very shy and inhibited. I was aware of slowly filling the sessions with a different kind of sexual energy, to give them the experience that it was safe, natural, normal, playful, and could be regulated—not just be out of control. I was proud of the work, I was very careful. But I also knew I wouldn't feel fully comfortable sharing it with my colleagues. [woman]

I work a lot with incest cases. So normally what I'm aware of [in terms of sexuality] is being horrified, angry, shocked, sad about what's been going on in a family. But you're surrounded by sexual material all day, and sometimes I've felt reactions I can't believe. Once I was doing an evaluation with a girl, about 5 years old, whose father had incested her. She was sitting on the floor with her legs apart, and I found myself looking up her skirt. Or, I've worked for several years with a guy, a recovering alcoholic, who'd been a wife beater and had molested his son several times during blackouts. He's slowly turning his life around, and I like him as a person. Sometimes I've felt attracted to him, and I don't believe it—with everything I know about what he's done. [woman]

Family-of-Origin Issues

How and whether we approach sexuality in therapy reflects how we approach sexuality in our personal lives—be it with shame, titillation, easy pleasure, or confusion. This often relates to images, messages, or experiences in our families of origin, of which we may or may not be conscious. Many family therapists invest hours in unpacking their personal histories, in order to understand themselves better as clinical instruments. Sometimes the connections between past and present seem obvious; at other times, their impact is both profound and incredibly subtle. I was made aware of this when one of my colleagues noted some discomfort I was experiencing as he discussed how his family's prurient interest in his sexual development colored the content he focused on with clients. He asked what I'd learned in my own family about sex, arousal, and flirtatious triangles. Taken aback, I realized a connection that elucidated a pattern relevant to my personal life, my clinical work, and these interviews themselves.

For many of the therapists, family-of-origin issues about sexuality—especially when they remained unconscious or unexamined—powerfully channeled how they recognized, evaluated, and worked with sexual material between themselves and their clients. But the goal of self-exploration is not simply to neutralize or contain sexual material; rather, it is to become aware of patterns that shape how the therapist perceives interpersonal realities, relates to her own sexuality, and intervenes most comfortably.

> You know, triangles have three parts to them. A while ago, I realized that it was easy for me to look at the dance between the couple as they vied for my attention, but it was harder for me to get in touch with my own role in maintaining the dance. I remember one case where there was this very nice-looking, sensitive guy married to this angry, pretty hysterical, overweight woman. I was younger than her, thinner, more educated. She was jealous of me, and I processed that in the therapy. It wasn't until a real stuck place occurred that I realized that I was competitive back with her. That was too familiar to me. It was me, my stepmother, and my father all over again. [woman]

> I see the world in sexual terms, always. I grew up in a house where there was no privacy. My parents slept in separate bedrooms, and Mom was always parading around in her underwear. But if I noticed, I was the dirty one. There were crazy, mixed messages. For years, I paraded around with a hard-on, defiantly. But it wasn't just rebellion: I also needed to feel such a basic part of me was good energy. I'm shifting that now. But I clue into this immediately with clients—the sexual shit in their families and in the room. Sometimes I am great, and sometimes I have to watch it. I'm learning I can feel it when it's not there for them. You know, it's not just my enemy. It also leads me to some real powerful, important work. [man]

> It is hard for me to raise sexual issues with clients. I used to attribute this to lack of expertise, to it not being the real issue, to their own inhibition. I used to make jokes about my Catholic upbringing. You know. You don't talk about sex; you do everything but do *it*; you never bring up sex in mixed company; nice girls don't; sex is dirty. I was aware of the havoc that caused in my private life, but it took longer to get how that totally blocked parts of my clinical work. [woman]

Gender and Power: Women as Sexual Objects

Cultural beliefs and sanctions dictate how men and women experience and express their sexualities. Cultural definitions of male and female sexuality and their "appropriate" manifestations exist in complex relationship with the inequality between men and women at the broadest social levels. An intriguing theme emerging only from the accounts of women family therapists was their acute awareness that male clients sometimes employed sexuality as an expression of power. In other words, women therapists' experiences were strongly constrained by their sensitivity to the social (and practical) meanings of sexually tinged male–female interactions. For some women, this related to feeling objectified, exposed, or invaded by men's sexual interest. For others, their discomfort was partially a function of the complicated knots of power and gender characterizing the treatment relationship. Notable is that the female therapist wields professional authority in the consultation room while living in a society that capitalizes on women's presumed sexual availability as one way of reinforcing men's control over women.

> On the days I lead the group [for male sexual offenders], I dress as if I'm a female eunuch. I wear no makeup, I wear sensible shoes, I tie my hair back. I'm sometimes irritated that I feel compelled to make such a choice, but this way I can insure that I can get some therapy done, rather than dealing with the men in the group flirting with me. [woman]

> I was treating a couple about my age and the husband was quite seductive with me. It seemed light and playful. But as a woman, I felt the timing of the teasing was no accident. Usually when I was close to hot material for the couple, he would compliment me or something, and I would get flustered or uncomfortable. It wasn't just that it was sexual. [This was how] he regained control when he was feeling uncomfortable, because he felt so confident in that arena. Even though I was the therapist, more educated than him, more in control, his coming on to me put me in my place. It's the same vulnerability I feel when a man looks me over on the street. I started out working with the sexual aspect of his teasing me, and that got nowhere—it was still on his terms. But things really started to shift once I began talking about it as a question of power. [woman]

> I was in a training class, and we were dealing with gender and family therapy. I played the therapist in a role-play interview of a couple. Afterwards, one of the men in the class told me he felt I'd been seductive with the role-play husband because of how I was sitting and how I leaned forward and pushed the hair back from my head. I immediately felt ashamed and embarrassed and shifted my entire physical posture. I told him I didn't feel I was being sexual. He disagreed. My male co-teacher then said that, as a man, he didn't see my posture as a come-on. I felt relieved. But then I realized that I was bouncing back and forth between how these two men were defining my sexuality for me! As a woman, that seemed second nature, and realizing that horrified me. [woman]

ETHICAL AND THEORETICAL CONSIDERATIONS

Because of my focus on therapists' positive sexual feelings toward clients, this chapter examines only one facet of how sexuality functions as an unnamed but powerful force in family therapy. As such, this analysis is not yet truly systemic, as it doesn't account for therapists' feelings of repulsion or neutrality, nor for the experiences of female and male clients, nor for the undoubtedly complex interrelationships among all human parts of the therapy system. Given the preliminary nature of this survey, it is beyond the scope of this chapter to address in depth the difficult ethical, theoretical, and technical dilemmas concerning whether or how to integrate explicit acknowledgment of sexual dimensions into the treatment relationship. Instead, I will highlight some major points in the hope of providing ways of orienting ourselves to some of the personal and clinical concerns.

Ethics and Human Dilemmas

To insure the safety and integrity of the treatment relationship, the ethical codes of all major clinical disciplines strongly forbid overt sexual contact or intercourse between therapist and clients (Margolin, 1982; Weiner & Boss, 1985). But this single prohibition does not provide adequate guidance through the murky intimacy of therapy. Most didactic training in our relatively abstract ethical codes doesn't prepare therapists for the presence and subtlety of sexual exchanges between clinicians and clients, or for the resulting human dilemmas (Edelwich & Brodsky, 1982). More important, outside of sexual intercourse or flagrant seductive contact, a wide range of behaviors are not even addressed by ethical mandates. Perhaps because of this, professional consensus about the ethical appropriateness of specific acts of physical affection between therapist and client decreases as the acts become less overtly sexual. For example, although over 95% of psychologists surveyed by Pope and colleagues (1987) believed that sexual contact and erotic activities with patients were unethical, about half viewed kissing as unethical and less than 5% believed hugging was clearly unethical. Furthermore, a significant number of therapists were not sure how to judge the propriety of certain sexually tinged behaviors in therapy. When therapists lack clear guidelines to aid them in assessing the appropriateness of their actions, solutions are created (perhaps haphazardly) at the individual level, without the support or constraint of our profession as a whole.

Given the current professional context, which discourages open, nonpunitive dialogue about sexuality and psychotherapy, therapists struggle in guilty, anxious, or confused isolation, specifically about ethical judgments concerning sexual fantasies or sexual attraction toward clients. Over 10% of surveyed psychologists believed that simply experiencing sexual attraction to a client was unethical, though an additional 10% evaluated such attraction as ethical under rare circumstances (Pope, Keith-Spiegel, & Tabachnick, 1986; Pope et al., 1987). What does it mean to believe that certain thoughts or feelings are unethical? This collapses the essential distinction between normal feelings and unethical acts. It is only acts that can be unethical, irresponsible, or dangerous. Feelings of all sorts have interpersonal ethical implications only when they are translated into behaviors that impinge upon, constrain, or influence the safety and integrity of another individual. Therapists experience a wide range of feelings. The goal is not to suppress the very experience of feelings, but to understand their genesis and to create mechanisms to insure that they are not acted upon carelessly. This seems to be a truism and, in fact, is something that most family therapists take as a fundamental point to be transmitted to clients. All feelings are appropriate; not all actions are. Thus, we must question why we have a double standard for the experiences of therapists and those of our clients.

Due to the wide prevalence of therapists who experience sexual feelings within the treatment relationship, blanket censure is no solution. In fact, significant dangers may arise when feelings are simply denied or hidden. Therapists turn inward, blaming themselves, numbing their feelings, or struggling with doubts about professional competence. As insidiously, therapists may unconsciously act out toward clients, or they may use their interpretive power to blame clients for supposed seduction or manipulation. Regardless, a context of shame and constraint is created which also may deny a very real component of the relationship for therapist and client alike.

What, then, can be the solution? It is imperative to address the fact that family therapists lack a protective and protected forum where these dilemmas can be addressed without professional risk. As long as sexual feelings are defined a priori as bad, wrong, or deviant, the safety of disclosure will be severely compromised, since any admission of these feelings seems tantamount to acknowledging a significant ethical breach. A different stance toward the issue is predicated on affirming the intensity and real intimacy of the therapeutic relationship, which may have sexual components for all involved. Rather than preempting discussion of intimacy and sexuality dynamics between therapist and client, this stance invites dialogue about normal feelings that all family therapists may experience and minimizes the likelihood of immediate censure and blame of those clinicians who are attempting to clarify their ethical positions and clinical practices. At the same time, the often abstract examination of the professional, moral, legal, and human responsibilities of therapists for their own feelings becomes grounded in the detailed definition and elaboration of the complex experiences of therapists. In this different context of inquiry and discussion, the major question then changes from, Why are these (bad) feelings here? to, How can we most ethically and responsibly handle these inevitable dynamics between therapist and client?

This second question is not easily answered. With the possible exception of sexual intercourse between therapist and client, no particular form of behavior is always associated with negative outcome. Some therapists will skillfully and comfortably employ nonerotic physical affection with clients in healing ways, while other colleagues feel constrained and cautious. Some clients will respond appreciatively; others fearfully. The gender of the therapist and clients, as well as family dynamics, significantly shape the meaning and impact of certain gestures and statements. Furthermore, therapists follow a variety of family systems theoretical frameworks that punctuate reality in different ways. Across these models, varying definitions of "correct" or "appropriate" therapist behavior lead to distinctively different ways of assessing and managing sexual feelings.

Too often, I have heard people respond to this position with charges of "moral relativism," as if it sacrifices all standards and thereby permits any and all behaviors. The task is far more complicated: We must discover how to honor sanctions that prohibit clearly abusive or countertherapeutic behaviors of therapists while also taking seriously the notion of multiple views of reality, in order to examine how sexual feelings are understood within a given clinical frame of reference. Untangling this complex web is not easy, but the contextualized description and analysis of various practices is a better solution than global ethical sanctions that remain silent on more subtle but more common experiences.

Theoretical Issues

Two major dimensions of the contextual analysis of therapeutic practice are (1) the treatment model and the degree to which it emphasizes the clinical importance of sexual material and (2) how the treatment model defines the preferred therapist stance (Kantor & Neal, 1985).

Treatment Models

It is a truism in family therapy that no single reality exists. We each organize the flux of experience through cognitive models or explanatory systems that are usually implicit, operating outside of consciousness. These models influence (if not dictate) our behaviors, emotional responses, and ways of understanding things. Models of reality are also created and perpetuated at the social level, for example, through religion. At the professional level, family therapists turn their allegiance to a given theoretical school, characterized by its distinct model of the clinical reality. This model defines the nature of change, the locus of dysfunction, the function of time, and the meaning of the symptom.

Currently, no family therapy model highlights sexuality as a crucial organizing dimension, in obvious contrast to Freudian theory, with its focus on sexuality and aggression. If one takes the notion of multiple realities seriously, any clinical model of reality can only be analyzed in its own terms, since there is no method or need to prove the "right" way of viewing the world. On the other hand, models can be modified or amplified. Clearly, it is part of my personal clinical model that sexuality, the internal experience of the therapist, and the emotional connection between individuals in the therapy system are all important factors in the change process. I simultaneously acknowledge that other family therapy approaches can function effectively and powerfully from different frames of reference, even as I suggest that therapy may be enhanced, deepened, or transformed through including sexuality as an explicit dimension of the clinical reality.

But when sexual issues are identified, how do we manage them in a sensitive, therapeutically productive way? Should they be ignored, interpreted, normalized, or employed? Family therapy models not only influence whether sexuality is deemed relevant clinical content, they also provide a repertoire of techniques for addressing sexual currents. For example, transgenerational therapists might seek out sexual information through structured questions in order to make links to family history, choosing not to reveal their subjective responses in the sessions to sexual reverberations between therapist and client (Berman & Hof, 1987). An experiential therapist could use free association about inner fantasies or impulses in order to catalyze repressed sexual energy between a couple, while a structural therapist might unbalance a couple system by very consciously flirting with the wife. A strategic therapist would use sexuality paradoxically (Simon, 1986), while a systemic therapist would examine meanings about sexuality (Sanders, 1988). These techniques, in turn, exist in different theoretical contexts concerning treatment goals and change. Thus, outside certain inalienable limits (such as that of prohibiting therapist–client sexual contact), we must include recognition of and respect for the assumptions of the treatment model, in order to best assess the appropriateness (or propriety) of different ways of naming or utilizing sexuality in family therapy. This perspective shifts the tenor of conversations between therapists. Instead of arguing whether it is right or wrong to acknowledge sexuality in the therapy relationship, we can focus on how our understanding of the clinical reality shifts when we employ a model that includes sexuality; that is, we can assess whether that model is a good fit with the models of the family members we treat, when to openly name the sexual dimension, and how technically to intervene.

Therapist Stances

Over and beyond the treatment model and the extent to which it directs attention to sexual dimensions, we must consider the experience of the clinician. As is obvious from the vignettes, some therapists seemed to experience sexuality in every encounter, while others reported several discrete incidents that had no major influence on the course of treatment. A concept that helps organize this diverse phenomenological material is that of *therapist stance*. Different family therapy models can be categorized by the degree of engagement they permit or require of the therapist. There is no one "right" therapeutic stance. The following description of the stances emphasizes how therapists—by virtue of how they position themselves with client systems—obtain or ignore qualitatively different kinds of personal and clinical information (Kantor & Neal, 1985).

Kantor & Neal (1985) define three therapeutic stances.

1. The *disengaged or detached* stance is one in which the therapist works from a fairly great personal distance, standing outside of the family. This maintains a certain kind of control over the system and minimizes focus on the therapists' own feelings.

2. The *professional* stance is one in which the therapist works from a neutral, middle distance, in order to maintain objectivity. This enables the clinician to have empathic experiences of the clients' feelings, while keeping his subjective experiences somewhat out of awareness.

3. The *engaged or informed* stance is one in which the therapist

works with the client system from a very close position and uses her subjectivity, feelings, and impulses as the primary gauges and resources of the therapy.

The following are examples of how these different stances influence the therapist's experience of sexuality and of how, consistent with this stance, interventions follow their own internal logic. The first vignette was reported by a therapist trained in the Milan systemic approach. She works from a detached stance, in order to remain "meta" to the system. Because of her theoretical interest in the belief systems of her clients and because she works to maintain a balanced neutral position vis-à-vis the client system, she tends to minimize attention to her internal experiences of sexuality. If she does feel something, she employs the techniques of the systemic school to address the issues without increasing the emotional intensity of the session or imposing herself upon the system.

I don't know quite how to describe it, but I am a cognitive person, and the systemic model is cognitive, too. When I notice sexuality in a meeting, it may be because of something that I sense going on in the family—a "daddy's girl" or a son that married mom when dad deserted the family years before. But I don't focus on my experience except to help me figure out a hypothesis or a new way of framing things to the family. I also don't want my experience to color my exploration of the family's understanding and ways of seeing things. [But let's say you did feel something at some point, how would you deal with it?] I might build it into a series of questions, such as, If Dad were attracted to me, who in the family would get most jealous? How would Mom signal what she was feeling? Who would move in to take care of Mom? Questions like that would address it, but with the goal of understanding how the family makes sense of it.

The next example is taken from a therapist who works from an engaged or informed position. He employs his wishes, fantasies, impulses, and eroticism as temperature gauges of the therapy hour. He is well aware of how his sexuality colors the clinical relationship, and he utilizes his internal experiences rather than containing or neutralizing them. His resulting interventions are evocative and provocative, as he spontaneously employs his personal reactions as a way of plumbing the depths of his clients' realities and transforming them. Coincidental with this, however, he seeks out careful supervision in order to heighten his awareness and control of his subjectivity, which is affected by how he orients to the world sexually.

Look, the charge is there. Sometimes I can't know whether it is there for the client or is my projection or is something between us, but I take the charge for granted and, in fact, notice and comment when it is absent. Because a lot of people just sit on their sexuality, attractiveness. It's totally closeted, and I'll look at that frame—about feeling pleasure and charged up and whether that's OK in people's lives. I work with that charge because it gives me information about critical images [of the client] and where to go. I want to register it in me, to know my own fantasies. When I work with it [the sexual energy], it discharges my own energy. I stay more juiced and charged. I love the initial projections between me and my clients, in terms of my fantasy. But when I work with it, usually kinesthetically, and with psychodrama, I use the sexual feelings to deal with sexuality between the client and their family of origin. When I do that, my own energy changes. It moves up from my genitals to my heart—which opens up when I better understand why they use their sexual energy in certain ways or don't use it at all. If I stay on the other level [of projection and flirtation], it [the sexual energy] remains. I get stuck with frustration—like not making love when you want to—and I can get punitive. If I work with it, it moves. I'm left with compassion. [So you address this with every client?] No, but I'm always aware of it and tracking it. But they have a right not to follow that direction once I name it, and, if they don't [want to], I have to watch out for my own reaction, so I don't unconsciously punish them.

Finally, the therapist who works from the professional stance blends objectivity, a careful assessment of his internal experiences, and a sensitive but contained responsivity to his clients' feelings and needs. He tracks his sexual feelings and those of his clients because sexuality is a conscious part of his treatment model. But, at least in this vignette, he addresses sexuality in a way that is both personal and bounded. He utilizes a dialogical but interpretive approach that acknowledges his own reactions while exploring those of his clients. In this way, he uses his subjectivity more than a therapist working from a detached stance, but in a way that is less vividly revealing than a therapist more comfortable with an engaged or informed stance.

The whole question of sexuality has to do with how you understand it in your own life and how you make it, if you do, a part of your treatment model. It's like with my daughter—I share an intense emotional space and connection with her. I've had sexual feelings with her and, at first, I was afraid and wondered about my boundaries. Then I had to face what to do about it. I could pretend it wasn't happening. Or I could stop hugging her. Or I could figure that sexual feelings are enjoyable and a natural part of life and intimate experiences and that I was not going to act on them but shouldn't totally repress what I was feeling. Because if I cut off those feelings, I'm worried that

I cut off other whole classes or sets of feelings. Or distort them. So, in therapy, I ask myself, What is so special about an entire class of feelings [sexuality] that we're so uptight? How is feeling turned on different from hating a client or being bored with them or being excited about them? With any intense feeling, I manage them carefully and with the well-being and safety of the client always in mind. I care for a lot of my clients, and I think it's impossible to have warm feelings and not have a sexual component too— if people were honest about what was going on. [And do your clients notice your sexual energy?] I'll talk about it with them. When I deal with the transference, I always include the sexual component. I mean, look at what therapists say. It's OK for me to talk to the client about how they are experiencing me as their father, but we can't talk about sexuality? We've talked about every other facet of the relationship, so why not talk about sexuality? In my experience, it makes the treatment relationship that much safer by normalizing the feelings. To my knowledge, no one has ever been offended or freaked out. [You mean you raise it that directly with them?] Why are you surprised? [What do they do?] Some clients feel awkward and will say they try not to think about it, but I don't think I've had any deny they knew what I was talking about. Sometimes they've been feeling bad, stupid, or vulnerable for having some feelings about me. We discuss it like any other boundary issue, and I always make clear: The feelings are OK; acting on them is not.

Without an understanding of therapeutic stances, miscommunication and diviseness will characterize clinical discussions of the propriety and management of sexual feelings of the family therapist. For example, therapists from the engaged or informed stance could argue that other therapists are repressed, while therapists of the professional stance could make the case that detached or systemic therapists lose important data by not openly utilizing their personal reactions. A different kind of dialogue and clarification of the issues results when careful attention is paid to the theoretical assumptions of the treatment model and to its prescribed or preferred therapeutic stance. From this perspective, we can begin to analyze the benefits and risks of each stance, based on the types of information about sexuality each stance promotes or minimizes.

CONCLUSION

Sex, eroticism, sensuality, lust, intimacy, longing—these passions exist in every human heart and are the stuff that dreams, as well as psychotherapy, are made of. Our culture both glorifies and vilifies love and sex. Families set the stage for the sweetest expression of intimacy and for its grossest abuses. Family therapy moves into the heart of this all: a clinical enterprise with deeply human meaning and consequences.

This chapter has made beginning efforts to illuminate that which is forbidden: the acknowledgment of an intense, difficult, hot, exquisitely vulnerable dimension of the psychotherapeutic relationship. Through the testimonies and formal discussions presented here, I have attempted to elucidate some of the professional and ethical dilemmas. A most difficult task is to build a bridge between these two realms of discourse—the poetic and the clinical. It is equally difficult—but even more necessary—to create compassionate ways of understanding the experiences of family therapists and their clients, while rigorously upholding standards that are unquestionably protective of those we serve.

It is essential that sexuality not be a forbidden word. We are called upon to make a radical but necessary shift, by assuming sexuality's understandable presence in the context of an intense, intimate therapeutic relationship, rather than acting as if its existence is deviant or anomalous. This does not give us license to act upon sexual feelings; rather, it allows us to examine and regulate them. Each therapist experiences sexuality in distinctive ways, adheres to a different systems model, feels comfortable with certain kinds of interventions and therapeutic distances, and will approach sexuality and intimacy with various treatment goals in mind. My wish is not that every therapist adhere to a model that integrates sexuality in formulaic ways. It is that all therapists at least think about this issue and make a conscious decision whether or not to include sexuality in their treatment model; whether or not to observe and utilize their subjective reactions; and whether or not to enable family members to articulate their own beliefs, thoughts, and feelings about their sexual selves. It is valid to realize as a family therapist that you don't know what you think about sexuality and its implications for your practice, but it is very important to know that you don't yet know. Without conscious choice and self-examination, too much that is out of awareness may influence the therapy and its outcome.

This self-awareness is a process without end. Our capacities for intimacy develop over our lives; our sexuality changes as we love and struggle with our intimates; our psychotherapy can only reflect who we are in all our intense relationships, built on pain and caring. In this chapter, although I began by defining sexuality in a complex and rich way, I chose to focus on material that revealed its more traditionally understood nature. But it is important to remember that, for many therapists, attraction and longing grow in a complicated unique relationship of caring and commitment. Without full acknowledgment of the intricacies of this professional but often profound connection, individual family therapists are left to struggle in isolation—only to discover that they are not alone, that another set of rules may *already* exist but cannot be openly named.

As this chapter has been dedicated to testimony, so may it end with one. A family therapist anxiously sought consultation after she believed she had begun to fall in love with an adult son of a family she was treating. She stated:

> This experience was hell for me. I tried to handle it with as much personal and professional integrity as possible. I got a lot of supervision and, with great qualms, talked to some of my friends. Almost all of my colleagues had a story of someone they knew who had dated or even married a former client. It was like this was all going on out there, but I had no idea. At the same time, people gave me incredible support; everyone was worried about me and my professional career. They urged caution about who I spoke to. Since I had decided to discuss what was happening with the family and then to transfer them to other therapists, I had to talk to a number of people. I was anxious, really stricken with self-doubt.
>
> It has been one of the hardest but one of the most important lessons of my life. No one blamed me, and the family appreciated my care and how hard I worked to deal with them openly and responsibly. I was expecting such censure and blame—at least as much as I censured and blamed myself. But, behind closed doors, I was met with so much understanding and care. More than I could believe at the time, my friends and trusted colleagues accepted that I was going through something very human—that the technical rules of our business can't always address the complexities we face, that the therapeutic relationship carries its risks, and that care can deepen into love.

PERSONAL RESPONSES

I have just put aside what I thought was the final draft of my answers to these questions. It had been well received by colleagues, who appreciated its candor and self-revealing nature. At the same time, they expressed concern about what it would mean for me to write something so personal in an edited volume for the family therapy community. Their comments brought me to experience more vividly and immediately the most important point I made more abstractly and academically in my chapter: The professional exploration of the sexual and intimate dimensions of family therapy must occur in a protected context of dialogue and collaboration. Without such a context, the personal testimonies of individuals are too exposed, without opportunity for clarification. Without dialogue, individuals can be singled out for adulation or censure, and this circumvents the need for us to discuss systematically how family therapists as a group address or ignore these topics. Because of this, I decided to modify my original comments, while being clear about why I was doing so. This, I hope, will suggest a different way to begin to handle questions about the context of safety and trust for the professional, rendering unnecessary the more common practices of simply silencing oneself or employing distancing professional language in order to guarantee the protection we all require.

Influence of Gender and Generational Socialization. It would be too easy simply to say that being a woman strongly influenced my writing of this chapter. It would also be too easy to employ a lot of political rhetoric, given my professional interest in the gender issues. The rhetoric would be passionate, accurate, and revealing and yet not really touch the heart of the matter. As I have integrated my thinking about gender into my clinical work, and as I have grappled with the ways that men and women fight and love together, I have become more and more aware of the places of profound confusion and loss. One of the major contributions of the women's movement has been the awareness of how the subordinate class is silenced. Discovering one's voice begins with defining one's personal experiences in one's own terms. Thus, the most important pieces of my chapter for me are the vivid testimony of the men and women, because they reveal some of the differences, the subtle distinctions that so powerfully shape how we live our lives. Holding onto the subtlety in my chapter was the hard piece, because it was tempting to make generalizations which, however accurate, seemed clichéd. Beginning to untangle the knots of intimacy seemed to call more for poetry than for professional discourse. As a woman, that made sense to me. Yet, as a woman socialized into the "right" ways of being professional, I also felt the need in my chapter for an "appropriate," formal, academic structure with the testimonies. That tension between rich testimony of the heart and conceptual structures and analysis was deeply informed by my being a woman.

My being a woman also strongly shaped my moral stance toward the expression of sexuality in the therapeutic relationship. As a professional who specialized previously in the area of violence against women, I am particularly aware of and outraged by the abuses of power and the sexual and physical victimization of women. It was striking for me to discover in my interviews how many family therapists knew of cases of sexual contact between therapists and clients, without having taken action or even known what action to take. This startling gap between our ethical codes and what we "know is going on out there" has special significance for most women.

More personally, I feel vulnerable as a woman, given the nature of the chapter. Why? Because its theme is sexual, because it uncovers much that is denied, because I am a woman naming these dimensions, I fear that people will dismiss this chapter because of my politics, my marital status, my personal characteristics—as often occurs when women dare to explore the unnamed edges of things. I fear this for good reason: The responses to my presentations and writings on sexuality and family therapy have been extreme, with many family therapists deeply appreciating the opportunity to talk about experiences that have never been openly discussed and others responding angrily, judgmentally, and accusingly. While I know that writing a chapter such as mine is the first step toward change, I have some anxiety about being its author. I don't know whether a man would feel the same.

I also think being a woman shaped how I began the "investigation" of the topic. My inquiry was neither academic nor formal, but personal. I was continually surprised to realize what I took for granted about being a woman. The talks were like excursions into foreign lands: I knew the language of women and was continually surprised by that of men.

In terms of generational socialization, though I was not conscious of this as I wrote the chapter, there is no doubt that my historical location strongly influenced the perspectives and values I brought to this chapter. I hit college at the height of the sexual revolution and grew up expecting a certain frankness and openness about sexuality. Since my own personal maturation was swept up in the quickly changing tides of our society's views toward sexuality, I am very aware of the contradictions, the conflicts, the paradoxes. I'm sure that this influenced my interest in the topic of my chapter, my sensitivity to some of the nuances, and my willingness to shed light on areas normally viewed as beyond the pale.

Influence of Personal Intimacy and Sexual Experiences. I am very aware that my chapter is like a projective test of how I currently shape, understand, and experience sexuality and intimacy. That is because I believe my psychotherapy reflects and transforms how I am, in my most intimate relationships. We talk as if we learn the skill of psychotherapy separately from our life context and as if, in fundamental ways, our professional relationships with clients are somehow distinctly different from our relationships with our intimates. The more I work and the more I supervise other therapists, the less I believe that is true. So, for me, my clinical work and, by extension, how I think about this chapter change as I change. When I first began doing therapy almost 15 years ago, I understood little about real intimacy. Having been through long-term relationships since then, with all the deeper connections and long-standing impasses that relationships of duration can engender, I am more aware (from the inside) of how gnarled the webs of intimacy and sexuality can be. The elements and their interrelationships are legion, and they include the themes I follow with my clients; the material they bring in (as if they could read my unconscious, and perhaps they can); the relationship dilemmas that seem most important to focus on in therapy; my boldness in addressing sexuality with clients; and the currents I feel in my own life that become currents in my practice. All of these have informed my chapter.

Implications for Family Therapy Training and Practice. The first implication is that subjective experiences of family therapists need to be integrated in different ways into training and practice, regardless of the specific systems approach being taught. For example, experiential family therapists would need to learn to track very carefully their spontaneous images and impulses around sexuality and intimacy, which they may weave into the therapy experience. Systemic therapists could be guided to explore how their beliefs about sexuality and intimacy in the family shape the hypotheses they develop. It would be very useful to examine the variety of ways that family therapists can choose to utilize, interpret, or ignore sexual issues strategically in the service of clinical goals, as variously defined within different systems approaches.

A second implication is that family therapy training should pay greater attention to therapy as a system of human relationships, a stance that requires that we go beyond our mechanistic language of pattern and function. In the long run, this entails developing and promoting a richer theoretical way of describing and tracking patterns of intimacy and sexuality in families. Obviously, as family therapists, most of us are already regulating and shaping patterns of intimacy in families, but our systems language and task-focused orientations can, at times, oversimplify if not obscure that we are working with humans and their hearts.

Third, sexuality needs to be brought into family therapy training. At present, most family therapists have no training in how to address and treat sexual dysfunctions, even though my clinical experience suggests that many couples struggle with issues of sexual adjustment or match. Although some family therapy approaches have a developmental dimension, we rarely integrate sexual development into our theorizing and interventions. Minimally, training should include a component on sexual themes, patterns, and strains in families. Maximally, training should also include a component that focuses on therapists' own feelings and attitudes toward sexuality and their own gender. This dual focus on family and therapist reminds us that sexuality and intimacy are not simply dimensions of our clients' lives, detached from us as co-participants in the therapy relationship.

A fourth implication, as elaborated in my chapter, is that family therapy training needs to expand the discussion of ethical and clinical dilemmas, specifically regarding the sexual dimension in therapy relationships. It is essential to make this discussion as concrete and personal as possible, to contextualize and humanize the difficult personal and clinical decisions. In order to do this, we will need to begin humanizing the role of the family therapist. Too often, trainees see only the polished, competent presentations of skilled teachers, thus depriving students of the opportunity really to understand the internal theoretical, technical, and personal questions even the most skilled therapists always face. If trainers and teachers take the risk of disclosing more of their own experiences in the domain of sexuality, intimacy, and family therapy, they will begin to create a fertile, protected context for trainees.

A fifth point is that changes must occur in more than training programs. To my knowledge, most family therapists don't know how to expose and adjudicate the ethically questionable sexual practices of family therapists with their clients. If a professional board exists (outside of those limited to our professional disciplines), its presence is neither well advertised nor familiar. Unless we as a field have a mechanism for morally and clinically assessing practices of family therapists, particularly in the domain of sexuality, we sanction (if only by default) inappropriate and dangerous acting out by therapists, regardless of what we may emphasize in our training programs.

Finally, whether we are addressing training programs, clinical practice, or ethical monitoring, I feel the crucial foundation rests on the basic acceptance that sexuality and intimacy are inevitable dimensions of the caring relationship between family therapist and client system. As I've made clear, currently most training programs either ignore sexuality and intimacy altogether or focus on them (especially in supervision) only when they are problematic. By accepting certain feelings as a given, training and supervision can then shift from engendering blame and guilt to a focus on how to regulate and protect the therapy relationship constructively.

REFERENCES

Berman, E., & Hof, L. (1987). The sexual genogram—Assessing family-of-origin factors in the treatment of sexual dysfunction. In G. Weeks & L. Hof (Eds.), *Integrating sex and marital therapy: A clinical guide* (pp. 37–56). New York: Brunner/Mazel.

Edelwich, J., with Brodsky, A. (1982). *Sexual dilemmas for the helping professional.* New York: Brunner/Mazel.

Gartrell, N., Herman, J., Olarte, S., Feldstein, M., & Localio, J. (1987). Reporting practices of psychiatrists who knew of sexual misconduct by colleagues. *American Journal of Orthopsychiatry, 57,* 287–295.

Kantor, D., & Neal, J. (1985). Integrative shifts for the theory and practice of family systems theory. *Family Process, 24,* 13–30.

Kardener, S., Fuller, M., & Mensh, I. (1973). A survey of physicians' attitudes and practices regarding erotic and nonerotic contact with patients. *American Journal of Psychiatry, 130,* 1077–1081.

Margolin, G. (1982). Ethical and legal considerations in marital and family therapy. *American Psychologist, 37,* 788–801.

Pope, K., Keith-Spiegel, P., & Tabachnick, B. (1986). Sexual attraction to clients: The human therapist and the (sometimes) inhuman training system. *American Psychologist, 41,* 147–158.

Pope, K., Tabachnick, B., & Keith-Spiegel, P. (1987). Ethics of practice: The beliefs and behaviors of psychologists as therapists. *American Psychologist, 42,* 993–1006.

Sanders, G. (1988). Of cybernetics and sexuality: Applying systems thinking to sex therapy. *Family Therapy Networker, 12,* 39–41, 79–84.

Scheflen, A. (1965). Quasi-courtship behavior in psychotherapy. *Psychiatry, 28,* 245–257.

Simon, R. (1986). Behind the one-way kaleidoscope: The strategic therapy of Cloe Madanes has a logic all its own. *Family Therapy Networker, 10,* 19–29.

Simon, R. (Ed.). (1988). The great cover-up: Sexuality and the family. *Family Therapy Networker, 12,* full issue.

Stiver, I. (1986). The meaning of care: Reframing treatment models for women. *Psychotherapy, 23,* 221–226.

Weeks, & Hof, L. (Eds.). (1987). *Integrating sex and marital therapy: A clinical guide.* New York: Brunner/Mazel.

Weiner, J., & Boss, P. (1985). Exploring gender bias against women: Ethics for marriage and family therapy. *Counseling and Value, 30,* 9–23.

9

CONVERSATIONS

David Kantor, Barbara F. Okun, Donald A. Bloch,
Peggy Penn, Maggie Scarf, and Carlos Sluzki

It started out as a whim. What would happen, we asked each other, if we expanded our dialogue about intimacy, sex, and sexuality in families and family therapists to include other male and female family therapists? Our contributing authors were certainly interested in these topics. Whenever and wherever we mentioned our project, we were struck by the enthusiastic responses and queries. Would we find gendered patterns? Were there differences based on the "school of thought?"

We tossed this idea around for several months and then decided that it was time to try it. And so we devised an open discussion format for inter- and intragender meetings involving the two editors of this volume and two female and two male professionals, five of whom are directly involved with family therapy. We decided to include one person who has studied and written extensively about couples, intimacy and sexuality, gender, and couple therapy but who has not actually practiced family therapy, hoping for a broader, different perspective.

We formed our agenda as we went along—via letter, telephone, and preliminary meetings—and in the process we learned a lot about ourselves, each other, and the subject, notably the frustration and difficulty of delving into the elusive domains of intimacy and sexuality in family therapy theory and practice.

David Kantor. Kantor Family Institute, Cambridge, Massachusetts.

Barbara F. Okun. Department of Counseling Psychology, Special Education & Rehabilitation, Northeastern University, Boston, Massachusetts.

Donald A. Bloch and Peggy Penn. The Ackerman Institute for Family Therapy, New York, New York.

Maggie Scarf. Fellow, Jonathan Edwards College, Yale University, New Haven, Connecticutt.

Carlos Sluzki. Department of Psychiatry, Berkshire Medical Center, Pittsfield, Massachusetts.

The results of these efforts comprise the chapter. We videotaped three conversations: (1) a conversation between the female editor and the two female participants, hereafter referred to as the women's tape; (2) a conversation between the male editor and the two male participants, hereafter referred to as the men's tape; and (3) a conversation among members of both the male and female groups. Excerpted segments of dialogue from the intergender conversation compose most of this chapter. The content of the other two conversations formed the basis for the third conversation and is often alluded to. (Carlos Sluzki was only able to be with us for half of the intergender conversation)

These excerpted segments, along with the participants' commentary, are intended to broaden discussion surrounding the basic issues of sex, gender, love, and intimacy in couples, families, and family therapy, and among family therapists. They are organized into the major themes that emerged from the dialogues, and they have been edited and modified by the participants.

The bulk of the chapter consists of excerpts of and commentary about the themes that emerged from these dialogues, pertaining to the stated subject matter. Following these is a section of excerpts and commentary about the process of dialoguing itself. All commentaries bear the initials of the commentator. Questions and implications for further consideration are taken up at the end, and some participants have chosen to write a commentary and/or make a final statement about our efforts.

The six participants were selected on the basis of their known interest in and willingness to explore these issues from their gendered personal and professional experiences. The female participants are Barbara Okun, Peggy Penn, and Maggie Scarf. The male participants are David Kantor, Donald Bloch, and Carlos Sluzki. Although all are in the same age/generational range and reside and practice in the Northeast, their professional training and personal family experiences differ. The three women had no previous relationship with each other, whereas the three men have been friends and colleagues for years. Two of the women currently have close working relationships with two of the men. We attempted to accentuate gender differences, but we caution readers to allow for other personal variables in whatever differences emerge; we are not suggesting that our intergender differences be generalized.

There was quite a bit of initial discussion about the purpose of the dialogue and what exact questions would be raised. Barbara suggested the areas that had been discussed in the previous same-gender conversations, and David set the tone of the intergender dialogue:

DAVID: I have the idea that this notion of conversations is a meta-phor for what intimacy is about. What goes wrong in intimate relation-ships is that men and women don't have conversations. They have, as discussed in an article published in the *Times* Book Review section 2 weeks ago, entitled "Sex Wars," discourse of an unfriendly kind. Unfortu-nately, that's what's been going on in the field. In my opinion, nobody has challenged men and women to develop a model for having real conversa-tions in which the gender views are intentionally amplified, not for the purpose of conducting a war, but for the purpose of discovering difference and what to do about difference, which in a true conversation is valued. Essentially that is what this meeting is about. So, even in the editing, the idea is to have conversations.

CARLOS: You want the amplification of difference. If I make a state-ment that really doesn't convey my own position, which might actually be more ambiguous or more on both sides, and I choose one side for purposes of the conversation, I may be doing a poor service to my own position. So when you ask us to be honest and to exaggerate our position, you are making a lot of assumptions. I can't be honest. By being honest I would maintain a position that would be absolutely in the middle.

DAVID: Yes, and perhaps that's one difference between you and me. I'm more honest when I amplify.

CARLOS: Okay, so the expectation is not to be what one is not, for the purpose of the conversation.

Comment: Carlos is establishing differences between himself and another man. An important point, as obviously all men are not the same.—D.K.

MAJOR THEMES OF THE DIALOGUES

We have identified several major themes of our dialogues. Some of these were explored more thoroughly than others, and we include those ex-cerpts that highlight the nature of the exchanges.

Definition of Intimacy

Peggy wondered aloud what a family therapy theory of intimacy would include. What would it be? How might it address and expand gender issues? Although the discussions about the nature of intimacy during the same-gender conversations indicated agreement among same-gender participants, we felt it necessary to begin our intergender conversation with the attempt to check out individual notions about intimacy. We were surprised at how difficult a task this proved to be.

CARLOS: There is the very complicated normative issue of, first, who decides what is intimacy and, second, who has decided that intimacy is good and that nonintimacy is bad? And what is sexuality that is good sexuality as opposed to bad sexuality? Are we talking about orgasm? In my view, it is slightly arrogant to state that intimacy is good and nonintimacy is bad. The measure of intimacy is absolutely subjective, and it's very difficult to establish any kind of normative statement about it.

DAVID: It's also gender linked. I understood the women in their tape to be contrasting men and women along dimensions that I thought were revealing of their definitions of intimacy. And one of the things I want to say is that I believe that I have a definition of intimacy that's different from theirs.

PEGGY: What is it?

DAVID: It has two elements that are and two that are not included in most of the definitions of intimacy that I've seen come from women. There are actually four parts to it. One is disclosure. To have intimacy, by my definition, you have to have disclosure of a profound and personal kind. Disclosing presupposes trust. Two, to have intimacy you also have to be able to do something like what the self-psychologists talk about when they speak of empathic mirroring. The person you are with has to be able to depend upon you to play back to them what is good about them. I think those two components, in adult relationships, are more characteristic of women's definitions of intimacy than what I as a man include in my definition of intimacy, so I add two more components. One is what I call constraint, which is very different from empathic mirroring. In fact, in some ways it's the opposite. Constraint is a way of saying, basically, if you are asking me to be what you want me to be or to play a certain part for you, I cannot do that. What I can do is serve as a constraining surface and put you back to yourself. Obviously, it has more to do with autonomy than dependence in relationships. I think that this third component is more a male characteristic, at least it's this male's addition to these other components that go into the women's definitions of intimacy. The last component has to do with the resolution of differences. There are four ways to resolve differences: the agreement to agree; the agreement to not disagree; the agreement to disagree, and seeking a transcending synthesis.

Both in my personal and professional experiences, women tend to prefer the first two resolutions, men the last two, as I, in any case, do. Hence, I include the agreement to disagree in my definition of intimacy.

Comment: Agreement to disagree requires symmetry and egalitarianism in the relationship, which is not enabled by our patriarchal society.—B.O.

DON: Does intimacy relate reciprocally to role performance? That is, the historical shift has been away from satisfactory role performance, as the gauge of the worth of a relationship, toward a set of attributes like the ones you just mentioned. The degree to which you help me actualize myself is essentially a whole set of affective and emotional components. Whereas, if you go back in time, and you go to other cultures, the measure of the goodness of the relationship lay in the ability of the other person to fulfill a role—to be a good wife, a good husband, whatever the set of attributes were—a good worker, a good earner, a good housekeeper. Roles defined relationships, and sexuality had no part. That is, the enjoyable sexual partner was sort of interesting, might or might not be there, but was never talked about except by inference. But what was really talked about was if the person did their job in life well, as a male or female. And, of course, the transformation over time and in this culture has been the one I'm alluding to.

PEGGY: So would you think that intimacy for David, at this time in his life, has the particular attributes he cites, but that it might have other attributes for someone at a different point in life? Is it dependent on age, personal constructs, and cultural time?

DON: Different historical context and a different ethnicity or a different developmental stage.

MAGGIE: We're talking about a certain point in time when basically we're in our relationships "by choice." And, in fact, most of us are not in them for economic reasons primarily. We're here, and that's why everybody's having to drop their game plan. Because, in fact, why are you here unless you want to be here? We have to find reasons why we're staying in. Now, if I were asked to define what intimacy means to me, I would say that intimacy is being able to say with safety who I am and what I want and what I need and to be heard by the intimate partner. Now that presupposes a lot of autonomy, because, in fact, to the degree that my partner forces me to be what his fantasy or what he needs me to be, I cannot be safe and be intimate. However, if he permits me to be autonomous, really be me—and I think that over the course of a long relationship, that becomes more and more possible. (Though, obviously, as anybody who's been married longer than 15 minutes knows, we all regress into places which make it seem totally impossible.) I really do feel that being intimate and authentically one's real self is one of life's great experiences. And I think we've all hopefully experienced jumps when more of that becomes possible in a particular relationship when suddenly the curtain goes up and there's another vista and there are things you can say, things you can say in the presence of your partner, which change things for you and for your partner. Now, why that happens and how that happens, I don't know. But again, it comes back to being truly you, in the presence of another, and [this] is really another thing from being truly you, all alone.

Comment: How does Maggie define autonomy differently from David and Don?—D.K. It seems like Maggie's definition is akin to Jean Baker Miller's notion of "self in relation" as the female version of male autonomy and individuation.—B.O.

BARBARA: Your definition sounds female, Maggie. It includes both autonomy and connectedness in interaction, as well as nonjudgmental acceptance of differences, which I, a female, believe to be a necessary component of intimacy. I agree with your concept of intimacy, that it is one of life's greatest experiences.

PEGGY: But do you know what a change those two definitions are already marking, just in this group? For a woman to think of intimacy as defined by autonomy is a big change from 20 years ago, when intimacy was certainly defined by complementarity, by some state of fusion, romantic or married, certainly for women.

DAVID: Yes, and I think it's still this way for many women.

PEGGY: Maybe still for many women, but, as Maggie points out, increasingly not. Just the definition of intimacy alone is a very good read on how things are changing. You can see it in the changing models of intimacy. It's one thing for us all to sit here and talk about intimacy, but if we asked our grown kids what they mean by intimacy, we might get a very different and surprising response. They are developing faster than we are.

BARBARA: So, in addition to gender differences, there are generational differences. And probably class, regional, and ethnic differences, too.

PEGGY: Don't forget political.

Comment: How do family theory and therapy reflect the kinds of differences that emerge from six different people's struggle to define intimacy? The men's and women's tapes were clearly different in that the women talked concretely about equality and partnership models of intimate relationships, while the men talked more about complementarity.—B.O.

DON: Well, my question is whether we as a group are addressing ourselves to the question of intimacy or to the question of the goodness of a male-female relationship. I think that leads to other questions about sexuality and the conditions under which certain kinds of sexuality prevail. But is the topic of our conversation to talk about good and less-good male-female relations? How are they judged? How do we judge them? How do we judge them as family therapists?

CARLOS: What is clear by your way of describing intimacy is that the only way to know whether a relationship is intimate is by asking. Because there is a subjective quality of intimacy that is the only answer that one has to the actual phenomena proper. I can be talking about very intimate things measured by social consensus and, nonetheless, not be in an intimate relationship. Unless one could say that therapy is an intimate relationship, which it's not because therapy is a pseudo-intimacy. It's not the same. So the only way in which I will know whether I was in an intimate moment with somebody will be if they ask me or if I ask them. And the other curious phenomena is that probably the experience of intimacy is retrospective, not prospective.

BARBARA: You and the other person may not agree about the same encounter. You may say, yes, I felt that I was in an intimate interaction, and the other party may say, no, I didn't feel like I was in an intimate interaction. Do you really think that one person can feel intimate when the other one doesn't?

MAGGIE: For me, the experience of intimacy is not primarily a retrospective one. It happens in the "here and now." Of course, I cannot know whether the other person is actually feeling as intimate as I am, but a combination of cues, empathic feelings, remembrances of past intimacies (heavily larded, no doubt, by fantasies and imagination) make me "know" that an intimate exchange is occurring at the moment that it is happening.

CARLOS: In my sense, the notion of intimacy is totally subjective and personal. So, up to a point, the phenomenon of intimacy is like a retrospective judgment that takes place on the basis of our behavior and on the effect of our statements on the other. That, therefore, becomes the basis of our relationship. It establishes the nature of a relationship that has to be evaluated. This evaluation leads one to define the relationship as intimate or nonintimate.

DON: From the little I've read in other cultures and in history, I think that this is an extremely new idea in human history: Intimacy is a new value and a new idea.

BARBARA: Because it's not functional?

MAGGIE: I find that very hard to believe, in one way. I mean, if you look at the span of evolutionary history and you know that recorded history, as we know it, is 1% of human time, I just don't believe we picked it up in that 1%. I believe it's part of the human reward package. We're wired in for something. We can put the name "intimacy" on it or we could call it something else—"bonding," perhaps. I don't think it necessarily has to be sexual. I suppose, when I was talking before about "those moments," I was thinking of a time that I had done some interviews with a friend of ours, a lawyer who was dying of a brain tumor. I was driving up to the Cape with my husband, and I started talking about something that was very disturbing to me about these interviews, and how upset I had been. And my husband picked up a memory from my life, which I had forgotten. We talked about it, and we both burst into tears. That was perfect understanding—intimacy—not sexual, but it was a moment at which I felt that we were truly together. I can't believe that this capacity just came to us in the 20th century. I don't believe it lasts very long, but I think . . .

BARBARA: Even talking about it and trying to grab hold of it is difficult because it's so elusive. We can't see it, and can only feel it.

DON: I think the value for intimacy is 50 years old at most in Western society, in Western middle-class society. I'm sure people have been close to each other, shared things, been moved by each other. I'm suggesting that intimacy as a value in a male-female relationship is almost an artifact of the psychotherapeutic times that we're in.

Comment: There seems to be disagreement or confusion among the participants about the nature and value of intimacy and whether it has something to do with models of male-female relationships and, as we shall next see, sexuality. Are there really qualitative differences in the way males and females define intimacy?—B.O. and D.K.

Does Intimacy Increase or Decrease Sexuality?

The relationship of intimacy and sexuality became the next topic for discussion as we proceeded to struggle with our definition of intimacy. Maggie responded to a question from Don and pointed out the differences that emerged from the women's and men's tapes.

MAGGIE: Do I believe that intimacy increases sexuality? Yes. I think the men did not quite agree. I believe that intimacy is scary, as we all know it is. And I believe it's scarier for men, who are trained not to open up and not to make themselves vulnerable.

DON: Yes, but Maggie, I heard you say that in the women's tape, and I want to come full tilt with that. If you follow the course of relations, many relations, the height of sexuality and of a fluorescent, burgeoning sexuality—which is inventive, imaginative, exciting, engrossing, and so on—is *before* intimacy seizes the relationship, not after it. If you just look at the connection between that kind of lustful sexuality, if you make the graph of everything from variations to fantasies, to exploration, to number of orgasms per unit of time—whatever criteria you use for a flourishing sexuality—it occurs before there is much intimacy.

MAGGIE: It ain't necessarily so!

PEGGY: All intimacy is the expression of a language of attachment. The biology Don refers to is a young man's reponse to his social, gendered learning about his body. Women, I grant you, have different biologies and therefore their language of intimacy has more zones, covers more areas, events, and relationships.

BARBARA: I think there are definite gender differences about the intertwining of intimacy and sexuality. Women are invested in and concerned about the relationship aspects of sex as well as the performance aspects.

MAGGIE: Well, Marc Hollander—you know, this guy who did the research on what women like in sex which later appeared in Ann Landers—found that women like a lot of cuddling and a lot of kissing. For women, feeling loved as a whole person is obviously a very strong motivator for sexual activity. Kissing and cuddling are important, I believe, because many women distinguish between being cared for as a full person and being "used" as a sexual object by a partner who, as she perceives it, has merely incorporated her into his own somewhat self-involved fantasy. Now, I personally would not rather have cuddling and kissing than sex; however, I will say that cuddling and kissing are highly erotic, highly erotic. And I think that a lot of men don't understand that slow and light are better than heavy and strong.

DAVID: Well, it depends on your sexual fantasy.

MAGGIE: Well, you know, a friend of mine is working on a book about which men women consider great lovers. The men devoted a long, long time to the enjoyment of lovemaking—to the process, not the end goal.

DON: Well, it's interesting; I have to certainly agree with you. As preparation for this meeting, I got a couple of porno tapes.

MAGGIE (*jokingly*): You shouldn't have worked so hard. What a wonderful student!

DON: I got the tapes because I wanted to compare a porno tape made by a woman and a porno tape made by a man. And I learned, to my astonishment, that Maggie was right. Light and slow is the name of the game for the woman.

MAGGIE: And the great male lover understands that.

DON: Really, it's so much more humane and nice. Humane and nice at the later "intimate" stage—but that is *after* the highly lustful coming together has been achieved.

MAGGIE: Not Rambo sex.

Comment: We are hearing some clear gender differences regarding the relation of intimacy and sexuality and the definitions of erotic sex. Barbara and Peggy are nodding in agreement with Maggie, and David and Carlos seem to be in agreement with Don.—B.O. and D.K.

Withdrawal of Sexual Interest

David commented that the women on their tape were really talking about low sexual desire, whereas on the men's tape, David was referring to withdrawal of sexual interest. He made the distinction by stating that the withdrawal of sexual interest is an intrasystem phenomenon, while low sexual desire is something impinged on the system by outside variables.

BARBARA: Both the men's and women's groups disagreed on what to make of lack of sexual desire in couples today.

MAGGIE: What did the men say?

BARBARA: Well, the men were talking about entropy in long-term relationships, and the women were talking about multiple role pressures on couples today.

MAGGIE: Oh, right, yes.

BARBARA: In their tape, the men were talking about the issue of novelty versus entropy in long-term relationships, and we were talking a great deal about the enormous pressures of multiple roles, on women particularly, but also on men. How exhausted you are—how can you have an active sex life when you're being super mom, super career woman, super wife, super house worker, and so forth and so on? And so we were talking more about the pervasive, widespread impact of social systems' pressures and roles on today's couples, as opposed to individual psychological or relationship issues. We were talking about the pressures on women who even aren't super women, because they're feeling a lot of discomfort from not fitting into that super woman modality that's stressed so much by society. We were talking about social pressures, economic pressures, the realistic pressures that make it not easy today for people to make a living, to be successful—whatever that may mean. The impacts of liberation on both men and women have really changed roles and expectations and perhaps the trade-offs have not been so liberating!

DAVID: I have a single word to account for this phenomenon.

BARBARA: What is that?

DAVID: Disappointment.

PEGGY: Whose, more?

DAVID: Well, one of those partners, probably both. But, whenever there is withdrawal of sexual interest, you will find disappointment preceding it. Not low sexual desire, but the withdrawal of sexual interest, which is different from low sexual desire, and it's also different from the loss of sexual interest or desire. These are distinctions that I happen to be making because I've been thinking some about it. But, for me, the key word is disappointment, and the disappointment is not just—you know—random disappointment. It's a very specific kind of disappointment, a process phenomenon that is characteristic of intimate relationships.

BARBARA: Disappointment of one or both partners? Perhaps disappointment in that their expectations for romance or passion are not met?

PEGGY: Do you think it's disappointment in oneself? Or disappointment in the other? One often sees disappointment in the other, rather than in oneself.

DAVID: The disappointment I'm referring to has to do with the breaking of mythic contracts. There are, I believe, three contracts that are made between men and women and, though sometimes they're explicit, they're usually inexplicit. These days they're more likely to be explicit, because people talk about relationships. But, for the most part, they remain inexplicit or unspoken. They are, nevertheless, actual contracts, mythic contracts, contracts about mythic aspects of the relationships between men and women. The first of these, the culture myth, has to do with images or models or myths about gender ideals and behaviors.

BARBARA: You Tarzan, me Jane!

DAVID: . . . about what the man is supposed to be that you married and what the woman is supposed to be that you married. The myth, for example, that I am buying into these days for myself is the myth of the Ulysses story.

Comment: A subtopic that comes up here deals with culture myths. These myths seem to underlie intimate relationships, and the participants attempt to describe the one or ones they or their friends subscribe to. The myth of Ulysses refers to the Greek hero Ulysses or Odysseus, who wandered for 20 years seeking new adventures and conquests after leaving Ithaca for Troy. He left his wife Penelope and his son Telemachus, who refused to believe he was dead, no matter how faint their hope of his return. Penelope waited and turned down all the suitors who requested her hand and Ulysses' worldly goods. Eventually, after many conquests, Ulysses found his way home to his wife and son.—B.O.

PEGGY: You mean with Penelope weaving and unweaving her "waiting" cloak?

DAVID: Yes; now watch this. I don't want the "waiting" Penelope as my mythic mate, but I want to be Ulysses. I think in every relationship there is, on some level, an agreement about what the culture story is that we are buying into in the member of the opposite sex. This is the first mythic contract, the gender myth. The second has to do with personal myths, those highly personal stories which I have been working on for all these years in the concept of critical images.

Comment: By critical images, I'm referring to my theory that each individual brings a small set of these images from the past into adult intimate relationships. Each is a powerful story, which describes themes and behavior repertoires that define our expectations of self and our partners. Inevitably, the partners fail to fulfill these expectations because to do so violates the behavior mandates of their own "competing images"—D.K.

DAVID: A third mythic contract has to do strictly speaking with sexuality. Each partner has a sexual fantasy, an image about the most exciting ways to make love. Often they are so private as to be communicated only in the sensual language of physical lovemaking. Often, they have naughty or perverse elements. In courtship, when we make this mythic contract, it's very easy for each partner to indicate to the other that the sexual fantasy will for all time be played out in the sexual relationship. It doesn't. Sometimes the sexual contract is broken because the culture contract isn't working or because the struggles over personal myths are unresolved. But, if any of these three mythic contracts—the cultural, the personal, or the sexual—is broken, the couple stands a very good chance, one or the other or both, of withdrawing sexual interest. If all three are broken, the likelihood is virtual.

MAGGIE: Does the Ulysses myth signify that you want to be an adventurous, wandering man who moves from place to place and discovers different aspects, different women, or himself on a different isle, so to speak, of life.

DAVID: Well, yes; I don't have to go very far. For me, it's from Cambridge to my farm.

Comment: This sounds all mythed up to me!—D.B.

PEGGY: That's your Scylla and Charybdis?

Comment: Scylla, in Greek mythology, was changed from a lovely nymph by Circe into a frightful monster, Charybdis, attached to a rock in the sea, a peril to all sailors who passed her. Circe did this because she was angry that Glaucus, a sea God, loved Scylla and not her.—B.O.

DAVID: Right; that's where . . . in the woods. But, you see, I think it's one of several currently available myths for me, and I happen to like that one.

MAGGIE: So, Don, what would your myth be for a male? I mean, if you were to name a myth. This game is called choosing a myth. It's a little bit like *Celebrity* or *Choose*, the game shows on TV.

DON: Well, I have to think about it. It's not a common language that I use, so it's not one that I . . .

MAGGIE: Nothing pops in?

DON: You know, I don't mean . . . unlike David, it's not a customary way for me to think, so I'll take a "bye" on that.

BARBARA: Carlos, you got a myth for us?

CARLOS: I have the myth of the Phoenix.

MAGGIE: You rose from the ashes? And when was that?

CARLOS: Constantly.

PEGGY: Daily? It's a little of Jesus. Always rising.

CARLOS: It's a mixture of a very open sexual and heroic myth. Some fantasies and myths are more apt than others to maintain a relationship by themselves. In fact, the fantasy that I was proposing was interactive. If I maintain—and I may be able to change it or reason it out—the fantasy of the Phoenix, the interactive bond gets revivified out of itself, not out of an external stimulation, so to speak. There isn't an outside role that is more or less specific that can titillate the Phoenix to rise from its own ashes.

DON: Well, the Phoenix doesn't know what it is. And some ashes are easier to rise out of than others.

CARLOS: The point that I am trying to explore in some of the fantasies and myths being proposed is, assuming that they can be guiding forces, how much of the actions of all participants may they induce or generate? When you were saying [that] there are mates that want to stimulate their partners and are unable to, I was thinking, I hope that the myth of the Phoenix isn't too dominant in my emotional and sexual life, for otherwise my wife would be stuck, as, what can the mate of the Phoenix do? Very little more than wait until the Phoenix regenerates by itself—to stick to the most literal version of the myth. I wasn't also too envious of the Penelope of the couple that would be guided by the myth of Ulysses: It sounds to me like, Let's open up the gate to allow Ulysses to go for adventures, and let's pray that he will ultimately return, as the stimulation for Ulysses seems to be for Penelope to do nothing except knitting and unknitting and be undemanding. Otherwise, I can see Penelope becoming more assertive and demanding, and there goes Ulysses for another 20 years.

MAGGIE: I'm still curious about what David raised initially. We have two happy wanderers in myth here, and one person who isn't committed to what his mythical character would be, and I'm curious about possible gender difference in cultural myths.

DON: You always get a chance to go first when you're asking questions, so why don't you just say what a common female myth might be?

MAGGIE: Well, a very familiar feminine fantasy is a daughterly one. Which takes us straight into the Oedipus myth, I suppose.

DON: Whose daughter?

MAGGIE: The real father's daughter, if we're speaking in mythic terms. But the women who embrace that type of myth seem to fantasize about older men, whereas many women I know have the opposite fantasy; they fantasize about younger men. Both are intergenerational fantasies. But going back to the daughterly one, I can remember something said by that same lawyer I was talking about earlier. Once, we were talking to him about his favorite sexual fantasy—I don't know how it ever came up—but he said to us, "My favorite sexual fantasy is a woman who's saying 'no, no, it's impossible', at the same time as we're having sex." Many women seem to identify with that. No, it's not a rape; it's just she's saying no, but she's doing it—yes—and I suppose the reason some women find that kind of myth agreeable is because of the lack of responsibility. So that I think that being ignorant and irresponsible sexually (like a young girl) is a particularly female idea. It's a notion of being cared for, protected, treasured by a knowledgeable, responsible "paternal" male. But can you think of a mythological figure?

DAVID: Why not Electra? Why not? And it *is* the Oedipus myth.

Comment: Electra was Orestes's sister, and devoted her life to helping Orestes return and avenge their father's murder by killing their mother.— B.O.

DAVID: It sounds like, in your mind, that the Oedipus myth is really a woman's myth, and Ulysses is a man's myth.

MAGGIE: Perhaps so, to some degree. The former has something to do with a nurturant yet erotic figure.

DON: You know, I realize that part of the difficulty I'm having with this is that I can't pull together one myth, because I really have a fair number of different role relationship fantasies, and it doesn't come together in a single mythic figure.

DAVID: Why does it have to?

PEGGY: I'm thinking of things that captured my imagination when I was a kid. I had read a book somewhere along in my youth, called *My Theodosia*, which was about the daughter of Aaron Burr. He was a man of very mixed reception, and he killed Alexander Hamilton in a duel.

DON: A duel, right out here in Weehawken.

PEGGY: Right. He was a man of great romantic attributes in government and in bed. And for awhile that was my favorite myth—*My Theodosia*—where this man might have to flee into exile, and I, of course, would have to go with him in an unending oedipal romance. I saw a couple of movies, like *Waterloo Bridge*, which reshaped the myth. Of course, my father did go into the Army in the Second World War, so that's not entirely unrelated, but, you know, this "through death and time and war and pestilence"— I think it was a romantic solution that would rescue my father and return him to me in the best oedipal display.

MAGGIE: Well, the female figure in this fantasy is—?

PEGGY: Theodosia turned into Vivian Leigh, but she was still pretty dependent, not yet able to aggress sexually on her own, like the woman in your lawyer's fantasy who kept saying no. She could only identify with his sexual aggression, in lieu of having permission for her own sexuality, permission women eventually gave themselves. Now I think more in terms of equality, like Anthony and Cleopatra, politically and romantically linked.

MAGGIE: That's very different.

PEGGY: Yes. Their worlds took them apart, but they came back together. It can be quite romantic . . .

MAGGIE: So it's built-in distance.

PEGGY: Distances permitted both safety and romantic fantasy. But, in general, myths for women are not so interesting.

BARBARA: They're very asexual, you know, like Joan of Arc. Or very romantic and tinged with yearning rather than conquest.

DAVID: It doesn't have to be. With Oedipus, obviously it is, but mainly what it does is establish a structure of the relationship between a man and a woman. To name the myth merely is to universalize what the gender structure of that relationship is. It's not so important to give me the name of it, as that there is a structure to the relationship and that there is a mythic component.

PEGGY: But you know it is true that women respond to men desiring them as well as from their own desires. That seems to be the reciprocity of it. You know, if somebody winks, it's hard to hold your eyelids still.

MAGGIE: Melina Mercouri, when asked what makes a man sexy, said,"if he likes you."

PEGGY: Chemistry!

MAGGIE: Well, you see my understanding of the oedipal myth is, treasured child, treasured daughter. Not child so much, but treasured daughter. The treasured daughter fantasy is certainly becoming a social reality, as seen in the common marriage between a younger woman and a more powerful, authoritative older man (who may be in his second or third marriage). The trade-off may be: You take care of me, says the female, and I'll be your good, protective parent and pave your way into the adult world, responds the male. So, what about you, Barbara?

BARBARA: Well, mine is similar to the daughterly myth, or it used to be, in terms of the oedipal themes. It's based on the loving, protective father. I used to fantasize about being taken care of, but I'm not attracted to older men as much as I'm attracted to men about my same age. I think more in terms of the brother, the playmate. My fantasy has more of a collaborative, playful—you know—let's run down the beach together and make love on the dunes or run through the woods, and be free together.

PEGGY: And I'll run as fast as you will.

BARBARA: That's right, there's an egality to it. And there is equality, so I don't feel the power struggle. There is mutual pleasing. But my choosing, my wanting it is important in my fantasy.

MAGGIE: Your wanting it knowledgeably.

BARBARA: Well, sometimes I've had that theme that resonated with me when you talked about it, about my sort of being irresponsible.

MAGGIE: This is happening, but I don't have to take responsibility.

BARBARA: That's right, but I think it's evolved much more into my initiating and my taking responsibility for myself and for my playfulness and freedom. The intimacy and trust allow for spontaneity and exploration.

Comment: What Barbara is describing at first resembles a gender myth but then slips into what seems more like a sexual myth—D.K.

MAGGIE: I have a question for you, David. Suppose Penelope had sex with her suitors; how would you feel about that?

DAVID: Penelope isn't the counterpart to my Ulysses image. It's more someone like Athena or Hera I want than Penelope. A more vital female mythic figure than Penelope. But I think a lot of what happens is that women marry Ulysses characters and pretend to buy into the Penelope counterpart and then discover that they really didn't want to. They made a promise they never wanted to fulfill, and they get very angry. One of the things the feminists did was to catch the attention of so many women who did buy into Penelope but hadn't bargained for so much male absence. They were given permission to get angry and began to ask, What did I buy into? I don't like this.

PEGGY: It wasn't just women who bought into Penelope. Men did, too.

BARBARA: And that's what some of the disappointment is. Expectations don't get met, so then you're left with this pain and sense of betrayal.

DAVID: That's one of the three disappointments that leads to withdrawal of sexual interest.

Comment: In this group, there do seem to be some gender differences in that the male myths are more defined by dominance, wandering, and conquest, and the female myths by adoration, equality, mutual initiation, and playfulness. If male and female partners' myths collide, leading to disappointment, then withdrawal of sexual interest and distancing may result.—B.O. and D.K.

The discussion of myths developed into ideas about subjective sexual constructs, intimacy, and gender premises. And the topic of differing male and female sexual opportunities was introduced.

PEGGY: No one has looked at how attachment premises are gendered, especially over time.

MAGGIE: You know, women go through a process of sexual disqualification as they age, so that many of them would probably not find partners if they wanted to wander or leave their mates, though I'm continually surprised by people who do find partners.

PEGGY: And I'm also surprised by people who don't, who seem qualified.

DON: A lot of the clinical problems provide some elaboration of that condition, where the woman becomes insistent upon lighting the fire of sexuality with her mate. And it just does not seem to work. One of the things that happens in those fairly dormant, . . . devitalized perhaps, or certainly de-eroticized marriages is that there is then for the woman a sense of increasing sexual interest, which the man can't respond to. That's the one way. The other way it happens, of course, is that the man takes up with a young thing and discovers to his total astonishment that he's able to have a very intense sexual life, that he can both have a lot of sex and enjoy it enormously, when he had long since given up on that notion. So that those two careers, if you will, challenge what I've been thinking of as the family therapy dogma or the lack of dogma in this area, because both of them are looked on as aberrated.

This led into a discussion about the nature of couple relationships, particularly the forces or actions against or sustaining a long-term relationship.

DON: There was a piece that I read by Helen Fischer, an anthropologist at the American Museum of National History (*The Four Year Itch: Do Divorce Patterns Reflect Our Evolutionary Heritage?*). She believed that there was a natural life cycle to human-paired relationships. The study of many cultures, of the patterns in agrarian cultures, where there was an economic reason to sustain the relationship over a long period of time, showed that they were the only cultures where there were, in fact, sustained, long-term relationships. But in all other cultures, relationships had a very natural cyclical nature based on producing and caring for the young during the early time. She said the 7-year itch is really the 4-year itch, and she pointed out that in many freely moving societies, new relations were formed and new couples were created about every 7 years and that this was the regular pattern. Divorce, in fact, was the common pattern, not the unusual pattern. And then she gives a lot of evolutionary support for this, in addition to this kind of cross-cultural related support. It's an interesting hypothesis, because it would certainly seem to conform to what we see, that is, that the struggle to maintain a long-term relationship in a single dyadic tie is really swimming upstream against enormous biopsychosocial forces, certainly sociobiological forces. But there are obvious other ways to play that, including the notion that one has a long-term primary partner and arranges other partners over the sustained span of that. And that, I think, is pretty much what, frankly, everybody does. It's what goes down, depending upon where you are in your life, whether you're young, old, or what have you. I think the reality is, that's what happens. I'm not asking you about your personal experiences, but I can tell you from what I've observed in this world, that's pretty much how it goes.

BARBARA: You're saying that a monogamous relationship cannot really exist?

DON: In nonagrarian societies specifically, where women are not economically subordinated either to the maintenance of the household or to the power of men. One of the interesting things Fischer describes, for example, is the change in what happened to the Roman marriages in the third century B.C. after Carthage was conquered and marriage became a civil rather than religious ceremony, with women controlling their own dowries. Women suddenly became economically powerful as inherited wealth passed from wealthy fathers to their daughters: If the women decided to divorce, they still retained their wealth. This changed the economic circumstances. The women became the possessors of the wealth, and the divorce rate went sky high because women were then, as they are now, able to "walk." So my point, very simply, is that family therapy does not take into account, first of all, this natural periodicity to human connectedness.

CARLOS: I must say that I agree with this. It fits very well, this sociobiological theory. Because, in our society, the contract of the marriage lasts the life. In fact, it's a very funny contract that never changes. The letter never changes, even though the spirit always changes and the situation is completely evaluated constantly. It doesn't. It is mandated, and the expectation from society is toward the maintenance of the relationship.

DON: The question we're asking is, Why the failure of desire? We don't say to people who come in: Look, for heaven's sake, your desires should have failed. It's gone on 12 years. Seven years is plenty long enough. Certainly, stay married to each other, but let's think about how you guys can get loose enough to get some other partners. How many therapists say that? Nobody says that. You're supposed to have new ideas [and] maybe those are important ideas. But we don't do it because we're not even thinking that way; that is, we're not defining the pathology. We're defining the pathology as either the itch or the failure of desire, but we're not defining it in terms of the fact that people are subordinating themselves to a maladaptive and nonfunctional arrangement, which may be true. I'm not saying it fully is. I really don't know, but it's an interesting question.

Comment: This feels like a very loaded issue, with the men questioning the viability of long-term monogamous relationships and the women responding in a subdued, incredulous manner. There appears to be reluctance among the women to bring out the different relationship and marital experiences of members of the group, namely, that each of the women is in one long-term marital relationship and the men had each experienced divorce and remarriage. The powerful connections between our own intimate and sexual experiences and our public and professional views and behaviors are difficult to surface—B.O.

The issue is indeed "loaded," and it is true that each of the men is in a second marriage; but what to me the men seem to be about is (1) agreeing that withdrawal of sexual interest is widespread in couple relationships and (2) considering explanations for this phenomenon which differ from ones the women, in this session, considered. Carlos is making an evocative point about the naïveté of contracts that "never change." Don is hypothesizing that the loss of sexual interest may be due to "natural periodicity" in human connectedness. I believe that the withdrawal of sexual interest is due to relationship factors.—D.K.

The women in this group were all in long-term first marriages, as Barbara observes. The men were not. What "male" responses, I wonder, would have been elicited from the husbands of the three women, who all remain (it is to be hoped) attracted to and by their original mates? Would they see the inevitable "entropy" in intimate relationships that these three males saw? (I hope not!) I was struck, on reading over this manuscript, with the vision of the woman as "other," as the "mysterious stranger," that was so appealing to the males in our group. What was sexy was what was novel. The "other" is not, in this situation, really known for who she is, and in that sense is not really an intimate—by which I mean an erotic best friend.—M.S.

Therapist Neutrality

In the context of a discussion triggered by Don on how possible the model of the long relationship is and what we are talking about as therapists, members moved into a discussion of neutrality.

DON: Family therapy speaks of a model of maintaining relationships. Is that anywhere near the truth of human circumstances? What are we talking about as therapists?

CARLOS: There are two polar attitudes by family therapists. One is a nomative attitude on the part of the therapist toward maintenance or nonmaintenance. And the other is a position of neutrality in the most literal sense of the term, in which, when we are set up as connected with a couple, we don't take sides, and if we don't take sides, it's ultimately because we don't operate with the assumption that the maintenance of a relationship is better than the nonmaintenance of a relationship.

DAVID: The women say there is no such thing as neutrality, and I agree with them.

PEGGY: The thing about neutrality is that it's been wrongly defined. Neutrality, rather than being nonpositional, is multipositional. You can enter and exit as you need to, and I think it's a much more operative definition of neutrality, particularly for a therapist, than the sort of cold, lofty, nonpositional definition.

BARBARA: So neutrality is more nonjudgmental.

Comment: Some of the discomfort here seems to come from the glaring interface of "theory of use" and "espoused theory." We don't always deal with incongruities between our personal lifestyle and the attitudes we project with clients.—B.O.

I don't read what's going on as "discomfort." It seems more like the excitement of discussing the undiscussable colliding with the constraints of unestablished trust.—D.K.

Periodic Recyclings or Renewal within the Same Long-Lasting Relationship

Comment: As the issue of therapist neutrality leads into a discussion about the possibility or probability of a monogamous long-term relationship, the group focuses on what they perceive to be the realities pertaining to the nature of such relationships.—B.O. and D.K.

DON: Well, you know, the observation that's been made by Carl Whitaker, among others, is that, under the best of circumstances, you're married to the same person many times. And that's, I think, probably relating to your concept, David, of the refreshing nature of the fantasies to rework the relationship with the passage of time. The empty nest is now another developmental marker, and, as such, it opens up a number of other possibilities which can be refreshing and revivifying for your relationship or for other relationships. So that the degree to which you can have a cascade of new dyadic relations with the same person as you move through life is highly desirable. People who can do that are fortunate. But a lot of people can't do that.

CARLOS: It would be interesting in that sense to explore whether in long-lasting relationships there are also those cycles of 4 to 7 years, containing certain rituals or remarriage that occur which allow for the next leg of 4 to 7 years. And at least it fits very well with my own experience, even though I've never been married more than 7 years with the same person.

DAVID: You might buy it this time.

CARLOS: I may buy it this time. I'm ready to do it now.

Commentary: Carlos leaves at this point. His later comments actually occurred in the first part of the taping but appear topically rather than temporally.—B.O.

MAGGIE: Ethel Person has a new book on the subject of romantic passion. She quotes Simmel as saying something to the effect that, in certain fortunate relationships, people merge again—they have this experience that you have during courtship—of merging again, of returning to that experience of high idealization and romance and then moving on. Because obviously nobody wants to be stuck in that kind of glue for huge periods of time.

BARBARA: When Don was talking about entropy being natural in a long-term relationship, I was thinking how I and many of my friends find that sex and intimacy flourishes each year of our marriages, not lessens. The empty nest is liberating, not constraining.

DON: The empty bordello!

The discussion of the cyclical nature of long-term relationships led back into consideration of intimacy and sexuality within the context of long-term relationships.

DAVID: What I say to the people who are dealing with the withdrawal of sexual desire in therapy, if I'm telling them something openly, is to conceive a new sexual fantasy. Usually what I think happens is that when the sexual fantasy runs out in an ongoing relationship, then there is the belief that, in a new relationship, whether it's an affair or a new marriage, that the old or a new sexual fantasy will make actual sex and the sexual experience between the partners better. What I say is they have the option of either going outside the marriage, having a new marriage, or reinventing the sexual fantasy within the marital relationship.

BARBARA: Within the marriage?

DAVID: Within the marriage. So that when I'm helping people to opt to stay in and they're having difficulty with withdrawal of sexual interest, I help them invent a new fantasy. But to succeed, we must deal first with the systemic consequences of the broken mythic contracts.

DON: Well, that's not a bad tactic to take, but the fantasy must be possible or its premise acceptable. Most people have to work very hard at finding a compatible new sexual fantasy. That's an extremely difficult thing to do, and it may or may not be attainable. The usual, much easier, way to do that is to find another partner. It's not easy to tap into another aspect of your sexuality with the same partner, because of all the entropy factors that are in effect and get the relationship stuck. You're really swimming upstream against an enormous entropic wind. What I'm saying, then, is that, in my view, intimacy and sexuality are interestingly opposed to each other. Intimacy builds entropy, it builds familiarity, it builds understanding, it builds sharing, it builds having visited the same thing until finally you know it in enormous detail or aspect. Those are valuable attributes, but they're in opposition to hot sexuality. They work against it.

BARBARA: But does intimacy have to be so constraining? Can't—as we help people to expand their sexual fantasies, can't we help them to broaden intimacy so they get a resurgence of energy in their relationship, which in turn can enhance their sexuality with each other?

DON: Sometimes you can, if there's enough struggle in the relationship. But, sadly, it's the good relationships that, in a sense, fail for this reason. When people are really in pain with each other, where there's some active struggling on each person's part to bring the other one into conformity with a particular set of fantasies, you've got material to work with that frequently can light up. But, of course, the good relationship is not there.

MAGGIE: I don't believe that intimate relationships necessarily run out of steam. If the relationship works, the partners talk, disagree, agree, fight, make up, make love, grow apart, reunite, rediscover each other, can't stand each other, fuse at times, distance at times. Relationships don't just sputter to a halt as a natural and inevitable consequence of long familiarity. To me, trust isn't boring, it's sexy. Intimacy, that is, to be truly known and to know the other, is a human wonder.

PEGGY: I just want to be facetious for a moment and then ask a real question. I actually wrote a screen treatment with Valerie Smith once, called "Flunking out Masters and Johnson," which was just that idea. This couple had to arrange a come-as-you-are party, and the man, of course, wanted to be Superman. But, unfortunately, he didn't take off his socks, so that when he stood on the dresser to sort of fly at her, as it were, he managed to wrench his back just as his parents, at the same moment, knocked on the door. They were visiting, to see how the kids were doing. And the old triangle was intact. Either Ma or Pa would balance the romantic duo, who were having all this trouble being sexy. But it was an attempt to do that same thing, which was to figure out that reinvestment within a comic mode. I was thinking about intimacy. The romantic fantasy has often been described as triangular. And there is a case to be made for tracking all the triangles when someone is having an affair: what it means to the person having the affair, vis-à-vis their system; what it certainly means to the "marriage" vis-à-vis, say, the man's relationship, let's add, to his mother and father, and new sister's husband, and the woman's baby, etcetera. You can really do a very interesting sort of configuration of all of the various triangles in a marital affair, in doing couples therapy.

DON: I'm trying to write a paper now for conference proceedings and the persistent title is "Sexuality, the Dark Side," and, when you think about what that dark side is, it is, of course, the triangular nature, the presence of imagined others or approving, disapproving questions of dating and a whole set of issues that are probably functioning in the system. There is a range in which it's a functional system.

PEGGY: But many times those romantic fantasies are quite dependent on one person sitting still while you have them, while you participate in them.

BARBARA: And that person can't intrude on those fantasies.

PEGGY: And, yes—that person either not knowing or not intruding. The dark side of sex is power. That, too, could be described as triangular.

Talking about triangles led us into the "rule" held by many family therapists that all sexual secrets must be exposed, that therapy cannot be effective without such exposure.

DAVID: There are some therapists who believe that every secret should be exposed and that they won't conduct a therapy unless the secret is exposed.

BARBARA: That certainly has been emphasized by two prominent male therapists—David Scharff, at his recent workshop at Harvard Medical School, and Frank Pittman, in his book *Turning Points*. I wonder if female therapists buy into that.

DAVID: If I'm to believe what Peggy is saying about the function of the triangle maintaining balances, then that view is off. It means that there are times when the therapist who insists on full disclosure always will unbalance relationships that mean to be balanced in the way Peggy was discussing and that's right some of the time or even much of the time. But the point is that some therapists are invariant in their theoretical and clinical views on the subject of secrets. They are in trouble, as far as I am concerned, in those systems that are balanced by larger truths to which the couple subscribe.

DON: The notion that there is such a thing as a clearly defined or unambiguously defined secret is purely a contextual statement. It's really an epistemological error to even talk in those terms. You can create secrets by the flock, you can have them by the thousands, so the notion that you're going to tell the truth is simply a highly politicized and obscure controlling operation.

PEGGY: Is it a way for a clinician to protect him- or herself against an uncomfortable alliance?

DAVID: That's another matter.

BARBARA: The clinician feels disabled in that uncomfortable alliance and may not know how to manage it.

DAVID: That's another matter.

BARBARA: But sometimes therapeutically it's necessary for the therapist to endure the discomfort of being disabled by maintaining a secret, to see if this is something that will correct itself and how it adds to the system. It's playing God to rigidly impose your rules on everyone, to insist on revelation of secrets no matter what.

MAGGIE: I'm not sure I would agree with the suggestion that there is no such thing as a noncontextual secret. I think that calling all secrets "purely contextual" robs them of their true power, which in certain instances is not too ambiguous at all. I do recognize, however, that there are instances in which what is "true" has to do with matters of value and may at times be highly politicized. But I'd maintain that there are such things as real secrets. At the very least, secrets can isolate a person enormously. Their effects are indeed real.

Comment: It's impossible to talk about the therapist role without alluding to the possibility or advisability of neutrality and the person of the therapist! The more emotionally laden and subjective the issue, such as sexuality and intimacy, the more vulnerable are the boundaries between the person of the therapist and the process of therapy.—B.O.

The other point I was alluding to is how knowing one partner's sexual secret disempowers that therapist and limits the effectiveness of the therapeutic process. Therapists sometimes confuse three issues: their need as clinicians to maintain freedom of movement, their personal views on the morality of sexual triangles, and their theories of intimacy. I believe that therapists need to avoid clinical traps, that morality is pluralistic, and that a theory of intimacy must consider the function of triangles in order not to be ignorant of pluralistic determination of adult relationships and naive about the complex nature of sensuality and sexuality. Ultimately, the therapist's view is an ethical one.—D.K.

Differences between Males and Females and between Male and Female Therapists

As the discussion seemed to evoke gendered responses, the participants turned their attention directly to gender issues.

BARBARA: Well, David, we've been talking about couples' issues, and maybe we need to bring it back to male and female therapists. Is it a gender issue? Do we look at these things differently, based on gender? In sexual affairs, for example, in couples? And all the kinds of issues that they bring in, including lack of sexual desire?

DAVID: Let's see. How are you putting the question again?

BARBARA: Do male and female therapists differ in the way they perceive couples' sexual and intimacy issues and also in the way they deal with their own sexual feelings about their clients? Those are really two different questions.

DAVID: And also what they do with men and women in therapy.

PEGGY: That's a huge mountain.

BARBARA: We talked in the women's tape about our absolute outrage when we hear about a client who has been involved sexually with a therapist. I don't even think we specified female client, male therapist, although that certainly happens more commonly than the other. And one of the questions we raised was, do male therapists have the same reaction when they hear that as women therapists do?

DAVID: I don't have anything like the violent reaction you women had on the subject. I don't approve of it. I've dealt with it a fair number of times in therapy, just recently quite strikingly, actually—15 years of rank sexual exploitation of a female patient by a male psychiatrist.

PEGGY: They had sex?

DAVID: Sex every session.

BARBARA (*wryly*): That's a long-term therapy.

DON: I want to know whether or not she paid.

DAVID: She paid. And the therapist also had the woman and her husband in couples therapy and maintained the relationship while seeing her alone in individual therapy.

DON: Well, talk about your triangular fantasies.

PEGGY: That's incredible!

DAVID: But then, let me be forthright about my visceral reactions. Viscerally, I'm "sort of" outraged, but I'm more theoretically outraged—I mean, outraged on an ethical more than a personal level. As pure fantasy, it doesn't seem like a shocking or strikingly terrible thing. As stark reality, it does.

PEGGY: Well, I am personally outraged. And I tell you, it's more than outrage. One person is in a dominant position in relation to another person and takes advantage of it. It's a terrible misuse . . .

BARBARA: It violates trust, and it's an abuse of power.

PEGGY: . . . terrible misuse of power. And it confuses what's reality, how real this intimacy is, etcetera. It's terrible to fuck around with somebody's head like that.

DAVID: You see . . . I don't disagree . . . I can never imagine my-self . . .

PEGGY: He should be drawn and quartered.

DAVID: The question came up in the couples therapy I'm doing with the couple now. The woman told her husband, after coming in for a half hour before the regular session on request. She was coming to prepare herself for telling him. She knew my rule about certain kinds of secrets that disable therapists, which I just won't have any part of when I am on top of things. In a later session, her husband was asking me what the ethics are here and was I required to do something about it. The therapist is a fairly well-known local psychiatrist who has been around for a very long time and is still practicing. The sexual violations stopped 4 or 5 years ago. But the couple has had miserable sex since the wife and her therapist stopped. I'm not claiming that the wife's loss of sexual desire and the stopping of sex with her therapist are related, but here's your triangle.

Comment: Here, the psychiatrist seemed to be a parent figure for the wife, a loving "Daddy." I'm not surprised that the couple is having a lot of difficulty dealing with this "intergenerational" violation of a professional trust. This is downright abuse, of course, on the part of a very narcissistic clinician. And the married partners are paying a very heavy price for the wife's "therapy."—M.S.

PEGGY: Without that other relationship, the "frame," they can't do it.

DAVID: She can't, as it turns out.

DON: You know—I mean—I basically share that view of outrage, but I think I'm a lot closer to David. I think the outrage needs thinking about. And I've a couple of different takes on it. One is that the only study that I've read where a number of psychiatrists who have had sex with their patients were interviewed was interesting because it showed that each of them was at some point of crisis in their own lives, that is, they were failing in some way. The study was done more than 15 years ago and was nicely systemic, even though I don't think they even knew the word *system*. What they did was take it case by case, and the psychiatrist either had a health problem or a career problem, or some failure in his own personal life or in his marriage, or something of that sort. The second thing is that that kind of hot judgmental stuff is not useful. It's like the same attitude toward incest or sexual abuse of children. Obviously, I agree with you—you have to be a maniac not to—but there is a way in which they are so easily turned to bad account, they so easily become the food for the antisexualists, for the repressors, for the people who use that outrage to wipe out any measure of the awareness of the legitimate and highly important sexual ties between adults and children. I think that sexual attraction between parent and child of the same sex, opposite sex, particularly the opposite sex, is an absolutely essential developmental feature. I think in a similar way that something of a sexual awareness and a sexual tie to a patient is also often there.

PEGGY: I am hotly judgmental and not confused about the difference between a sexually exploitative therapy and normal sexual attractions in families that are appropriate. They are NOT the same.

DON: But then once you open the door to be so judgmental about it, it seems to me that the door is slammed shut. It really speaks for the fact that all this is like a really horrible thing, horrible. Sure, you shouldn't do it, and if you do it, you may go on with a happy, healthy life afterwards, and everybody may survive. And I've known lots of cases like that. So I think you guys [*the women*] came down too hard. I read that piece of the womens' transcript, and I think you came down much too hard on that, and I thought it was really a very genderized political move.

PEGGY: Very genderized. It is hot. But I also feel there are ways built into the therapeutic situation to deal with a therapist's crisis and sexual attraction to a patient, without its getting out of control. There are ways to deal with that sexual attraction without acting out on it.

Comment: The women therapists are clearly more outraged when they hear about a client who has been sexually involved with a therapist, and their pain is revealed more on the tape than in the transcript. I am anxious to keep the record straight. Although my phumphering there seems clumsy at best, I did not exercise the right that all participants had to edit embarrassing, censurable, or incomplete representations, because I feel so strongly that sexual abuses will occur less often in therapy when therapists acknowledge that they have real feelings and fantasies and are given opportunities to share these with peers. My outrage was less personal than that of the women because I couldn't identify with the women's sense of bodily outrage as they did, not because I identified with the man. It seemed right that the women were more outraged. In another case I've dealt with indirectly, a male psychoanalyst sexually engaged his male patient over an 8-year period. I was less outraged here than with my woman client, not because I have homosexual leanings, but because of my chauvinistic inclination to protect women.—D.K.

We women react with incredulity to the men's statements. In later discussion among us, we processed our disappointment that we did not forcefully coalesce to rebut the men's assertions. I know that I personally felt my emotionalism would prevent me from being heard or being logical, a not uncommon feeling for women in disagreement with dominant cultures. I cannot imagine any situation where sexual engagement between a therapist and client, an adult and child, a teacher and student, to name a few, is not sexually exploitative and an abuse of power and trust. I have treated so many women who have engaged both willingly and unwillingly in these relationships and find the effects to be pervasive and destructive on many levels.—B.O.

If these clinicians had started shoplifting or embezzling because they were at a point of crisis in their lives, would we find their behavior excusable or understandable? Or would we believe that their deeds merited societal compensation of some kind? It is my belief that "attraction" and "acting out" exist in vastly different moral realms.—M.S.

DAVID: Let me say how I come at it a little bit differently from Don, though essentially we're on the same political platform, I think. Because I have been training therapists for so long, I have seen so many subtle crimes in therapy that go unnoticed. For example, if I refer a couple that's on the edge of a separation to one particular therapist, that couple is going to separate. If I send a depressive to another therapist I know very well, well known in the field, then that person is more likely to attempt suicide, than if the client goes to someone else. I've been watching for many years the kinds of decisions people in therapy make about their lives, through the influence of therapeutic interventions that alter the "structures" without scratching the surface of meaning that clients invest in those structures. Very close observation of what therapists are doing, quite apart from what they officially say they are doing, frequently reveals subtly coercive pressures on clients that are insidious because they go unnoticed. I am very much concerned about such hidden intrusions, because they are not as dramatic as literal sexual tyrannies, but they either go unnoticed or they are accepted without alarm as part of therapeutic realities. I agree with Don: If the heat of moral indignation drives healthy "sexuality" out of therapy from a fear of the witches' broom, we lose the perspective Don is calling for. I would only add that raising the temperature of moral indignation about these other therapeutic indiscretions might help put the whole subject of dangerous therapist influence in sharper perspective.

BARBARA: Bravo, David. The therapeutic guild does collude and conspire to cover up and hide the crimes.

DAVID: One of the reasons I'm so interested in opening these questions up is that I don't think the field is opening them up. We're training people, and we have no idea where they are in their sexual development. We send therapists out to deal with complex sexual realities without helping them to know when or whether or how their own sexual realities are creeping into their work.

BARBARA: Exactly. I am terribly concerned about the harm that results from these "therapeutic" crimes to clients. Many of them occur without therapist awareness, and there is no mechanism of check and balance built into the therapeutic system, particularly after training is completed, if it is indeed ever completed. Too many therapists deny their own relationship issues and can only relate from a controlling, powerful professional stance.

DON: Not only that, David, but even to inquire into that is a no-no at this point. In other words, the whole obliteration of any interest in the person of the therapist is, you know, almost complete—just a few vestigial cells rest here and there.

PEGGY: We don't even ask the people to have experienced therapy themselves. We don't really ask that.

DAVID: We don't ask a lot of questions.

BARBARA: We make a lot of assumptions, and we don't check people's blind spots. There are all kinds of blind spots.

PEGGY: But we accept it all in good will and with no investigation. We're hoping that our hunches will prove right in training selections, and they all . . .

BARBARA: And there's the whole economic aspect, too. We all need trainees, right? So let's be honest. We need to fill this training group, and then once you get somebody in, it's very difficult to get them out, to screen them out. Everybody says, oh well, we'll have loose admissions policies and we'll screen people out, and I can tell you that that doesn't work, either. You know that, because you just can't.

MAGGIE: Well, you know, in a sense I'm sorry about what you've all been saying, and it puzzles me a little. I think that there's never been a successful prosecution of a faculty member for abuse of that privileged *in loco parentis* role. But there have been prosecutions of psychiatrists. So the capacity for screening therapeutic abuses is actually there.

DON: I am sorry to say I've been an expert witness against a psychiatrist in a case of that sort. And this was a most peculiar man whose distinctive feature was that he never gave the women any pleasure. What he did was to have them perform elaborate acts upon him, but he never did anything for them at all.

MAGGIE (*jokingly*): Well, what was the crime, Don?

DON: That was the crime—malpractice.

MAGGIE: But it seems to me that I can think of a dozen situations where a therapist could collude with a very difficult situation by assuming a neutral position, vis-à-vis that situation. Now maybe what came out on the women's transcript was too much passion for you males along this line. But when I think of what Peggy suggested [on the tape], the case of a father who is seducing each daughter as she comes of age, and I think of that family coming into therapy, I think that the therapist is indeed placed in a very awkward position. I mean, should the therapist intervene to get the three next girls out of the house? You know—where's the point at which you take a stand and intervene?

DON: I think we're clear on that. I don't think that there's any dispute.

MAGGIE: But you've already objected to people coming down in an antisexual manner.

DON: But there are numerous prosecutions for fondling. Divorce laws now include charges of sexual abuse. They may include, sadly, the kinds of things that might involve normal affectionate caressing and physical touch. I mean, I'll go on record—I haven't got a child whose fanny I haven't patted with great enjoyment.

BARBARA: But I think that's different.

DON: I agree it's different. I'm not suggesting it's the same thing . . .

BARBARA: We were talking about the cases where there is overt sexual acting out, not just the innuendoes. Although, in a therapy situation, I think it's a lot different than the parent who pats the kid's bottom or who's feeling turned on to them—everybody's turned on to their kids. It's not the feeling that's the problem, but acting out inappropriately on the feelings.

DON: Okay, well, let's see what it is we're talking about. I mean, clearly there's a line where the fantasy turns into an act or where the casual action turns into a serious one. And we all agree about that. I guess we'd want to monitor it. I think what we're perhaps disagreeing about is the permeability of that line or the degree to which it's a jagged line as opposed to a rather sharply and clearly drawn one. I think David and I, maybe from a male view, are a bit more inclined to see the line as having a wavy or jagged quality and be semipermeable. I mean, I do know therapists who have had sex with a patient. And, you know, that seems to be an isolated incident. If, in that particular case I'm thinking of, it had really gone on to some kind of a major confrontation, I think it would have been harmful to everybody.

Comment: Once is okay? Or what?—M.S.

BARBARA: Well, maybe what was happening with the women when we made our tape was what Maggie termed a gender flash. I mean, we were really all reacting in a gender identification with the victim, the female victim of this, and it sounds like, when you're saying yes, it's wrong, but you have compassion and let's not overreact to it with such passion, you're having a gender flash with the male perpetrator. But I'm still outraged when I think about it, whether or not it's an isolated act or a therapist's crisis. I can't imagine a situation when it could be in the patient's best interests.

DON: Well, I also know, for example, of a woman therapist situation . . .

BARBARA: There are those cases.

DON: And where in many, many respects, it looked quite exploitative, not just sexually but otherwise.

MAGGIE: But that doesn't change the situation. We're still talking about the same situation. And, you know, if we thought that every father, say, who was having a career crisis or having a problem, decided that maybe he'd have intercourse with his 15-year-old daughter until the problem worked out—I mean, that doesn't excuse it. I'm sure that we can all find reasons for the scuzzy things we've done in our lives, but that is a real breaching of a boundary that is very serious.

DON: I'm totally in agreement with you, so I want . . .

BARBARA: But I think what's important that you raised—that both of you raised—is the importance of the person of the therapist. It's like David said, there are certain people who, whether they're aware of it or not, helped the couple get divorced because that's a reflection of some of the issues that they're going through now.

DON: I think David's absolutely right about that.

BARBARA: That's right, and how do we deal with that?

DON: People selling divorce, who are selling some version of that for reasons which entirely . . .

BARBARA: Or selling affairs, giving permission, colluding—and it may not be a conscious collusion on the part of the therapist.

MAGGIE: That's true, I've seen that happen.

DAVID: The person I was thinking of is someone who, in his bones, does not have confidence in a long-term relationship. He just doesn't believe it's possible.

BARBARA: You mean the therapist doesn't believe it's possible, and so his beliefs contaminate the therapy?

DAVID: Yes.

Comment: A later segment of the tape returns to the issues about gender differences in family therapy. We are talking about several very sensitive subjects at once: our different personal reactions to sexual abuses in therapy; the blurriness of lines on what is abuse and what is not abuse; confusion and concern about what ought and what ought not be called abuse; therapist influences on therapy outcomes such as divorce, affairs, and even suicide; legal and moral liability of therapists when it is clear that sexual rules have been violated, as well as the need for guidelines when the rules themselves are not clear or when definitions are and perhaps should remain unclear; and the field's negligence in the screening and preparation of therapists for informed judgment and the use of self in sexual domains.—B.O. and D.K.

The discussion (God knows it is a grim failure as true conversation) is not very fruitful. In its clumsy way it nicely defines parameters. Without question, gender differences divide the group.—D.K.

I see the "clumsiness" emanating from prevailing male-defined assumptions and models of sexuality, sexual abuse, morality, therapy, and so forth. Until those assumptions are examined and reformulated by both males and females, no "true conversation" can occur. The women understand clearly what the men are saying, having been raised in a male-dominant culture; but the men do not seem to want to question their basic dominant-culture assumptions.—B.O.

BARBARA: Don, do you think that there are implications for differences about the way male and female therapists would deal with sexuality with couples?

DON: I think that this is not appreciated enough. First of all, I think we all agree with David's belief that there is very little good, useful talk about people's sexuality in family therapy. I don't mean that nobody talks about it, but that there's much too little. We don't teach much about it and, if you look at our students, they are not helped in any way to talk much about it. But then, within this, I do think there's a gendered response. I think that women are much more appreciative of this aspect and men tend to blend it out or blur it out or not notice it. What do you say, David? I think there really is a gendered awareness about this.

DAVID: Oh, yes, I think there's a very serious problem for therapy. I think you're talking about women's images and not about men's images. When I deal with men and women in therapy, I no longer try to get men to buy into women's images, because I don't think it works. There is a couple. To ask the man to sacrifice the image that's guiding his behavior in this relationship, his sexual behavior, and to call it wrong may imperil the relationship. What we want to do is to open up an interchange in which his imagery about sexuality is valued as much as hers, so that they can negotiate the interchange, not to ask the men to be what the women want them to be. It doesn't work.

MAGGIE: But if you get into the cycle of, You did something lovely for me, so I'll do something lovely for you, it's a lot different from the male image, which says, Do it this way, my way; I'm the guy in charge. She often goes away from the sexual encounter angry, doesn't want it next time. While, in the other cycle, you are really always thinking in terms of who's patting who on the back and what's going to happen next. Now, how about the male in the you-pat-my-back-I'll-pat-yours interchange? Let's say he gets into the position where the woman is doing a lot of stroking and caressing of him. That's not a Rambo posture, but it might be an awful lot of fun for him, even though it doesn't correspond to the male-dominant (or "sexually dominant") image he might have.

Comment: Reciprocity, yes, but in the feminine vogue. I'm not endorsing a "do it my way" model; I'm saying that women are more aware and men should catch up, know what they want, and then emerge in discourse.— D.K.

BARBARA: You're talking about opening up possibilities for both men and women.

MAGGIE: It might open up a different side for him. I don't mean to sound as if I think that female images are the only images in town. But I do think that, as people grow sexually, we try each other's roles and try to move around in places. He gets more, not less, by playing along with that image.

BARBARA: They both get more, don't they, if we're "opening it up" and broadening and exchanging the images?

DON: What's implicit in David's comment is that, by accepting the fact that you're not going to align the fantasies, maybe you have to construct something fairly elaborate that will accommodate them both.

DAVID: Absolutely.

DON: Then there is a built-in tension. To the degree that a dominance–submission fantasy is a shared fantasy—a no-no-no as you yes-yes-yes; well I'm going to make you while I'm going along with your wishes; I'm going to touch that part of you that can't say no—to that degree you're dealing with an enormously complex set of matching and presumably fitted or complementary fantasies. But, if those fantasies stray or get out of alignment, which they do all the time, they include breakdown in one form or another or spill over into violence, rape, or various kinds of sadomaso-chistic things. We're choosing the particular path we propose to thread through all of those dangers. But it's a goddamn narrow path. It's a sort of accommodative ethic—you rub my back, and I'll rub yours, but part of my rubbing your back is spanking you, or . . .

MAGGIE: Obviously when you go into sex, you go into certain regressive fantasies. Whether or not this could spill over into dominance-submission or spanking, I don't know. But I'd view the "treasured child" fantasy as very different from the "beaten child." In any case, what I'm really saying here is that this vision of a good lover that most women have is of the slow and gentle and related lover (and, interestingly, lesbian relationships are like that, while male homosexual relationships are usually not). I think that when men try the sense of relatedness, they can discover aspects of themselves that they're often too anxious or defensive to discover while they're into the Rambo number. I'm not saying that men and women aren't different. I believe that we are very different, but I'm not sure that this is a necessary difference in our sexual relating.

Discussion of gender differences led us into a discussion about the ideal of androgyny.

PEGGY: My original question was, if the sexual revolution means that women are moving toward independent stances and are less interested in connection, and men are moving more toward dependence and more connection, what will happen to the nature of romantic love?

DON: It's a fascinating question.

PEGGY: Yes, and how will that change, since historically the man has been more the pursuer unless, as Confucius says, man chases woman until she catches him? It seems to me that that's only true up to a point, that what Maggie was saying before about the feedback loop that can be created between men and women where men participate in a different kind of sexuality only to discover that it's as pleasant as whatever the sexuality was that they participated in before. Androgyny is true up to a point, as everything is. I don't think there is a basic way to redefine differences, nor do I want to.

MAGGIE: Do you know how I would see the difference, if I were to make a quick and dirty summary? It would be that, indeed, men and women are both interested in connection and both interested in mastery and control; however, if we were to layer those, I think that women set more store by these relationships.

PEGGY: Without sacrificing the mastery. But androgyny is your word. My word—mine might be just equality.

DON: No, it's a big difference.

DAVID: It's a very big difference.

DON: Equality is a matter of judging things to be of equal worth, but they could be quite different.

BARBARA: Androgyny means that males have the capacity for attachment in relationship, for the relational skills that are gender specific for females; and that females have the capacity for mastery and achievement, gender specific for males.

MAGGIE: Women will sometimes sacrifice the mastery, in fact, in favor of maintaining a relationship. In fact, they will often do it, and men are not totally uninterested in intimate connections at all. But, in fact, for men, mastery and control are layered above intimacy. Men and women are marching to somewhat different music. If you ask me, the notes are the same, but the way they're being played out is, in fact, where the difference is.

Comment: Not true. Women must listen to men and how they achieve intimacy.—D.K.

Perhaps men and women need to listen to each other and become aware of the different meanings and definitions of intimacy and eroticism, to expand opportunities and experiences for both without the intrinsic power struggle of a win–lose battle.—B.O.

Is the suggestion made in this segment that if women listened to men—truly understood the ways in which men seek intimacy—then the inevitable waning of desire in long relationships would NOT occur, that Ulysses would not sail off in search of adventure and novelty, that is, to the other women on the strange islands out there? Or is the idea that women MUST understand the male need for novelty and not respond with bitterness to what is inevitable anyway? This isn't quite clear to me.—M.S.

MAGGIE: When I was doing my depression book and watched and talked to women to find out what the depression is about, I found as depression researcher Myrna Weissman has said, that when you get above the top level, it's relational. That's really what it always is. And if I looked on the wards at the men who were hospitalized with depression, usually they were older and it tended to be a career issue.

BARBARA: So it's loss of identity, whether it's through a relationship or through a career.

Comment: This reminds me of Don's excusing male therapists' sexual acting out with clients on the basis of their career or life traumas and not attending to the meaning relationally for the woman. There is a striking gender difference in our basic constructs and concepts.—B.O.

On this point, we come to a place of promise, but also to a place of danger. Danger because, conversationally speaking, we do not stand on firm ground yet. We can retreat to our military-like encampments and waste our strength on gendercidal verbal war, or remain "at the table" for further dialogue. In my opinion, we are on the verge of learning something vitally important about gender-different responses to one of the hottest subjects of all. Had time not run out, had we, in the time we had, trusted more, we would have learned something new. The faint outlines are there—"gender flash"; "body identity"; the surprising scope of "clinical injustices" that go beyond the heinous ones; and, as in Barbara's and my very different sightings on what Don and I were saying, "gender screens." These are promising beginnings for new understandings. But, time did run out. Having followed the rules, we risked, and find ourselves exposed. If, in 9 hours, we got no further than we did, what can we expect of our readers? Should we censor, as is our privilege?—D.K.

MAGGIE: What's the basic sense of self? Where have you really failed? Not that I don't think there's a biological component to this—the development of a clinical depression, I mean. Not everybody will get depressed if they flop out on a relationship or on a career.

DON: We need to consider the hard-wired issues, things that are related to basic neurological organization. There are differences, therefore, in the kind of responsiveness.

MAGGIE: Yes, the whole ethological argument about mastery for males and connectedness for females can be made in a very elegant fashion. How that plays out now, as we go home to our separate lives and our separate bedrooms, is what we're really struggling with here.

DON: How do you evaluate Eric Erikson's work? Peggy worked on this in terms of child development. What about the gender differences of children, the kinds of buildings they construct?

PEGGY: Eric Erikson really felt that there was a biological difference in terms of spatial understanding and expression between boys and girls. If you had a penis, you were likely to build towers, and, if you had a vagina, you were likely to build gates and doorways and enclosures. And, by God, you know, maybe it's because that's what we were looking for, but it seemed we saw, counted that.

DON: What do you think about it now?

PEGGY: Now I think that probably, yes, there are biological differences and men still may be more spatially expressive in terms of verticality and women of enclosure. But I think that there are so many different educative norms toward being a boy and being a girl. Now—I mean, little boys are allowed to knit now and have a doll, if they want it, at last. And little girls are allowed to play fireman or firewoman or fireperson, or whatever—garbagewoman . . .

DON: Firefighter, mail deliverer.

As our group continued to struggle with biological and cultural differences, we reached the end of our time together. The best summary came from Peggy, in response to David's query about where we should go from this point.

PEGGY: Well, Helen Singer Kaplan and Masters and Johnson have provided a wonderful answer to Freud's definition of male infantile sexuality. They are the proponents, the teachers of how to solve problematic sexual events in terms of the low-slow method. All of the sensate foci exercises, all the getting to know each other is much more in the female genre than in the male. If you send somebody for sex therapy to a sexual clinic, it's a female genre. Even Charlie Fisher, who does all the REM studies on erections, tried to do the same study on women, and he put the electrodes on the woman right inside the vagina, in order to see if they had the same kind of arousal from REM sleep as males did. And he said it was impossible to calculate. When he did the interviews before and after, he found that sexual responsiveness is contextualized for women. There was obviously a biological difference!

Comment: The gendered differences in defining terms and in values or ideals about relationships, intimacy, and sexuality have enormous implications for the ways that therapists assess, interact with and treat clients. If we could get beyond the reactive politicization that Don refers to, we could really learn about these differences together and be clearer about their impact on our personal and professional functioning. I agree with David that we don't need agreement but can agree to disagree and respect variant positions.—B.O.

THE PROCESS OF DIALOGUING

We have two objectives in this section. One is to provide excerpts and comments about the experience of these three taped conversations and the second is to excerpt segments illustrating the actual group process.

Comment: The women perceived that the women's tape was the most harmonious of the three tapes; that a trusting, open climate was set for relaxed interchange. They experienced support as well as permission to agree or disagree. They found the men's tape to be more frivolous, and the women felt that they deferred to the men in the joint tape and were covertly subject to the men's rules. The men do not necessarily agree with this, although, when you see the tape, it is more evident than when you read the transcript. Most of the members agree that David tried the hardest to create an intimate environment and that the women seemed more cautious and the men more incautious about revelation. This tendency seemed more protective of others than guarded about self, a distinction of interest that very probably is gender based. It seems that, in the intergender dialogue, there is a question as to who more often initiated new directions.—B.O.

It seems to me that the men, who knew on another well, discussed touchy issues more openly when they met without the women. They expressed doubt then as to whether discussion could be expanded and deepened in the cross-gender meeting, due to the lack of trust and intimacy among all the members of the group.—D.K.

DAVID: I think that the first thing to do is to set the agenda we want to follow in the next couple of hours. We may have different ideas about what we want to do this afternoon. I want to say what I want to do, and then you can react to it and modify it. I think we should choose the hottest issues that we have from the two tapes. What I think the issues ought to be about is their capacity to call into play different gender voices; that is, men should feel differently about the issue than the women do. If we agree with one another too much, I don't think we're going to have too much fun.

Comment: David is trying to set the rules for the gender conversation.— B.O. and D.K.

DON: David, when I do something like this, I have to have the end product more firmly in mind. We're building a chapter in a book?

DAVID: Yes, and I think it's going to be a substantial chapter.

DON: What is the book?

DAVID: We are trying to enlist mainly family therapist people who would be willing to extend their thinking into the whole question of intimacy and sex and sexuality and gender in family therapy—to be talking about these matters in families, rather than the culture.

BARBARA: And in the practice and the process of family therapy.

Comment: Don is trying to define the terrain and its product. An interesting example of how the group process operated appeared during the initial agenda setting.—B.O. and D.K.

DON: I started to read through the transcripts of the men's and women's tapes and found some common areas of . . . I guess concern would be a good word, of interest.

DAVID: We started it. This is one of them.

Comment: David is referring to the discussion of cultural myths underlying withdrawal of sexual interest.—B.O.

BARBARA: Yes, well, we sort of started on how we would explain or what we think about the lack of sexual desire in couples. So David presented his three contracts and the women had said they thought, in their transcript, that a lot of the lack of sexual desire has to do with the social pressures on both men and women, particularly the impact of liberation on women and the impact of liberation on men, the fact that roles and expectations have really changed and, perhaps, not been so liberating in their trade-offs.

Comment: There was some sharp division around the issue of family therapy's removing sexuality from consideration and Nate Ackerman's role as a proponent of sexuality.—B.O. and D.K.

DAVID: I wanted to ask Peggy something, though. How many of the leading figures in family therapy—the people who are writing the theory that guide what most of our therapists think they're doing—would know what you're talking about when you refer to the importance of intimacy and sexuality?

PEGGY: One school would say that people look at sexuality only developmentally. I thought about Don's remark on the men's tape about how many pioneer family therapists sanitized family therapy—dipped it in an acid bath and took out all the dark grain of sexuality by throwing out so much of psychoanalysis, rather than critiquing it. Perhaps it was somewhere at that juncture that we forfeited our own claim on a theory of sex.

DAVID: We lost the sex.

PEGGY: And it would have been a very interesting challenge to have struggled with that tradition and looked at it very differently. Instead, family therapy organized around communication theory and boundaries and hierarchy. And so we all assumed, as long as the hierarchy was intact, the sexuality was supposed to flow. That must have been the idea.

BARBARA: It didn't work. When you get finished restructuring and reorganizing the system, there may still be intimacy and sexual difficulties!

DON: You wouldn't remember this, but I have a personal memory of the enormous antipathy Jay Haley had for Nate Ackerman.

PEGGY: Oh, I do remember. I mean, I don't remember, but I heard it.

DON: Ackerman was extremely interested in the place of sexuality in the family. Forbidden sexuality, permitted sexuality, and how to work with that therapeutically. And that all just became moves on a chessboard.

CARLOS: But he was interested in the sense that he was operating with disturbed families.

DON: I think he was personally interested. I mean, he was personally interested and that's how it happened that he did that kind of work. But I think it's another aspect of this that is the degree to which a personal predilection influences one's theory and practice.

CARLOS: Well, did he use that content for any kind of therapeutic move? He would use it for content, for exchanges.

MAGGIE: There's actually a discussion in this book, *Object Relations Family Therapy* by the Scharffs, about an Ackerman tape where he moved very fast on a family and the Scharffs felt that it had caused certain problems. But I've seen his tapes and, in fact, he does move into these issues with great rapidity. He's certainly on them, and I'm not sure . . . not too rapidly, at least in some things I've seen . . .

CARLOS: Well, he was talking about it. That was the main semantic field. But what interventions around that? It was my impression that he was a very skilled structural intervener, and a good part of his moves can be described in those terms and not in terms of the effect of interpretation or of making the explicit implicit, or whatever—or the mystifying, or whatever family myths may have been in terms of sexuality. In which case, the fact that he talked about it didn't make it more interesting, or it may have made him more interesting in the naughty sense, but not in the therapeutic sense.

DON: I think it's not hard to think of any therapeutic structural language.

CARLOS: I'm defending the . . .

DON: In other words, it's another language.

Comment: There are many segments of the transcript where one gender is trying to convince the other gender that there is one view. Competition to be right ensues, as well as the implication that there is something wrong in disagreement. The interaction stalls somewhat, but not, I submit, because we are impaired individuals, but because we were not an intimate group.—D.K.

I think that there were some double messages in the group. On the one hand, we were instructed by David to be open and revealing, to amplify our differences, but when the women interjected differences, they were not heard. The rule was "Be authentic and disagree, but don't disagree." In order for across-gender group to be intimate and have the type of conversation David desires, I think that there needs to be true egalitarianism among members and that members cannot work for one another, have been trained or treated by one another, or have any type of previous acknowledged or unacknowledged dominant-subordinate relationship.—B.O.

PEGGY: But Carlos was pointing out a difference between the sexual fantasies, which was that one set was more interactive than the other set, in that it depended on response. Women tend to be very responsive to the response they generate in men.

BARBARA: Women resonate to the relationship context.

DON: I'm not so sure that there's much male-female difference.

Comment: Or another example of the process of gender difference.—B.O. and D.K.

PEGGY: I'm looking for disagreements about women being responsive to responses they get from men.

DON: I really don't think it's gender as much as you do.

CARLOS: I agree with you.

DON: It's part of the common mythology that the female is presumably just objectified.

PEGGY: No, I wasn't saying it clearly enough. I don't think that women go out on the "make" as much. A man can go to a party and think, "that one"—and really I don't think women do that as much.

DON: And you know what I've seen? I've seen, just as they were doing that, there was a little flicker of "that one" that let them know . . .

PEGGY: Well, we're not going to get very far in terms of our research here.

Comment: Another example of the gender difference process.—B.O. and D.K.

DON: What's really troubling me a lot is that we're agreeing much too much. And that's not true gender lines, so what are we going to do here?

BARBARA: Maybe that says something, though.

MAGGIE: We disagreed about the incest thing; come on!

Comment: Note how this does not get picked up by anyone. It's too loaded an issue, one that will reappear in the next section of this chapter.—B.O.

PEGGY: I wonder if females and males get along better as family therapists when they're actually somehow tied by a model or some ideas about therapy that they share.

DON: Maybe we're being seized by entropy.

BARBARA: Maybe what we think are gender differences are a lot of differences at certain points in one's life stage. Maybe things aren't as simple as solely gender differences.

QUESTIONS AND ISSUES

In this section, we will try to summarize the persistent questions and issues that emerged from the more than 9 hours of dialogue taping. While the process may have evoked more guardedness than anticipated, the very fact that six people attempted to address and discuss issues of gender, intimacy, sex, and sexuality in families and family therapy is noteworthy in itself. The disagreements support our contention that there is much to be learned and thought about in these areas.

One of the critical questions raised by Peggy concerned what a family therapy theory of sexuality and intimacy would be, what it would have to include? Peggy contended that it certainly would have to address gendered issues:

PEGGY: I think that some of the more interesting questions that family therapists, who have an ear to the gender ground, are asking are questions like, What was it like to grow up as a male in your family? And was that similar to other males in your family? And how does that fit this family of males? And their differences in the wider world of males? And what kind of anticipations do you therefore have toward females? I think that the kinds of questions that the notice of gender is eliciting in the treatment situation are very important.

DON: There's something about the discussion of gender and the politicization of gender that has effectively blocked out meaningful and useful discussion of those questions. The reason for that, in my view, is that those political discussions of gender have always tended toward the equivalence of sameness with equal rights, power, and the ethical position. What that's done is to obliterate any kind of meaningful discussion of the differences between males and females, and it has tended to obliterate the central question, which, in my view, is the question of mate selection. . . . Our awareness of gender has also hindered us. And that, plus the other source of a kind of antisexualism that we were talking about earlier, the lack of interest in psychodynamics of the individual—those have really made it very hard for us to pay attention. . . . I think this makes us rediscover some of those roots of family therapy, but it's not fashionable to speak about the differences between male and female sexualization as being something valuable and necessary for the new family formation. Androgyny is the banner we're all supposed to sail under. Well, I don't believe it.

DAVID: Nor do I.

DON: It's the banner in the American family therapy field. Androgyny is the aspiration that family therapists have.

These segments highlight the question underlying this meeting: If family therapy has ignored or minimized attention to intimacy and sexuality, is it because of a strong cultural undercurrent of antisexualism? Is it because of a lack of interest in individual dynamics, including individual sexual and gender identity and sexual dynamics between parents and children? Have the meaning and richness of individuals been lost to a fascination with the structures and organization of the system? In other words, have some schools of family therapy, in reacting to psychoanalysis, lost awareness of intimacy and sexuality issues? We all agreed that our clinical experience confirms that, if boundaries and hierarchies are intact, sexuality does not just automatically flow! And what about the notion of androgyny? Do women therapists espouse that as an ideal more so than males?

PEGGY: It is important for family therapists to understand the complicity between sexual constructs and premises around intimacy. They are extremely complex and very interconnected.

We asked the group if they think family therapists are prepared to deal with this complexity. Does it matter if they are not prepared? Does family therapy's technology protect therapists who remain innocently uninformed about adult sexual complexity? The question was raised as to how many of the leading family therapists, the people who are writing the theory, would agree that what we are talking about is vital? Our conclusion was that it would depend on which of the different schools was responding. One school would say that these issues about gender, intimacy, and sexuality are too content-oriented or subjective, whereas another would look at these issues only developmentally. Our question then became, Can this omission continue when we might be falling out of step with what our increasingly sophisticated clients are asking for? The group talked about varying groups of clients, referring to working-class clients versus those from the middle and upper classes. We referred to two different studies turning into two truths about whether the basic desires and expectations differ or just appear to differ. It became clear that the evidence of class differences in these areas is inconclusive and that much of our thinking is based on incomplete stereotypic impressions.

One of the most productive interchanges that occurred emerged from a heated discussion of gendered responses to therapist–client sexual involvements. The women were unequivocally outraged, and this was viewed by the men as being overly reactive. The men considered themselves to be more open and reasonable, and the women found the male responses unacceptable. It is apparent that more extensive dialogue among a wider spectrum of male and female therapists about this particular issue is necessary, despite the intense degree of discomfort for both genders. However, as the focus shifted to selection and training of therapists, it became clear that the sexual development and identity of therapists must be considered and addressed in a systematic way. For, in fact, the personal views of the therapist relate to the types and formats of therapist "rules" and influences that occur in actual therapy, which may differ from the therapist's official or public position and posture. The notion of therapist neutrality comes in for examination and needs to be studied in greater depth. Is there such a construct? Is it possible? Should we strive to defend the notion of neutrality? Under what circumstances do we substitute another construct? Should we invent a new concept?

How do the suggested gendered differences about definitions of intimacy, erotic sex, and requirements for arousal affect couples therapy? One question that emerged from this discussion relates to the ideal or possibility of long-term relationships. Is there an assumption by men and/or women that women are committed and monogamous in long-term relationships, while men tend not to be? If some males and some females have this assumption, does it mean that most do? Obviously, attitudes of liberation combined with realities of the greater economic independence of women are major contributing factors to changing relationship mores. How do these changes affect family and couples therapy? How do the assumptions of one particular therapist impact a couple differently from what their experience might be in someone else's office? Is it just the "luck of the draw"? Are there gender differences in the way women and men look at affairs and other issues couples bring into therapy, including their loss of sexual interest or desire? Do we line up differently in the couple's politics when the woman has pulled out sexually? When the man has pulled out? If we've had an affair or experienced loss of sexual interest in our own relationship, do we act differently at crucial times than our model mandates us to?

The dialogue suggests that we consider whether or not women have a greater appreciation for and gender awareness about intimacy and sexual issues than men. The women referred to their parenting experiences as shaping their comfort with dealing with bodily functions and intimate relationships in a noncompetitive, empathic manner, which in turn transfers into their therapeutic comfort in dealing with the subjective nature of intimacy and sexuality. How have the gender awareness and role changes of the past decade impacted both genders in these areas?

In considering gender issues, do we ignore or take into account the arguments about neurologically based differences between males and females, put out by the sociobiologists? These theories are derived from experiments with nonhumans, do these models provide some input that helps us explain humans?

In the end, it seemed as if our dialogue had raised more questions than answers, leaving us with somewhat of a dilemma: Where do we go from here?

SOME FINAL STATEMENTS

MAGGIE: Looking over these excerpts, which have emerged as the most important parts of our conversation, I would say that there are three major areas for future discussion that can be discerned. One is the mythic character of what "turns us on" sexually—a subject that would have to be explored by people who were feeling very comfortable and ready to be open and honest, for it is a scary subject indeed. The participants might want to remain anonymous, using pseudonyms.

The second topic that strikes me as quite important is the subject of "secrets." No one has dealt with this subject adequately, and I think that our discussion never got fully developed. Questions related to basic values, politics, and so forth intruded. It's too bad, because secrets—especially sexual secrets—are something that every therapist has to deal with.

The third important topic, which David raised, is a closely allied one. This has to do with the therapists who act out their own agendas when they are working with a particular client. We all know the "divorcing therapist" and the "therapist who encourages affairs" (otherwise known as "personal growth"), as David mentioned. What is or is not an acceptable therapeutic stance? I was surprised by the lack of consensus, even where sexually abusive behaviors, such as incest, were concerned.

There were, in a number of instances, sharply divergent views, constituting a psychological fault-line dividing the women and the men.

The group as a whole was, nevertheless, able to pinpoint certain key areas of interest, certain questions worthy of being readdressed far more extensively as the dialogue on intimacy and sexuality continues.

PEGGY: My hope for this book is that it acts like a flare at sea for the field, reminding us we are drifting away from our core understandings about human connections. I believe the feminist theorists responded first to large social and particular familial inequities for women, and their important critique brought the proverbial house down on conventional stereotyped roles for both women and men. The most recent work on violence and abuse has challenged gender stereotypes regarding how a social order is maintained by the fixed behaviors of women and men. It is interesting that an early by-product of the work on violence was the evolution of a new curiosity toward gender definitions, gender constructs in individuals, and gender constructs in families and how all of these were similar to and different from cultural definitions of gender. These researchers began to explore how men and women think differently about ideas like abandonment, commitment, competition, autonomy, play, love, and so on. New questions are being developed that underlie the significance of gender issues in work with families, questions about our experiences as males or females in our families and in larger society and culture. These are our new frontiers.

DON: This process helped me clarify my own thinking, and it convinced me that intimacy and sexuality are two separate tracts, for males, anyway.

This inquiry represents what the field of family therapy could bring to the neglected areas of intimacy and sexuality, a fine-grained look at their inherent gendered contexts—personal, social, and political. That would be a unique and valuable offering!

10

MYTHIC CONTRACTS AND MYTHIC JOURNEYS IN INTIMATE SEXUAL RELATIONSHIPS

David Kantor

> The question then is: So why does everybody persist? If love
> cuts them up so much, and you see the ravages everywhere,
> why not be sensible and sign off early?
>
> —Saul Bellow, *More Die of Heartbreak*

In working with adult couples as they struggle to realize their goals for intimacy, I am struck by a question the complexity of which baffles the imagination: What is it that makes intimate partners keep trying to make their relationships work when that very struggle may strip them of sexual desire? And yet, that desire lies at the center of most people's wish to be in an intimate relationship in the first place. The paths which lead dedicated couples into sexual dysfunction, sexual impasse, and loss of sexual desire are part of a rich mythology of men and women in ongoing relationships. Buried below consciousness, like many myths of modern society, the gender patterns of a couple's relationship must be uncovered before they can regain their sexual intimacy and passion.

The sexual impasse is possibly the most devastating symptom of all of a family's struggles for intimacy. Beneath most problems brought to family therapists lurks a sexual dilemma, which eventually leads the

David Kantor. Kantor Family Institute, Cambridge, Massachusetts.

couple to this point of impasse. Yet mainstream family therapy has undertaken no serious examination of the origins of the sexual impasse, of its workings in the couple's life, or of its effect on children. In ignoring the sexual origins of family dysfunction, the field has tolerated a critical oversight.

Perhaps family therapists have balked at the enormity of the task which looms ahead, once they accept that family dysfunctions are frequently rooted in sexual dysfunction. For a theory of the family system's evolution and development cannot exist without a theory of the couple system's development as its central thread, and any such theory of the couple's evolution cannot exist without including a theory of the adult sexual development that takes place within the intimate relationship. In this essay and the other chapters in this book, I and my co-authors set out upon an arduous and important pursuit—to uncover the evolution of sexual development in couples and, subsequently, in families. As my tool in this endeavor, I use the time-honored medium of myth.

THE IMPORTANCE OF MYTH

Although our culture no longer celebrates myths formally in poetry, drama, and religion, they wield no less force in individuals' lives today than they did in ancient times. Today myths penetrate our consciousness via films, television, and newspapers. Whatever their vehicle, once myths take hold in a culture, they become standards for its members and influence individuals' definitions of normality. Thus, the child whose makeshift "S"-emblazoned cape emboldens his superhuman flight from plush armchair to stuffed couch gears himself for any of a variety of Superman myths his culture amply supplies.

Can we choose the myths we live by? Ultimately, yes, although few people, even among those who successfully choose their myths, can tell of the process by which they did so. Oftentimes unaware, individuals choose intimate relationships according to the myths that give meaning and structure to their lives. These choices show up in the form of tacit agreements between the two partners as to how each will behave, as man and woman, in relation to one another. The fate of many intimate relationships rests upon the mythic contracts that partners make during courtship and beyond. Serving as the bases for the relationship, these poorly understood contracts are typically fraught with many complex interpretations and damaging distortions of meaning. Sexual desire eludes the couple when the reality of the relationship violates the terms of the mythic contract.

"What *is* sexual desire?" Robert Stoller, a psychoanalyst who has probably contributed more to this important subject than any contemporary writer, points out that almost no professional literature discusses *why* a person becomes sexually excited. "About 'sexuality'? —yes, we have innumerable studies. But about 'sexual excitement,' not much exists" (p. 32). Stoller insists that prevailing belief holds that a sadomasochistic element underlies all sexual excitement. In my opinion, this explanation lacks any constructive, creative possibilities for human growth and understanding. If, instead, we look at sexual excitement from an interpersonal perspective, we find that sexual fantasy offers ready access to the nature of the sexual desire and to its vicissitudes in the intimate relationship. The sexual fantasy, a key factor in the creation of erotic excitement, is, in my conceptual vernacular, a *sexual myth*, an image from which we shape our particular sexual realities. And sexual myths when negotiated by two people in an intimate relationship, set down the conditions of the couple's mythic contract. In this tacit agreement, each partner decides how to build the sensual and erotic into his or her life and experiences—or whether to deny them outright.

Mythic ideals also determine sexual desire and the health of the mythic contract, because mythic ideals not only define one's sexual identity for the other, but also furnish an arousal coming from within the self for the self. (*When my friend Arthur C. used to hitch up his belt, throw out his chest, and perceptibly grunt, I knew somehow that he was feeling his masculine/imperious sexual identity in a form of self-arousal.*) Alternately, the mythic ideals which others present and which we find attractive, trigger the sexual arousal and desire for the other that plays so central a role in the making, keeping, and breaking of sexual contracts.

THE NATURE OF SEXUAL DESIRE

As a journeying clinician and dedicated student of couples' intimate relationships, I have developed this hypothesis: The withdrawal of sexual desire occurs when there is a *breach of contract*, a breakdown of the intimate partners' prior (but usually unspoken) agreement that each will continue to endorse, support, and idealize three types of mythic images that the other holds. Both partners have incorporated these images into their self from experience, and then present them to the other as integral parts of their self- and sexual identity.

The first mythic contract is based on the mythic ideals the man and woman use to define their gender arrangement. Thanks to the feminists, men and women today have considerable choice in the gender ideals available to them when they negotiate an intimate relationship. Couples now can choose models in which the man and woman share equal dominance and responsibility for both mothering and providing. These ideals result in a very different gender arrangement, with very different sexual consequences, than when the woman has primary responsibility for mothering and the man primary responsibility for providing.

Thus, though not an attractive couple, Zeus and Hera offer a more viable source of gender ideals for some modern couples than the more frequently chosen mythic couple of Odysseus and Penelope. A stormy marital pair, they contrast sharply with Odysseus, the wandering hero who provides, and Penelope, the faithful weaver patiently tending the hearth who obediently awaits her husband's return. The marriages of both mythic couples survived because the partners based their sexual contracts upon openly understood gender arrangements. Hera, for example, knew of Zeus' premarital profligacy and fought his indiscriminate promiscuity after they married with a matching vengeance. Both knew the drama and the roles they each would have to play.

The first threat to a couple's sexuality occurs when either partner (or both, of course) becomes disenchanted with the existing gender arrangement and challenges it. Disappointment lies at the foundation of such challenges. If a Zeus cannot tolerate Hera's confrontations over his compulsive profligacy; if a Penelope discovers that she chose a Zeus rather than an Odysseus; if an Odysseus finds his Penelope is not the faithful, patient weaver but a Hera who matches his dalliances during his 10-year journey home after the Trojan War with dalliances of her own, we can predict the onset of *disappointment*. Whether the tone is of anger or despair, this disappointment provides the impetus for the breaking of the first mythic contract.

The second mythic contract is based on personal myths that originate not in the culture, but in the intimate environment of each partner's original family. Personal myths are the humble myths of the child's imperfect world—imperfect because no parent, however good and well-intentioned, can completely fill the needs of the helpless infant or the dependent child. The mythic themes of protection, abandonment, loss, lack of recognition, etcetera are large indeed. Yet, the narrative storylines that accompany them contain innocent memories that seem, under cynical adult scrutiny, surprisingly commonplace and trivial: An eager 12-year-old brings his first "A" home to please his distant father. Preferring his newspaper to the news of his son's hard-won achievement, the father cruelly crushes a budding intelligence. The boy's mother reinforces the young one's despair with a telling, disdainful, silent glance at her inattentive husband—a divisive message to the child. Inevitably, these painful personal memories are tremendously significant for every child who so helplessly depends on the all-powerful parents for personal and emotional survival.

At the outset of an intimate relationship, the man and the woman each bring into their intimate interaction a set of personal myths that they have internalized from childhood experiences. These myths define their separate realities and set their expectations of how they and the other will interact in meaningful situations. In fact, the man and the woman become attracted to one another in the first place because of the conviction that the other's qualities and actions will be compatible with those of key figures from these myths.

Through the interaction and integration of the two sets of personal myths, a new family is born and thereafter evolves over the lifetime of the relationship. Rarely, however, does this scheme for growth occur without struggle, for inevitably the myths clash and compete for the right to prevail in defining reality. Both partners, believing their own myths to be superior, defend them with a fierceness they would only use to defend life itself. And when painful, early childhood experiences are repeated in the adult intimate relationship, with the very one chosen as the mythically ideal figure to redeem the past, the individual experiences an anguish of disillusionment and nonfulfillment. The breaking of the second mythic contract also inevitably leads to the process of disappointment.

The third mythic contract hinges upon sexual myths, images, and fantasies that the man and the woman bring to and use in the actual sexual experience. The sexual myth offers hope, possibilities, the freedom to adventure in realms that are often mischievous, mysterious, forbidden, and even "unsavory," "satanic," or "animalistic." This mythic contract does not resolve the ambiguities of sexual attraction, arousal, and inchoate sensual consciousness. In fact, for some couples a key condition of the agreement is that neither partner speak or recount the secret of their own sexual fantasy or demand that the other reveal theirs. Despite this secrecy, in the actual sexual experience, the other must often act as if he or she knows the partner's fantasy. (*Keeping the secret is not an element of all sexual contracts; my personal preference for silence in these matters may bias my perception, so that I find the secrecy condition in most couple arrangements. Some part of me believes that sex becomes a little better by being a little bad and that by keeping the secret of the sexual fantasy, we preserve the mystique of rapture.*)

Through the third mythic contract, we come to understand the politics of desire. One of the central issues for an individual is: Under what conditions will I incorporate, sustain, or deny the sensual and erotic in my sexual experience with a long-term intimate partner? Common wisdom suggests that sexual disappointment results from too much familiarity with the partner's physical characteristics. Along this line of reasoning, physical boredom and the need for change result in disappointment and the breach of the mythic contract. And to be sure, of all the realms in which men and women negotiate the ways and means to sexual intimacy, the realm of bodily politics proves the most mysterious. But if desire indeed arises as a systemic or interpersonal phenomenon, then a suppression of the sexual fantasy and a withdrawal of the promise-to-comply in the mythic contract by one or both partners could explain the couple's loss of excitement.

Psychological justice does not follow legal guidelines; the contract breakdown dramatically effects the couple even though they make the three mythic agreements in the form of an unconfirmed understanding. Most sexual relationships survive reversals in one, or even two, of these mythic spheres. However, a breakdown in any one sphere can become the impetus for a sexual withdrawal by the partner heavily invested in the mythic image of that sphere. A partner, for example, whose sexual excitement, or worse, whose basic sexual satisfaction is contingent on access to fantasy-fed, sexual primitivism may panic when the other refuses to comply, and thus reneges on the implicit sexual contract. If broken contracts in all three mythic spheres wreak extensive disappointment and loss, the withdrawal of sexual interest is a virtual certainty. In any case, the triple threat puts sexual intimacy in jeopardy for many couples.*

THE FIRST MYTHIC CONTRACT

Certain myths, both ancient and modern, serve as the primary sources for gender behavior. They are the models the culture provides us with for knowing, deciding, or discovering what it means to be a man and a

---

*A book in progress will examine in full the mythic contracts of the three spheres. In this chapter I will discuss only the first mythic contract.

woman. These myths help us face and resolve, in the different ways that men and women do, the issues of sexuality that unmercifully haunt anyone who chooses love and intimacy as the lifeblood of family relationships.

The Odysseus Myth

The Odysseus myth, depicted in antiquity by Homer, offers *one* (but not the only) ideal definition of maleness and femaleness. Although women thinkers have criticized and challenged its ideals, the Odysseus myth remains appropriate and acceptable to large numbers of modern-day men. Large numbers of modern-day women also accept its ideals as did the figure of Penelope in the *Odyssey*. Those of us, both men and women, who object to the depiction of women as the ideal helpmate would hardly care to admit the extent to which many women welcome that role.

Of course, in the instances where Penelope appears to be women's ideal choice, one wonders whether these women are choosing between two negative alternatives. By buying into the Ulyssean* wanderer–provider arrangement, they don't risk forsaking a marriage or the intimate heterosexual relationship altogether.

Odysseus, on the other hand, is decidedly a man's *choice*. Odysseus appeals broadly to men as an archetypical mythic figure spanning many hero types—not only the explorer–adventurer types, the men of action, but the adventurous scholar, an Archimedes or a Galileo, for example, whose journeys take them into realms of a sort different from the ones Odysseus enters but, like him, outward and into unknown places. It is also not uncommon for one individual to combine two or more mythic ideals, take Sir Walter Raleigh, for example.

The point I wish to make is that men and women select heroic archetypes (or imbue ordinary people with heroic, larger-than-life qualities), use these archetypes as gender models for themselves, and present them to potential partners when negotiating intimate contracts. If men are to evolve a new male psychology comparable in substance and depth to the new psychology of women, they might start by analyzing the character types of their mythic heroes. Instead, men today seem to meekly accept and adopt a definition prominent in current-day therapy culture. This definition, while not entirely inconsistent with some versions of the Ulyssean ideal, involves, in Robert J. Lifton's words, " . . . an experimentation with a more gentle ideal, that of an open, non-combative self-explorer, willing to inhabit formerly 'female' areas of concerns" (1987,

*I shall use "Ulysses" and "Ulyssean" and "Odysseus" and "Odyssean" interchangeably.

p. 26). Both male and female therapists, responding to feminist revisions of human developmental theory have, too insistently and too soon I think, urged men to experiment with these softer, more gentle attitudes, behaviors, and concerns.

It bodes well, of course, that American culture and its therapy subculture are consciously promoting new gender models for men. Women and men both may well feel heartened too by the appearance of various versions of psychologically dominant, physically assertive, self-assured female ideals. But if my hypothesis about the mythic contracts made between intimate partners holds true, therapists may be doing some couples and families a disservice by advocating new gender ideals to men without them first discovering what their own ideals are. In their zeal to experiment with new gender roles, therapists may unfairly make use of their power to interpret and influence reality. People simply do not change their ideals like a suit of clothes. By denying gender differences and condemning masculine ideals we happen to disapprove of or cannot fathom, we may be confusing and disrupting some couples' politics. The clearest example of an unfathomable model for most therapists is a modern perversion of the Ulyssean ideal—the Rambo or Rocky, a tight-lipped sexual conqueror, tough, and capable of brutality and violence for the "right cause." Should therapists support this near caricature of the male ideal or dismiss it because of its extremeness? The question cannot easily be answered.

For one thing, the John Wayne phenomenon, a gentler variety of Rambo, appeals to very large numbers of American men and women, few of whom are violent or in favor of violence. Its emphasis on strength, cunning, protectiveness, courage, and absolute loyalty to fellow group members translates readily into numerous Ulyssean variations, from pioneer efforts in space or science to the less glamorous efforts of the factory worker or miner. Neither John Wayne's super-masculine wartime bravado nor his breadwinner role as protector and provider can be dismissed. We might even ask, can the "John Wayne thing" explain why hordes of hardworking, sedentary psychotherapists as well as hard-hatted, physical construction workers gather with other men to watch the Superbowl, the NBA playoffs, or the World Series? In these domains, male athletes dramatically symbolize for so many men the supermasculine power of their sex.

(I remind the reader, not for the last time, that I am speaking here not for all men nor for all men and all women. Every man's and woman's theory of the human relationship is an elaborately externalized system of

very personal explanations. My view, then, is admittedly biased in that it arises out of my own experiences and my experiences as a male in particular. Whenever it is clear to me that some personal, and particularly some male, bias is obviously impinging on the text, I try to reveal this through italicized comments. I invite other men to join me in this exploration of male bias, in order to decipher from the weight of many male perspectives and explanations a generic male view that invites conversation, especially with those women who have been doing this very same thing for their gender. It is good that women have been developing new explanations; they must acknowledge, however, that these explanations are grounded in female bias. Historically, men have presented explanations about both men and women from an unacknowledged bias. Our task as men now is to develop our theories of maleness from a position of acknowledged bias. When we do our work or enough of it to catch up to the women, a true conversation will be possible.)

Odysseus: A Myth for Family Therapists

To illuminate the effects of sex and gender relations on the family's sexual development, family therapists would do well to look to the myth of Odysseus rather than to that of Oedipus, which has dominated the practice of psychology for 50 years or more. For in comparison with Oedipus (which a colleague, Anne Peretz, called "a woman's tale, a tragic story of love between mother and son"), the Odysseus story offers more inclusive possibilities for the family therapist as well as a rich array of family stories: It is about a woman and her conflict between faithfully tending the hearth and catering to her own passions and interests; it is about a son who, his father presumed dead, has the power granted by patriarchal rule to barter his mother in marriage to the highest bidding suitor, yet chooses not to exercise this power; and it is about that same son's search for the father who, when he does return, enlists his son's help in killing off the suitors.*

The story of Odysseus is also a multigenerational story spanning three generations. Odysseus's mother, Anticleia, dies of heartbreak while he is fighting in the Trojan War. His father, Laertes, is still living in Ithaca when Odysseus returns some 19 or 20 years after leaving home. An intriguing gender issue clouds the relationship between Odysseus and his father, who inexplicably handed over his throne to the vigorous and

*A. Peretz (May 1988), personal communication.

shining Odysseus. Once a brave warrior and still capable of fighting by the side of his son, Laertes remains at home and makes little attempt to protect Penelope, the kingdom, or his grandson's rights from Penelope's suitors. Instead, he retires to the life of a gentleman farmer while his son proves himself as a remarkably brave and cunning hero.

Thus, the *Odyssey*, a story of how the prolonged absence of the wandering Odysseus affects a whole family's destiny, is a mythic fountainhead and its central metaphor of the absent mate and father is painfully apt for these times. Today, of course, not the physical absence, though that may be a part of it, but the psychological and emotional unavailability of the male defines the parameters of what I call the "absent father syndrome" (see Kunitz, 1987). In attempting to shed some light on how this pervasive, but little understood, phenomenon has such toxic effects on sexual intrigues within the family, I have chosen here to concentrate on the part the syndrome plays in male–female relations—specifically, on whether or not male absence leads to withdrawal of sexual interest.

From the plethora of possible themes which the Odysseus story offers, I have selected four that I think are relevant to the making and breaking of sexual contracts:

- *the psychologically absent father*, which deals with man's search for transcendence in work.
- *the son's search for the father*, which attempts to tie the man's capacity for work and intimacy to the vicissitudes of his own father search.
- *the woman's dilemma*, which raises the crucial question, What do I do about work, sex, and passion while my mate is absent?
- *the culture of waiting*, which highlights the relationship between how women resolve this perplexing dilemma and the survival or withdrawal of sexual interest.

How intimate partners manage these themes is crucial to the survival of sexual vitality. When partners "mismanage" them, a troublesome sequence often occurs which begins with conflicting gender ideals, leads then to the breaking of gender contracts, and finally results in the potential withdrawal of sexual interest. Recall that one broken contract, or even two broken contracts of the three, may not undo a couple's sexual vitality. Each broken contract, however, does result in disappointment, and disappointment proves a crucial factor in understanding any partner's loss of sexual interest.

Odysseus Reenacted

If men model their gender identities upon cultural myths, we might begin our more sympathetic exploration of a man's character by turning to the Ulyssean myth to find the origins of stereotypical male behavior. The Ulyssean male prefers *action* (striving, exploration, adventure), *hardness* (activities that require muscular strength, endurance, the refusal to give up), and *individuality* (being on his own and doing things by his own effort). The allure of individuality, in particular, continues to puzzle many women.

These Ulyssean qualities, at their worst, set the stage for violence. In earlier times, action, hardness, and individuality prepared a man for survival and enabled him to gain critical knowledge of unexplored worlds. The fact that these traits may be unnecessary for explorations of a modern world doesn't rid man of his attraction for them: Although typical male gender behavior has continually undergone modification as time proceeds, men continue to seek expression in action and in strong character. Though these ideals remain essentially the same, the locus of their expression has shifted from the domain of geography to that of work. Indeed, as my colleague Michael Miller has pointed out, the idea that having a strong character (which he defined as one incorporating determination, will, individualism, and striding) limits, rather than enhances the possibilities of intimate relationships is, on close inspection, suspect.* If men speak washed words only, voices scrubbed clean of the lion's roar, do they deny their wives and children what is valid in their core, and, more importantly, do they deny women the shape of difference?

Most of the men I have worked with are men who are absorbed. They are absorbed with ideas, with making money, with computers, etcetera. Some men are only comfortable with machines such as cars or trucks and tools; others with sports, animals, or guns; and still others with guns that kill animals. All this can be considered work, men at work. Men are comfortable at work. Even when they use words, many communicate best in the silent language of acts (and for some men words are acts). When men feel comfortable with each other, they are bridged (metaphorically speaking) by work—by a shared interest in the act of making money, playing with computers, using or repairing machines, engaging in sports or watching sports with other men, etcetera. Connections form through joining in actions; rarely are they direct, emotional, or expressed. Whereas

*M. Miller (June 1988), personal communication.

women revel in the freedom to express, even those men who have the words and feelings prefer to speak the more silent language of acts. They express in characteristically male ways—a nod of acknowledgment, the locker room swat on the ass, the boylike bumping of shoulders, a hip to hip (avoiding the touch of genitals) embrace, etcetera. Acts and man's expression of himself are one. Acts and work are one. Absorption and work are also one. All this comprises the male equation. Yet, where does that equation begin?

Seeking Transcendence Through Work

At the heart of a man's compulsion to work is his impulse to explore, to adventure, and to know. Although not all men embark on "adventure" in a strict sense, most men do set sail on a hero's journey when they give work a central place in their lives. A sense of wonder about his own humanity fuels a man's impulse to explore and adventure or merely to venture. A sense of terror about mortality feeds the impulse to achieve. In contemporary man the two impulses often fuse, and achievement becomes equated with adventure and the need to know. At its best, a man's compulsion to work is a compulsion to discover himself. His search begins with, and simultaneously is, a search for the absent father, the man distanced either physically or psychologically from his family.

The Absent Father

The mythic image of the absent father haunts the modern imagination, breaking the heart of families and plundering the dreams of wives and children. Whether he has died of natural causes, suicide, or the whimsy of war; whether his absence is a consequence of divorce, illegitimacy, or abandonment; whether he is separated from his family by the fatigue and anxiety rendered in the workplace; whether the gulf between him and his family is because of voluntary absorption in ideas, cars, computers, or money-making—wives, daughters, and sons of these absent fathers have borne the burden of a deep-rooted ambivalence about whether to love or denounce the unreachable father.

  1. Often, he has been denounced by sons:
       "My father never told me he loved me until 2 years ago when I
          was 34 . . . since then—one awkward embrace, never a kiss."
       "In a dream I called out to him . . . he never came."
       "He was never really there for me . . . and it was lonely."
       "One word? My father was *cold*."

2. Wives have also denounced him:

"His work has been a killing ground for this relationship."

"If *he* is proud of his invulnerability, it turns *me* off."

"He's never cried except in secret when watching a mawkish movie."

"He 'knows' so much, but so very little about himself."

"His attention is always outward—never to birthdays, doctor's appointments, new shoes . . . it is lonely."

"One word? My husband is *cold*."

"Cold" is a recurrent epithet in these statements—cold-hearted, cold grief, cold death—a litany of estrangement. Sons and wives excoriate and vilify the man for his psychological, as much as his physical, absence. I heard these words, and many more like them, from women in couples therapy about their husbands and from these husbands about their own fathers. In a curious paradox, men and women who come to therapy disagreeing in so many ways along gender lines, agree about one thing—the significance of an absent father: In this chorus of both men and women ring ghostly echoes from the distant past—of the husband, as a son himself, crying out for his distant father; and echoes from the disturbing present as that grown son invokes the wrath of a woman who cries out for a deeper connection with her man. When a son is born between them, the chorus weeps in sad division; the son, like his father courted by the waiting woman, cannot give up the search for his own absent father.

Of all the players in these family dramas, sons have suffered the greatest injury by far. In the worst cases, their mothers, out of the anger and deprivation brought on by having absent mates, unintentionally sacrifice the sons to their own pain, which further mystifies father absence. Even in the best cases, where such pain does not exist or is kept private, the sons themselves mystify the absent father, which intensifies the need to find him. In either case, something of the son is surrendered, offered up, condemned, as in some ancient ritual in which humans are sacrificed to appease or court a deity. Here, the son is sacrificed to a remote and disinterested deity, the absent father. Later in life, their own women, in seeking or giving up seeking intimacy, either vilify or ridicule them. (*It is a mistake for women, and men riding the feminist wave, to ridicule the psychologically absent male. As a son of an absent father and as a father who is sometimes blamed of being absent, my sympathies naturally go with these men, not more than with daughters and wives, but with a difference steeped in gender identity.*)

We might begin by construing father absence not as a travesty but as
a core happening from which male identities in intimate family environments are bent, forged, and shaped. Pursuing this course may reveal some
of the puzzling mysteries of sexual fortune and misfortune in adult male-
female relationships and thus in all of family life. To embrace the mythic
male ideal is to embrace the father ideal. Work, and the man's journey in
general, then becomes the arena in which the son can pursue his father.
And the successful search for the father through work ends, spiritually
speaking, in the discovery of self. The father's absence, however, renders
him intangibly, implacably, and intractably elusive. Because of the tenuousness of the connection with an absent father, the man's journey
through work, ultimately becomes the search for transcendence.

The Tenuous Paternal Connection

If we are to understand, rather than condemn, the father's defection from
his family, we must begin at the beginning. For the child of either gender,
the maternal connection is held together by biological bonding through
the processes of gestation and nurturance, then by the constancies of
primary "mothering," and finally by the intractable gender definitions of
the dominant culture. In contrast, the paternal connection has little basis
in biology and human development. Biological differences between man
and woman make bonding, nurturing, and "primary mothering," occupations suited better to the woman than to the man. Despite modern
paternal disguises, the child "knows" the difference between a male and
female's caregiving: Mother's breast, either wet or dry, has a woman's feel
and mother's arms a woman's reach. Mother "stays" and father "leaves."
In those experimental families where father "mothers" and mother "fathers," the child seems to end the experiment when the parents themselves do not.

Do biological imperatives or cultural ones persuade the child to
revert to gender norms? Will we ever know? Need we? What we need to
know is that the maternal connection serves to clarify the male child's
gender identity: The connection is *there* for the having, and it *defines*
through difference. In contrast, the tenuousness of the boy child's paternal
connection burdens the formation of gender identity: It is not there for the
having. By being out of reach, the boy tends to *mythologize* the father
rather than realize him as a person. The proof of male identity, then, is in
the son's search for the absent father.

When a man's journey is deeply probed (in therapy, for example), we
find within the man a son who seeks atonement from a transcendent or

transcending father. In the spiritual realm, Christ-the-son reconciles God-the-father and man, the imperfect son fashioned in His image. In the secular realm, work reconciles father and son. Most men offer their work as an expiation to the distant father as if a wrong or an injury had been committed. But what is that wrong, that injury? Who has been wronged and who injured—the father who then demands reparation and/or the son who then demands satisfaction? I would answer each—each is injured by a separation forced on them by an immutable biology, which establishes a critical distance between them. For many this separation spans a lifetime.

(As I have come to understand man's work as a search for transcendence and reconciliation, I have added enormous conceptual breadth to my clinical efforts. Fallout from the collision of the two psychic energies, the father's and the son's, does less damage when understood in this light. When I remember the history of my own father-son struggles, I can both keep in check and put to better use my own intuitive sympathies as a father and as a son. Just as importantly, this understanding has subtly advanced my ability to help women/mothers help reconcile fathers and sons without adding insult to their own injuries.)

The Son's Search

> I called out to him to pay some attention to me, to
> give me counsel on the conduct of my life.
>
> "Father!" I cried, "Return! You know the way. . . .
> Instruct your son, whirling between two wars. . . ."
>
> . . . oh teach me how to work and keep me kind.
>
> —Stanley Kunitz*

The theme of father-son relations has crept up on us over the last 3 or 4 decades. We find it in the novel, in film, and extensively in poetry. Stanley Kunitz, speculating on the reasons for the spectacular increase in father and son poems since midcentury, points out that it is a peculiarly American cultural phenomenon. "In their richness, strength and power," he says, "these poems provide an insight not only into existential sources, but into the mythological heart of a culture in crisis" (1987, p. 36).

*From "The quest for the father" by S. Kunitz, 1987, *The New York Times Book Review*, p. 36. Copyright 1987 by *The New York Times*. Reprinted by permission.

In attempting to address the crisis in intimacy in our culture, I shall rely on Kunitz in at least two ways. First, his *Times* article lead me to regard Odysseus as an important mythic source. "The predominant syndrome of male psychology," says Kunitz "is not Oedipal rage but the more elegiac theme of the quest for the absent father" (p. 36). The theme of the absent father now occupies a central place in my thinking about men and their intimacies. Second, his own father–son poems, as well as others he refers to, get to the heart of the father–son relationship as only the poetic imagination can. These poems helped to shape my views on the importance of the son's search for the father and on the symbolic equivalence of man's work with the quest for the absent father. In my opinion, man's success or failure in intimacy with women is linked to how he conducts the search for the absent father and to how his mother, and later his women lovers, manage the environment of waiting created by the father's/man's absence.

When I consider how different men I've known in life, the arts, and therapy have conducted their search, I can clearly discern three major motifs. The motifs of "patricidal obsession," "futile flight," and the "hero's journey" show up in poetry and in literature eloquently reflecting my experiences from life and from therapy. The underlying themes may vary in each, of course, and may overlap in some male psychologies while remaining obsessively distinct in others. For the therapist or anyone else exploring gender relationships, it behooves one to listen for these different motifs and, in so far as is possible, to know one's own.

Patricidal Obsession

A few of the poets, and the men they represent in the culture, are consumed by patricidal obsession: "I spit upon this dreadful banker's grave/Who shot his head out in a Florida dawn." Or "Father, whom I murdered every nite but one." The first poet, John Berryman, could not forgive his father for killing himself when he was still in his teens; the second, Howard Moss, murdered his father often in a recurrent dream (quoted in Kunitz, 1987, p. 37).

In therapy, when their search is not going well, these men seem self-destructive, as in the following case. I saw Joseph R in three different therapy sequences over almost 20 years. During each, we dealt with a new crisis: law school stress and sexual problems early in his marriage; his and his wife's decision to divorce following his discovery that his wife was having a serious affair (8 years after the first sequence); and a morbid dissatisfaction with his career (7 years after the second sequence). Joseph

R's father, like Berryman's, also "shot his head out" when Joseph was a boy. Following his father's footsteps, he had become a "successful" lawyer by his fortieth year, but felt tortured daily by work he hated. To break the spell of "love and yearning" and bitter hatred for his "absent guide" (these are the poets speaking for my client), he turned to women who, like his "selfish mother," disappointed him with "promises they did not keep." (These are the words of my client, which extend father hatred to include mother hatred.) When his second marriage began to falter, Joseph realized that the themes of love and yearning and bitter hatred, which had haunted him since his father's suicide, persisted in his relations with women and with work.

Working with his patricidal obsession in therapy, I tried to discourage rather than encourage or endlessly tolerate the venting of his patricidal rage. I speculated about whether his father's own search necessitated his absence, and whether neglect of his son was a by-product of a failed search and, perhaps, marriage. I meant, ultimately, to shift attention to Joseph's own search. In negotiating with men like Joseph R over ways to conduct the search, in order to help them transcend patricidal ideation for example, I join them in their struggle and undisguisedly offer them "counsel on the conduct of their lives."

Futile Flight

Some sons, attempting to escape from their father, shape their lives around a futile flight. All their lives they may yearn for the approval of the father through a gulf they have made too wide to bridge. Franz Kafka, one of our best known literary figures, adopted the futile flight model. Kunitz writes that Kafka "wanted to group everything he had ever written under the collective title 'The Attempt to Escape from Father.' Nevertheless," he notes, Kafka ". . . confesses in the devastating letter to his father, 'My writing was about you. In it I poured out the grief I could not sigh at your breast'" (quoted in Kunitz, 1987, p. 37).

Sartre took another but still very similar path. He cut short his search altogether in what Robert Lifton (1987) calls Sartre's ". . . celebration of fatherlessness: 'There is no good father, that's the rule. . . . Had my father lived, he would have lain on me at full length . . . and crushed me. . . . I left behind me a young man who did not have time to be my father, and who could now be my son.'" (p. 19). Lifton here refers to Sartre's liberation through his father's early death. Sartre, Lifton writes, "raised fundamental contemporary questions not only of fatherlessness but of mentorship and authority and reversals in both," questions central to our search theme (p. 19).

Most sons are not able, as Sartre was, to let their estranged or dead fathers go. Kafka, it seems, was neither able nor willing. Although Sartre's search motif seems the better one, I think that for neither author was the search successful. Would the successful journey not end in forgiveness?

Some sons follow a variation of the "escape" or "flight" motif, which falls closer to Kafka's solution (attempting to escape the father while craving his approval), than to Sartre's (celebrating fatherlessness while fearing the father's power to crush). For these men, self-value cannot be high and their very being complete unless and to the extent that the god-the-king-and-father approves of them. Haplessly, however, god-the-king-and-father is not at hand to approve. He is, like Odysseus, off somewhere; or he is absorbed; or, more malevolently, he withholds. Saul Bellow's masterful short novel *Seize the Day*, offers a priceless example of malevolent withholding. The tale portrays a 45-year-old man whose life is unraveling. A lost soul, he keeps reaching out to his father for spiritual guidance, under the mantel of seeking financial support, but is cruelly rebuffed instead of validated. Transparently weak and shamelessly needy, he looks repeatedly to the pitiless father rather than to the self to find himself. Thus his search collapses before it even takes off.

The Hero's Journey

The following outline of the "One Story," Joseph Campbell's synthesis of many myths (described in Klaven, 1988), is an apt introduction to a discussion of the hero's journey:

> First, the hero is called to adventure. If he accepts the call, he encounters a protective figure, usually an old man or woman, who supplies him with charms and instructions.
>
> "With the personifications of his destiny to guide and aid him," the hero overcomes the guardian of a threshold and moves into "the regions of the unknown," which are "free fields for the projection of unconscious content." Here, "incestuous libido and patricidal destrudo" are . . . reflected back against the individual and his society in forms suggesting "threats of violence and . . . dangerous delight."
>
> These regions, however, are also the womb of the hero's rebirth, because now, "the hero, whether god or goddess, man or woman, the figure in a myth or a dreamer of a dream, discovers and assimilates his opposite (his own unsuspected self). . . . One by one the resistances are broken. He must put aside his pride, his virtue, his beauty and life and bow or submit to the absolutely intolerable. Then he finds that he and his opposite are not of differing species but one flesh."

If he is fortunate, these trials prepare the hero's consciousness for the ultimate adventure. This could be his atonement with the Great Father, or his own apotheosis; sex with the mother of all things or with an immortal god. Then, if the hero chooses to accept the challenge of returning to the world of light, and if he succeeds, he brings with him a boon or elixir that restores that wasted plain. He is now "master of the two worlds," able to "open his soul beyond terror to such a degree that he will be ripe to understand how the sickening and insane tragedies of this vast and ruthless cosmos are completely validated in the majesty of Being."*

For his unique contribution to our understanding of myths, rituals, and legends, Joseph Campbell will rest forever in the company of Sir James Frazer, Jesse L. Weston, Robert Graves, and Mircea Eliade. Campbell undertook a truly monumental search—a synthesis of all myths—in his books *The Hero with a Thousand Faces* and *The Masks of God, Myths to Live By*, the shining results of which I have used for my own (and I hope not too dimming) purposes: an equating of the "hero's journey" with man's search for transcendence by finding the father in work. *The Hero with a Thousand Faces* is Joseph Campbell's attempt to decipher that "one shape-shifting yet marvelously constant story" (quoted in Klaven, 1988, p. 60). To illustrate the unity of many diverse tales, Campbell gathered together myths and legends from all over the world and, from an analysis and synthesis of the content and structure of these myths, forged the universal tale of the hero's journey.

In its broadly generic sense, the hero's journey, with its themes of descent and transcendence, is the most universal and therefore the most "normative" of the three solutions to the son's search for the father. By using Joseph Campbell's term "the hero's journey" for this search I am at once glorifying it (*it is, after all, my preferred solution*) and depathologizing it (*it is, after all, a term Campbell invented to encompass all myths of a certain category*). We might even view the other search designs (patricide, flight from the father, and fatherlessness) as subcategories, or specifically, as unfortunate diversions from a universal norm.

The mythological symbolism of Campbell's synthesized hero's task applies readily to the themes of the absent father, the man's search, and the son's search. In the modern hero's journey, each man follows his own uncharted map in the search for the absent father through transcendence in work. In setting out upon his task, the hero feels a "call to adventure." If

*From "Joseph Campbell, myth master" by A. Klaven, 1988, *The Village Voice*, pp. 57-64. Copyright 1988 by *The Village Voice*. Reprinted by permission.

he "accepts the call," his work takes on a significance that threatens his place at the hearth. Seeking guidance as he attempts to find satisfaction in, and come to grips with, his gender identity through work, the hero encounters an older protective figure who supplies him with charms and instructions. Bearing with him the golden bough which, on the advice of the protector, he has plucked from the sacred grove, the hero overcomes the guardian of the threshold and moves into the "regions of the unknown."

Many interlocking demands impede the hero's task and slow his journey: He must provide for those he leaves behind; gain a sense of his own value as an individual, as a man, and as a worker; overcome the dragons that appear in his path as inevitable hazards of the workplace; and overcome also his own unconscious projections, that is, whatever "incestuous libido" or "patricidal destrudo," he carries with him. Throughout this part of the journey, the father remains totally illusory yet prominent. Ironically, by becoming absorbed in the search for his father through work, the son also becomes an absent father.

To explore the "regions of the unknown," the modern hero must deal with abandoning the hearth and those who warm it while he is battling the forces that befall him; and for so absorbingly dedicating himself to that battle that he neglects his need for the hearth he believes he is protecting. Nonetheless, attracted by the heroic role, he plunges further into the perilous deep in search of the "boon," the father, and the self.

The region of descent, while confronting the hero with its perils, encourages his rebirth as well. For the perilous deep is also the transcendent deep; here "the hero . . . discovers and assimilates his opposite (his own unsuspected self)." Transcendence cannot take place without further trials, however. In his wanderings, the hero faces the forces of his own underworld, "reflected back . . . in forms suggesting threats of violence and . . . dangerous delight." He must also stave off the seductive temptations of the marketplace: competitive meanness (the "brother battle"), ruthless ethics ("patricidal destrudo"), and the feckless affair ("incestuous libido"). When he can acknowledge his desires (to destroy, plunder, and rape), he may find the atonement he seeks, an atonement for what he fears he is but knows he must not be. As the hero faces his weaknesses one by one, his resistances break. To be strong, "He must put aside his pride . . . and bow or submit to the absolutely intolerable." He finds his real value by stripping himself of his conceits, disowning his most fiercely held doctrines, and denying nothing. "Then he finds that he and his opposite are not of differing species, but of one flesh."

For the fortunate hero, these trials prepare his consciousness for the ultimate adventure. "This could be his atonement with the Great Father or his own apotheosis . . ." For the modern hero, it could be an atonement with the father, establishment of equality or identity with him, or expiation finally made for the ill-defined wrong or injury. Simultaneously, the modern hero finds satisfaction, rank, and oneness with his self in his work. Thus, he exalts in the effort.

Finally, if the hero accepts the challenge of returning to the "world of light," he brings with him "the boon or elixir," which restores the wasted hearth he left behind. He is now "master of the two worlds" and able to "open his soul beyond terror . . ." Our modern hero returns from the deep bearing a baffling wisdom, a circle of paradoxes. Causality has become indefinable (his father has committed no crime that cannot be forgiven), duality extinguishable (the son and the father are one), and authority replaceable (the son can empower the father). Now great work is that which inspires and illuminates this circle of paradoxes.

Though each man gives his own "accidental shape to the narrative," the hero's journey remains an unchanging, ever repeated story. Recognizing that this story without an end empowers only those who take the journey, the hero will speak of the journey to his own son with the hidden voice all men possess.

THE WOMAN'S DILEMMA:
AN IMAGINARY CONVERSATION

The absent man will inevitably be "mythologized," draped in mystery and power for the wife and mother, as well as for the son. Is mythologized power the issue, really? I don't think so. Power, aggression, and hierarchy by themselves are not the chief issues; what is relevant is how they are dealt with. For the man, absence does not represent a problem in itself, but rather what the waiting one is doing about the spiritual and psychological self during his absence. For women and sons, what matters is not waiting itself, but how those who wait define the father's/husband's absence, what they do about their own spiritual and psychological selves during the waiting, and what each brings to the relationship when the wandering one and the waiting ones rejoin. In contemporary relationships, these issues are frequently identified with man's compulsion to work and woman's response to that compulsion. How a woman waits and how she defines for herself that waiting period proves critical to the male/female relationship.

Dealing with Sex, Passion, and Work during the Man's Journey

I am aware that what follows in this section—fragments from an imaginary conversation between a feminist activist named Pamela and two
Penelopean women—puts me at certain risk. After all, how can a male
interpretation of a female discussion about women's issues be taken
seriously in a world no longer tolerant of men's right to speak for women?

Women friends of mine who know I know better cringed when they
read this section of my chapter. "You will be creamed," they said. You will
be attacked as a simplistic oaf who has not kept pace with developments in
the women's community. However clearly you present your reasons, you
and they will be misunderstood. Your guileless claim that intimacy can not
survive without reflective gender conversations, men and women speaking in their own voices, exploring the depth and consequences of difference, will be dismissed as an insincere prevarication. The main point of
your paper—the man's journey with its indisputable contribution to the
woman's dilemma, and what women do about the "loneliness of waiting"
when facing that dilemma—will be lost in the furor.

Why then do I persist in the face of such sensible and compassionate
advice? Because to play it safe is to forfeit a game worth playing. Yes, my
rendition of a women's conversation is fraught with errors of male
interpretation. Yes, it barely represents and reflects the rich research
women have done on the shaping influence of myth on women to make
psychologically and spiritually healthy decisions in their lives. Yes, this
account of a woman's discussion is prejudicially modified by a particular, a
male, perspective.

But that is my point. If the rules of gender conversation between men
and women can be altered, if gender bias and difference can be used to
bring forth rather than nullify the best of these sexual worlds, a new age of
intimate relationship may get the boost it sorely needs.

Many sources contributed to this imaginary conversation. It would
serve no purpose to cite them all. Their influence on me, on a self-
consciously masculine perspective, on a male perspective willingly constrained by differing feminist perspectives that all began seriously over 20
years ago, is more in my bones than in my head. However "imaginary" I
claim the conversation to be that follows, it is not quite so. I called upon
old and new texts as sources for the two most extreme women's voices. My
source for the ideas, attitudes, and words of the ancient Penelope, the
traditionalist, was, fittingly enough, a book (*The Women of Homer*)
published 90 years ago by the scholarly Hellenophile, Walter Copeland
Perry (1898). Perry's unintended (and I would hope forgivable) chauvin-

ism is lost in the author's genuine love and passion for Homer, the epics, and Homer's women. Pamela's voice was influenced by what is now considered foundational positions of the feminist movement (as I interpret them). These positions have been articulated and elaborated over the past 15 years by feminist theorists in the fields of anthropology, sociology, political theory, and women's history. All differences aside, these varied voices do come together—as a fervant commitment to changing gender arrangements, like the classic Penelopean one, which feminists consider damaging to individuals and dangerous to society.

To further exaggerate their differences, I have introduced Penelope 2, a 1980s counterpart of the ancient Penelope, who rephrases the words and ways of her prototype with a modern twist; a woman when all is said and done, who has chosen the Penelopean myth, incorporated some of its major features into her gender identity, and used it in the gender arrangement she has with a man.

This conversation has a twofold purpose: It shows that, in spite of the differences in times, the Penelopean myth remains a popular mythic choice for modern "Penelopes," those very women whom feminists must reach if they are to speed the winds of change. Second, and most importantly, this contrived conversation allows us to contrast more sharply the positions held by two women who share the same mythic "preference"—one in response to a "choiceless" tradition that she happens to buy into, the other as a "choice" resulting from a weighing of options, one of which—the rejected one—is the option to wage total war on patriarchy. What women of all three persuasions do about sex, passion, and work while their mates are "away on a hero's journey" is the focus of this section. The answer to the question, which is dealt with at the end of the chapter is crucial since the way in which women define and handle the "culture of waiting" has much to do with the survival of sexual desire and intimacy. What I have learned in my personal, as well as my professional life, is that how men who are sojourning respond to their women's journeys, counts just as much. When all this is understood, a truly reflective gender conversation may ensue.

A Shakedown of Basic Positions

PENELOPE 2: I have heard your line of argument many times. Of course I agree that women should not be "Oppressed" by men, but I completely disagree with how you offer to change the situation.

PAMELA: It's been my intention to clarify the reasons why people continue to accept existing gender relations even though those relations have caused such pain.

PENELOPE 2: It's my understanding that feminists want to undermine the entire system of gender relations. You're against "sexual conservatism"—meaning support of the sexual status quo.

PAMELA: My aim and that of other feminists has been to uncover the emotional sources of male–female conservatism in order to completely subvert the status quo.

PENELOPE 2: Yes, I understand that in this aim, you and others like you are on a hero's journey of your own.

PAMELA: Yes, a lifetime journey.

PENELOPE 2: This I admire—envy might be more honest. But the insinuation that I might fit your definition of sexual conservative because I do not want to change my basic gender arrangement leaves me bristling. You imply that any woman who does not actively undermine the dominant gender arrangement is for "oppression." This does the women's cause a grave injustice.

PAMELA: I believe that any serious inquiry into the cultural and emotional sources of dominant gender arrangements will lead to that conclusion.

PENELOPE: But that's the problem. How can I put aside what you feminists call "systemic inequality," which I don't even perceive? Maybe I just accept the system unawares—but for me it isn't a problem, it's just the way things are. And the way things are certainly isn't one-dimensional. In my culture, alongside the women who resignedly accepted their lot were those like the powerful goddesses Hera, Athena, Artemis, and Hecate. Indeed, you remind me of Hera, whom I admire.

PAMELA: I'm not so sure that I can take that as a compliment. Feminist scholars have discovered that stories about the very goddesses you name have been changed and used in the culture to assimilate and disarm previously "untamed" female characters. But I'm really not interested in urging my project on you, Penelope, but in examining the resistance of so many of us to analyzing our conservatism. I do believe, though, that the prevailing mode of "interdependence" and "emotional complimentarity" characterising relations between men and women must be changed. If not, it will mean the destruction of our species.

PENELOPE 2: You may find, Penelope, that Pamela uses terms whose meaning may be unfamiliar to you. By "dominant gender arrangements," she means a gender status quo where women have primary responsibility for the care of infants and young children, while men have primary responsbility for history making and shaping the world. When she refers to psychological interdependence, she is refering to a psychological symbiosis that leads both men and women to support what is in her opinion, a malignant gender arrangement.

PENELOPE: But why should one want to relieve women of their primary care of infants and young children? My life is a privileged one, I admit. But less privileged women thoroughly and happily accept the responsibility to educate the children about their places in community life. My memories of family are joyous, and they were even more so for the children of our time.

PAMELA: In our time, a time very different from yours, there has been an impulse to redesign existing gender arrangements. Explosively accelerating technological changes have taken place, accompanied by equally great changes in women's needs, expectations, and desires. These changes have clearly made our ancient sexual arrangements increasingly obsolete.

PENELOPE 2: Many women in our time do experience pain, fear, and hurt about being trapped in motherhood with unavailable mates. Seeing new possibilities for themselves, they do not accept their lot with resignation. They hurt with longing.

(Two background facts about Penelope 2: First, she originally trained as an architect, but interrupted her career to marry and begin raising her children. She maintains ties to her profession through a passionate involvement in various forms of architectural preservation. Second, we know privately that for a brief period she had an affair and gave it up— not because it was morally unacceptable but because it was sexually unsatisfying.)

PAMELA: Thank you, Penelope 2, but I don't believe that this pain, fear, and hurt is new. A sense of strain and opposition between men and women has predominated in gender relations as far back as recorded history allows us to trace human interaction.

PENELOPE: What can I say, Pamela? I do not recognize this strain between men and women. You must understand; my life was not intolerable in ways that I was aware of. Should it have been?

(*In Pamela's terms both Penelopes are sexual conservatives. Pamela here might describe the ancient Penelope as a woman apt to think of the dominant gender system as natural. The modern Penelope might be seen as a more culturally informed individual who consents to the prevailing gender arrangement, not because it is "natural" or "ordained," and not*

because it is tolerable without some modification, but because of consid-
ered "choice." She has made a mythic choice that works for her, whereas it
does not for Pamela).

Sex and the Double Standard

PAMELA: Haven't you, Penelope, found the double standard to be difficult? You have been held up to countless generations as the very prototype of a loyal, faithful wife.

PENELOPE: There were exceptions, of course, but in my time the woman was faithful to her husband.

PAMELA: And husbands were not always faithful to their wives.

PENELOPE: Hector, Menelaus, and my own husband were all regarded as faithful husbands.

PAMELA: In spite of the fact that while you were mourning your absent lord and desperately holding off the clamorous and persistent suitors, Odysseus consoled himself in the arms of Circe and Calypso!

PENELOPE: Certain things were not considered dishonorable. Concubinage, for example, was quite common, but I do not believe that Odysseus indulged. Besides, what was important to me was that during his journey, Odysseus yearned to see "the smoke leap upward from his own land" and "his face was ever turned homeward." So great was his longing, he refused the nymph Calypso's offer of immortality. For a Greek, to whom youth and beauty were sacred, to turn down an offer of eternal youth and beauty had the magnitude of a sacrifice.

PAMELA: You and I do not seem to pay attention to the same details. For example, Odysseus had no scruples on your account: He dallied with Circe for a whole year and remained with Calypso a full 7 years. He even fathered children with her. You don't blame Odysseus for these infidelities, but if you were guilty of the same conduct, it would have been regarded as altogether shameful. What I mean to say is not only that the double standard rule applied in your time as it does in mine, but also that in both our cultures women who consent to it suffer the most perfidious of all fates—lack of choice. They are denied the expression of autonomy, and therefore sexual freedom. Women now are beginning to question the double standard.

PENELOPE 2: Some of us, Pamela, who think of ourselves as women free to "withdraw" this "consent" do not merely consent, we choose. What we do with our longing is another matter.

(The question What is Choice? is no doubt the stickiest of all in the
conversation. My raising it in a format that denies it the full treatment it

demands is in itself a problem. Worse still would be to fail to say something about my own perspective on the matter.

I agree with those who hold that until there is a fundamental shift in the locus and distribution of real power between men and women, the question of "choice" in women's gender arrangements makes a mockery of political logic. Also, I feel that women who, over the past decade, have reexamined the psychological origins of traditional sexual arrangements have issued an open invitation to men to follow suit. My reeducation about women's issues began 20 years ago. But only recently have I begun to reexamine the psychological and political sources of my own choices. It is late, but not too late, to prepare for a truly reflective gender conversation. In the meantime, my having given the edge to Penelope 2 in this imaginary conversation should be considered suspect.)

PENELOPE: If women in my time had such longings, I was unaware of them. Those who consented, consented and those who didn't—the goddesses and demi-goddesses mainly—didn't. Don't forget Lysistrata, arguably the most famous mortal withholder of sexual favors during antiquity.

(There is a sexual difference between Penelope 2 and Penelope 1 would like to point out. In keeping with the psychological spirit of her times, Penelope 2 is romantic, sentient, and sexually demanding with men. Homer's women completely lacked what we call romance and sentimentalism. True, Penelope and Andromache, who happened to have husbands they could love, did express strong emotions, but even these were constrained when compared to those of Penelope 2 and other modern female gender types. Penelope even argues that she did not suffer sexual deprivation.)

PAMELA: Still, Penelope, what interests me is that although men were sexually freer, they acted more possessively than women.

PENELOPE: As a rule, yes, but there were important exceptions. Beautiful, stately, and regal Hera held her own in the sexual realm. She was the consort of Zeus, the supreme god of the Olympians, who ruled over the heavens and the earth. Time and time again Zeus was unfaithful. But with the powerful Hera, he met his match. Her stormy conflicts with Zeus were famous in mythology. Yet we solemnly revered and worshiped her nonetheless as a powerful goddess of marriage.*

PAMELA: Homer also portrayed her as a vindictive, quarrelsome, and jealous shrew. Though I am not a mythologist, I know of numerous stories

*In the discussion about Hera, I have borrowed ideas from Jean Shinoda Bolen's *Goddesses in Everywoman* (1985, pp. 139–142).

of Hera's wrath. And she did not direct her rage at her unfaithful husband, but at "the other women," at children conceived by Zeus, or at innocent bystanders. Surely her misdirected wrath is a further sign, only a bit more subtle, of the persisting double standard.

PENELOPE: All this is as you say, Pamela. But in spite of Hera's humiliation and vindictiveness, she is for me a figure to be revered. Three times during the year we worshiped and celebrated her—as Hera the "Maiden/Virgin," as Hera the "Fulfilled One," and as Hera the "Widow/ Crone"—each time representing the three stages of a woman's life.

PAMELA: Penelope, you seem intractable. Ultimately, you fully buy into the double-standard rule.

PENELOPE: My father and Odysseus "bought into" this marriage and what you call its sexual rules. I "bought into" nothing; I had a marriage which was favored by the gods.

(I am stopping this part of the conversation short because of stalemate. Pamela cannot scale the wall of convictions that Penelope has erected around the question of fidelity and the double standard.)

Sex and Passion

PAMELA: Pure physical pleasure and the expectation of pleasure— being fucked when one wants and for as long as one wants—is more problematic for women than for men. Again, because of crippling gender arrangements, women have not been well-fucked.

PENELOPE 2: That's quite a mouthful, Pamela.

PAMELA: Yes, the "culture gap" is getting to me a little.

PENELOPE 2: Penelope implied that she neither expected nor desired intense sexual pleasure. That, however, is what I expect and strive for from emotional and sexual intimacy with men, from my husband.

PAMELA: Yes, here we agree. For us, sexual feeling is experienced inwardly and holistically. It connects our inner worlds with those of the men who attract us. But despite the significance of sexual feeling for us, I'm sure you'll agree that our society's gender arrangements aim to curb the female erotic impulse.

PENELOPE 2: The suppression of female sexual impulse does concern my community—the Boston-Cambridge academicians and professionals. But no, I don't find any "rule" stating that female erotic impulse must be curbed.

PAMELA: Do I understand you? Are you saying that you have not had to suppress or renounce your sexual passion?

PENELOPE 2: Yes and no. I have had my share of experiences with men who seem to fear a genitally demanding woman. With them I've run like a scared rabbit.

PAMELA: Men fearing their mothers' powers?!

PENELOPE 2: Not necessarily! I know that theory: Men fear the power of women over them, especially the power of the mother. Thus, women's sexual demands, deeply felt and explicitly stated, reinforce and recreate this childhood fear. And because the man's fear can make coitus virtually impossible, the woman tries at all costs to avoid provoking it.

PAMELA: To soothe the fear, we deny and devalue our lust, but this cure only makes the sickness worse. Denied, our lust is more frightening still.

PENELOPE 2: I am getting to know you better. You would say that, inevitably, woman's sexual impulses, like any other supressed force, comes to be seen by men as uncontrollable, overwhelming—the ultimate threat to their masculinity. And inevitably, this makes it more imperative to suppress these forces.

PAMELA: I would take this even further: In addition to this practical and realistic concern, there is a different, nonrational kind of fear, a deep, fantasy-ridden resentment directed against female impulsivity itself. A woman's own bodily pleasure in sex, independent of the pleasure she gives her partner, is the essential threatening fact.

(*Pamela and Penelope 2 are discussing a rather broadly supported feminist view, psychoanalytic in nature, of male–female sexual intimacy and the origins of its problems in childhood. This view is the result of recasting psychoanalysis and object relations theory from a feminist perspective. My main quarrel with it is its fiercely deterministic edge. If the model for adult gender arrangement is irreversibly set in infancy and childhood, what room is left for choice? In my opinion, gender and other myths that play a central role in adult sexual relationships are "chosen," and therefore can be "unchosen" and replaced, not easily but with a great deal less than totalistic effort.*)*

PENELOPE: I've been silent for a while—listening, learning more than I imagined possible about the distinctions you "moderns" make between feminist and feminine ways. For us, passion was inspired by feminine beauty. Helen, the pink-cheeked, white-armed, fair-haired, nobly-born daughter of Zeus, whose name one shudders at, was the most feminine of creatures.

PAMELA: My god! Helen was the world's original sex object.

PENELOPE: You misunderstand, Pamela. Although she was the apparent cause of a war devastatingly fatal to Greeks and Trojans alike, she is generally spoken of with sympathy, compassion, and awe because of her entrancing beauty.

PAMELA: Sure. Helen's place in history, literature, and culture has been shaped by countless generations of men—men like Homer who have raised our conception of her to unsurpassable heights of admiration, adoration, and mystique. It's possible, though, to form very different, far more cynical and critical views of her.

PENELOPE: It is impossible to speak of her entrancing beauty in adequate terms. Even Priam, who had the most to lose from the war, addressed her in affectionate terms: "Come hither, dear child, and sit by me, that thou mayst behold thy former husband, Menelaus; kinsfolk; and friends. I hold thee not to blame; nay, I hold the gods to blame who brought on us this dolorous war of the Achaians."

PAMELA: So what, if Priam, and as I understand it Hector too, whom she bewitched, treated her with kindness and respect.

PENELOPE: Helen's actions were dictated by angry gods, not by herself.

PAMELA: Like the men of Troy, who succumbed to and suffered from her almost demonic influence, you can see nothing but her dazzling and bewildering beauty.

PENELOPE: Helen was what she was—a woman of radiant loveliness. Given her consciousness of the extraordinary fascination she attracted, she responded with touching humility.

PAMELA: Is she not the supreme example of the femme fatale?

PENELOPE: . . . the treacherous, seductive, inscrutable siren who lures men to their doom?

PAMELA: My real critique is not of Helen, but of the blind worship of female beauty for the wrong reasons. I am not saying that Helen was a depraved character. I do not agree that she was the female counterpart of the weak, grimy Paris, who made her an adultress under her husband's roof and as his houseguest. I do not revile her for her enjoyment of sensuality; if anything, I applaud her for it. Helen's only crime is her own rapturous mythic beauty. The real wrongdoers are the people who keep her there. A culture like ours, that humiliates women, as it does through our famous Miss America Beauty Pageant.

(In 1967, I participated as a group leader and resource person in a Boston-based conference on women's issues, which was organized by men. The experience shot to shreds my conviction that I had developed a gender awareness mature enough to deserve a leadership role. By midafternoon on the first day, that assumption had come under serious question. All hell broke loose as a group of women, led by wringers from New York, Betty Friedan among them, halted the program in violent protest because of its male-dominated directions and demanded that the men turn the running of it over to them. By 10 P.M., dinner forsaken, the bloody takeover succeeded. Before the din and smoke of battle settled, however, one of several men who had "lost it" emotionally, had been taken away from the conference grounds in an ambulance to a hospital. The others left on their own feet.

In the vernacular of the times, the lessons in female degradation I learned that night and the next day "blew my mind." They are as vividly fixed in my mind today as when they were delivered more than 20 years ago. In one of the most memorable exercises, designed by the new (women) leaders, men willing to participate in a "beauty pageant" were told to strip down to their underwear and keep a wary eye out on their competitors, who, of course, were out to win. About 20 of us stripped and stepped forward. When it was apparent that our bodies were being circled, measured, and compared by the inscrutable standards of six preliminary judges, the ground felt soft beneath my naked feet. What should I do with my hands? Should I smile? Were my genitals showing in the jockey shorts that had seen too many washings? Was letting them show part of the rules for winning?

"Before admitting first round winners to the second and final round of the pageant," one of them announced, "we would like you to take the place on this line that shows us and the other contestants where you want to be in the ranking, and what you are willing to do to get there." We were urged to be honest with ourselves. If competitive feelings had been invoked, we must act on them, as we normally did, using guile, seduction, aggression. A new set of questions arose: Should I play it straight and try to win? As a conference leader, was role playing a less-than-truthful participant permissible? Did I want anyone to know how ruthless my streetwise competitiveness could get? What was I to do with my judgment that my body ranked pretty well—third or fourth maybe out of the 20 male bodies? The six females looking on inscrutably were gaining power as I got the message, but only after bumping head-on into myself, that I was in this experiment, trapped; and once in it, I wanted to win. This first wave of humiliation caught me off guard. Why, in spite of the ridiculousness of it all, was I aggressively trying to establish a third or fourth place.

The second wave of humiliation hit me like an oven blast, lasting longer than the first by far. I was one of seven who had made the second round—the finals. I was surprised by how humbled we all already seemed, by how obedient we were as we took our instructions in silence. The spit was out of us. Others, too, were bumping into themselves with new awareness. We were to introduce ourselves to 12 new volunteers from the 70 or 80 female conference participants. They sat in two rows. We could say anything that came to mind. Then we were to perform, again doing anything that showed off our talent, while simultaneously parading our beauty before the judges, whose final act was the announcement of the first three winners. I was ranked number two. It was unfair, arbitrary, and meaningless. My performance, I knew, was a complete wash out. By the time my turn came, I was a wreck, an actor with no ego. I hated the exercise with a wrath heated by the half hour of ritual degradation that I had just put myself through. The game had become real, and so, too, had the humiliation. The man ranked number one felt, I would guess, even more vulnerable than me. He had an embarrassingly uncomely physique, and performed no better than the average.)

What Women Do with Power and Work

PENELOPE: In my time, men were absorbed in war, the chase, and the struggle for existence. Upon women fell the responsibility for training the children and transmitting our national customs and traditions from generation to generation.

PAMELA: As in the modern world, civilization was mainly fostered and advanced by women.

PENELOPE: You say that so strangely, as if you reproach us for it.

PAMELA: I don't disapprove of our contributions to civilization, but rather our lack of material contribution to the arts and to the making of history. In your world and in mine patriarchial rule is ubiquitous, and women are wooed away from autonomy and competency.

PENELOPE 2: If I may interpret, Penelope, Pamela proposes that your patriarchal upbringing made you amiable, well-behaved, and moderate and correct in every word and action. And because of these characteristics, men can control any inclinations you might have to freely act in a world dominated by them.

PENELOPE: I did not have those inclinations. Patriarchy, as you put it, reinforced the sanctity of family life—a good thing.

PAMELA: Controlled by the sanctity of family life, you could not even imagine having such inclinations—a not so good thing.

PENELOPE: My purpose was to prepare the children for their futures. Of course, the education of the girls was the simplest. They grew up in their mothers' apartments where they learned, without any formal, intellectual training, everything that seemed necessary for their future career: a modest bearing, skill in needlework, the management of a household, and, above all, reverence for the gods.

PAMELA: By training them in that way you also trained them to unquestionably comply with the brutalities of men. When men rule history, barbarism is inevitable.

PENELOPE 2: But that's not your basic point, Pamela. I agree that there is a great deal of barbarism in the world, and that patriarchal rule is probably to blame. But I don't see a link between patriarchal despotism and the traditional division of labor between the sexes.

PAMELA: I do see a fundamental link between the incessant waves of cruelty that engulf every corner of this earth and masculine rule over the historical process. My second objection to Penelope's views is that such training teaches girls that they have no place in the making of history.

PENELOPE: For children, the early years are full of play and mirth, as they should be; childhood is a time for music, song, and dance for both boys and girls. A strong and enduring mutual love between parents and children comes out of them. Is this not as important as history making?

PENELOPE 2: That explains my decision to leave the domain of work.

PAMELA: . . . For the exclusive responsibility of nurturing.

PENELOPE 2: . . . temporarily and not without attention to my own projects, which I admittedly filtered down in order to leave me free to devote myself to my family. I've had problems with my choice, no mistaking that. I've had uncertainties about my loss of freedom, and I've had my share of battles with my husband about child-care responsibilities. No one option is perfect. But I had an overriding investment in my family, and I wanted to have a controlling hand. Also, I knew the nature of the man I had chosen, and I accepted his limitations, though reluctantly.

PAMELA: What limitations?

PENELOPE 2: Several—the most relevant one here was an irritating, no, an infuriating tendency to trivialize me and my intelligence when he was lost in his work.

PAMELA: Look, Penelope 2, you know my position—this aspect of our sexual arrangement is most obviously unfair. I simply cannot tolerate this overt male monopoly of public power, nor female compliance with this outrageous arrangement.

PENELOPE: We Greek women accepted that men went to war. We did not seriously question our patience, support, and suffering. As a woman, I was vulnerable to the suitors. As a man, he was vulnerable to the vicissitudes of war. When he returned, he demonstrated his old skills and resumed his old authority.

PAMELA: When he returned, you fostered the illusion that he had all the power and control, a reward for his militarism and abandonment. And as a part of the deal, you abandoned your sexual passion.

PENELOPE 2: You say it harshly. What does that have to do with sexual passion?

PAMELA: It's just one more example of how the man gains protection from his vulnerability by forcing the woman to deny her powerful sexuality and desire. In their intimate relations, he is in one very important respect more vulnerable than she is: She can more readily reinvoke in him the powerful and overriding fear of the mother. If he lets her, she can shatter his sexual sense of power and control. She can bring out the helpless child in him. Men try to handle this danger by excluding women, by creating rigid sex roles and sex-segregated institutions, and by devaluing women's contributions. In cooperating with the cover-up of this vulnerability, you assist them in renouncing the opportunity of deep feeling. One way to do this is to keep love superficial, both emotionally and physically, another is to disassociate its physical from its emotional possibilities.

PENELOPE: We took the first course. Sexual passion was not a priority.

PENELOPE 2: We "moderns" take the second course: Sexual passion, emotional depth, and continuity are disassociated from one another, and all from useful work. But not for all of us: My work is important to me and his participation in child rearing has become important to him, though the imbalance you abhor is definitely there.

PAMELA: There have always been women who have coped with this imbalance. But for mother-raised males and females alike, it's hard to view female authority as completely legitimate, even when women are the "bosses." Unable to erase this bias, most women give in and deny themselves power and worldly contribution.

PENELOPE 2: Women I know relinquish claims to authority and accept the supportive role, not because they are forced to but because they choose to.

PAMELA: You say "accept" and "choose." Don't you mean "accede?" Don't most women view the roles men "offer" them as honorable alternatives because they have no real alternatives to speak of?

PENELOPE 2: Not all women and not as many as you think, Pamela. In these times, as more and more women feel free to exercise their creative selves in the world, more and more women will also actively and freely choose a version of the Penelopean role, by balancing contributions to history with nature, community, friendships, play, culture, and meaning.

PAMELA: And primary, if not exclusive, responsibility for early child rearing.

PENELOPE 2: In my case, primary but shared responsibility. Besides, as I keep saying, my individuality is not disregarded or degraded, and I do have projects of my own.

PENELOPE: As I did, but more.

PAMELA: Not to insult you, Penelope, but it seems that you had to listen to men's opinions and keep your own pretty much to yourself.

Odysseus hogged the limelight, and you offered yourself as an audience. Our situation has not changed much. Today a "traditional" woman allows herself activities that nurture a man's projects. She is seen as merely selfish and odd if she insists on pursuing her own endeavors. And if she allows herself an autonomous, competent, and competitive voice, she knows she violates the rules. Some strong and intelligent women manage by guile or heroic tact to find some way of nonetheless allowing the man the position of leader and instructor. When that rule works, both can enjoy the triumph of necessary but complementary roles. The imbalance persists, however, because he is unquestionably boss, leader, teacher, and the one who makes history.

PENELOPE 2: Though my work appeals to me wherever I do it, being "out there" making history by itself does not. I happen to believe that women who want overt power "out there" in the man's world will behave as men do. I don't choose to join that rat race. Don't you see I have no inclination whatsoever to be a leader out there?

PAMELA: Aren't you deliberately playing a trick on yourself? Aren't you making a deal where you delegate your fate to a despotic power, while trying, always vainly, to see it as benevolent and competent?

PENELOPE 2: I am not "dodging" responsibility, and I am not venting my anger, indirectly or unconsciously. When I vent my anger, I vent my anger. Can't I enjoy my competency without "enterprise" and history making? Two things interest me—passions of the moment and emotional connection. If you were to ask me if I would relinquish my competency, in the family and the world, for those two, I would have a hard time of it. Probably, however, I would, though it does not occur to me that I have to. My "Ulyssean" husband has never asked me.

PAMELA: But your gender arrangement requires you to split competency and what you call "the moment." Our society demands that we separate our engagement in the "moment" from our focus on "enterprise." The more sternly we renounce the moment, the more we hate the enterprise for its inevitable failure to compensate for that renunciation. Work is constraint: We lose our direct pleasure in it, we start pushing against the restrictions it imposes, and we idealize and long for the moment.

PENELOPE 2: I recognize that longing.

PAMELA: We handle it by adopting a belief that the world-making enterprise is in some essential ways destructive to us as women. The man takes the main responsibility for keeping that enterprise going, seemingly for the woman's behalf as well as for his own.

PENELOPE 2: Yes, I feel as strongly as you that much of the enterprise in the world can rightly be considered destructive. But I don't feel that the yearning for "the moment" must be segregated from whatever "enterprise" I build into my own life and into my identity. I, or rather we, think of our division of tasks as different but equal contributions to the stability of the family.

PAMELA: In modern times, the status this agreement preserves is becoming increasingly shaky.

PENELOPE 2: Yes, many women find it deadening and for these women, I'm sure, it IS shaky. I've heard them carp, mostly harmlessly, since they remain in marriages they condemn as "deadly."

PAMELA: As that deadliness increases, it becomes less and less possible to keep their running critique harmless and peripheral. It is forced into focal awareness.

PENELOPE 2: When awareness is flooded with discontent . . . .

PAMELA: . . . they may have to leave the marriage.

PENELOPE 2: Yes! Some should. All power to them.

THE CULTURE OF WAITING

What happens when a modern-day Penelope and Odyssesus become intimate. All too often, the man's inaccessibility for sex, according to the woman's schedule, and his unavailability and ineptness as a nurturer for the woman and her children, lead to the withdrawal of sexual interest. What I call the culture of waiting becomes, between today's Penelope and Odysseus, a source of chronic and potentially toxic tension in the male-female tie. The man's psychological absence during periods of intense absorption in his work, and the woman's peacemaking or war-making responses to this absence and return, generates this tension.

I am well aware that, as a male describing the different directions women take in resolving the dilemmas of waiting, I walk on thin ice. To understand how men and women construe the waiting period, we must first understand the role of choice. The conversation between Pamela, Penelope, and Penelope 2 has illustrated and contrasted different approaches to the woman's waiting role. Armed with this understanding, we can then explore the three options available to women and men in dealing with the sexual tension that threatens intimacy during this crucial waiting period. But first I wish to discuss a central question: What factors determine whether men and women, once they discover gender difference, avoid, overcome, or give in to disappointment and its destructive effects on sexual intimacy.

The Hero's Search: The Transcendence of Difference through Compassion

The Odysseus–Penelope myth, the most traditional of gender arrangements, is a metaphor for the search for fulfillment. If unimpeded by the psychological quandary of loss of other or sacrifice to other, that is, if both do what they do *by choice*, each reaches a deeper metaphysical level, one step closer to self-realization. It is a lonely psychological journey, much of which must be done alone. Because the man's and the woman's spiritual trajectories pull in different directions, the separation can strain commitment and the sense of mutuality. Yet if each agrees to the mythic contract, and gives his or her blessing to the other's search, neither need be entirely alone.

At a second level, the myth is a metaphor for transcendence; for ultimately, the searcher encounters his or her self in the depths and experiences self-realization. But this is not enough. In order to deal with an intimate other and to rejoin the outer world, one must transcend the self in coming back. One must also transcend difference, for both have been waiting, and the waiting other is more different at the time of ascent than descent. Upon greeting Odysseus on his return, does Penelope recognize her husband as the man who journeyed afar? She does, but with difficulty. She also needs the help of her servant. My suspicion about the validity of their mythic contract rests with the fact that Odysseus does not face the same dilemma in greeting Penelope and fails to ask whether she has been on a journey of her own. The ancient patriarch did not need to, of course. Nonetheless, Odysseus does find that Penelope has not been idle during his absence; her weaving and her suitors occupied her night and day. Are these the symbols of her sexual self-interest? By slaying the suitors, does Odysseus stamp out the passions of Penelope's self-interest? Homer's story is metaphorically weak at this point. The modern couple cannot afford to be.

Today, men and women, both *together* and *alone*, must face the challenge and the threat to intimacy that hangs over the waiting period. The culture of waiting is not a curse visited upon women by absent men. It is an environment naturally created whenever two people attempt intimacy. The culture of waiting, then, comes with the territory of love.

Although the man and the woman have little command over the advent and haunting presence of waiting, they do have a hand in the quality and texture of their lives while they struggle for love's survival during it. They can at least positively shape the nature of the waiting by being compassionate. As each embarks on his or her own spiritual journey in the search for self-realization, this compassion for difference serves as an ever-shining beacon to help guide the way. During each partner's own descent and return, the other is expected to be there with a particular look, feel, and presence, different for each partner and different from other possible partners, but with a loving hand, the hand of the companion, the hand of a gender opposite. Over the course of the journey, terrible questions inevitably arise: Is this the hand I took? Is the feel of it really right for me? Is it stronger than I wished? Softer? Too desperate in its hold? And why did it seem to let go when I needed it most? These are the challenges to what I have called the first mythic contract—the gender contract.

Not all partners set out upon a hero's journey, and it matters beyond measure to the survival or failure of intimacy whether both, one, or neither partner does so. The worst cases of failed intimacy are ones in which neither the woman nor the man embarks on a hero's journey. Boredom and a passive waiting for (spiritual or physical) death are two of the ill-fated consequences of this disastrous arrangement. Problematic, although not to the same extent, is the arrangement in which one partner, but not the other, pursues the hero's journey. The confusion men, women, and therapists experience about this arrangement does indeterminate damage to intimate relationships. If they themselves are devoid of the concept of the *search*, they misconstrue the searcher's intellectually, spiritually, or psychologically important behavior as mundane, vacuous, or emotionally maimed.

Tests of Adequacy

Certain searing questions confront each partner during the period of waiting: Am I satisfied with my choice of mate? With his or her mythic characteristics? With the gender contract I have made? In all, I have identified three criteria, call them "tests of adequacy," that help to answer these gnawing questions about the gender arrangement, and which influence how couples (primarily women in the "traditional gender arrangement") resolve the dilemma posed by the culture of waiting.

The first test questions whether the couple is matched or mismatched in their gender ideals. An Odysseus and a Penelope are matched and a Helen and a Menelaus are matched. A Helen and a Paris, however, are mismatched. This test of adequacy has no societal standard of measurement: The individuals decide, alone or together, what a good match is. Although individuals base their gender ideals on choices provided by the culture, these external standards are irrelevant to the partners' private perceptions of the match. Matching can be "complimentary" (unbalanced) or it can be "synchronous" (balanced). Which type an individual chooses is determined by inner constraints only.

Under the best of circumstances, each partner has fully examined his or her own inner-directed gender ideal and the gender ideal of the mate, and found the match to his or her liking. Unfortunately, this is not what happens in most intimate relationships. Most people are not aware of their gender ideals when they sign on. (I say "sign on" rather than "choose" because people often stumble into choices.) Some people respond to societal pressures; others simply accept where they find themselves in life; and, of course, some are moved by the force of a personal or sexual fantasy myth that holds sway over the gender myth.

The second test of adequacy naturally follows the first: Does the chosen gender arrangement excite each partner sexually? I believe that there are three distinct sexual contracts that couples make and though all three come together to form the totality of any couples' sexual experience, they make separate contributions to that experience. Some couples sustain sexual interest solely on the strength of matched gender ideals, when the other two mythic contracts (personal and sexual) are either under siege or have been dissolved.

I have already discussed the third test of adequacy: the undertaking of the search itself. Individuals who, in the quest for intimacy, commit themselves to a long-term relationship, with its golden promises and deep purple trials, face a characteristic dilemma: Whether to set out upon a search for self-realization outside the relationship (in work, for example) or within it (in the family, for example), or to forego such a search because of the demands it places on the self or because of the threats it poses to the relationship. I have made my bias clear: If neither partner undertakes such a search, boredom or *death-waiting* results.

If only one partner undertakes the search, the one who does not must decide what to do about his or her sex, passion, power, and competency during the period of waiting. While the searching partner "descends into the depths," and thereby becomes psychologically and sexually absent, the mythic contract is put to its severest test. Few such gender arrangements escape without some cuts and bruises. Stress arises from the uncertainty of whether the romantic spirit of unity will be so compromised during the journeyer's search for self that the partner's love will have dissipated. When both partners independently undertake a search for self (in work or family), the relationship is similarly stressed, but less so than when neither or only one partner undertakes the journey. The couple does create an environment of waiting, but one more likely to be characterized by a tolerantly intolerant sense of postponement than by stridency or death-waiting. For ideally, in this gender format, support is available for each during the descent into the depths, and the return from the depths prepares each for a mutual appreciation of differences. When both partners undertake a search for self, the sense of satisfaction and adequacy each feels with the mythic contract receives a boost.

Three Resolutions to Waiting

Couples must eventually resolve the dilemma they face when struggling to maintain intimacy during the time of waiting. Three ways of defining the experience are open to them: This period can be described and experienced as a culture of abundance, a culture of adequacy, or a culture of deprivation. How the couple fares with the three tests of adequacy plays a decisive role in which of the three descriptions they will use to view their relationship. Insofar as these descriptions work so does the mythic gender contract, and sexual interest will remain intact.

The Culture of Abundance

The ancient Penelope of the earlier conversation and Odysseus lived in a perfect mythic *culture of abundance*. Penelope endured her husband's long absence, remained faithful, and, on his return, welcomed him to his rightful place. As for Odysseus, yearning for wife, home, and family, but driven off-course by fate, the whims of competitive gods, and his own need for adventure, it never occurred to him that his place would not be waiting there for him.

With regard to the first test of adequacy, Penelope and Odysseus pass with high marks—they are well-matched in a complementary gender arrangement. Odysseus wears well the garments of patriarchal power and authority, and Penelope honors and respects this authority while wearing her own as educator, guardian of culture, and manager of the household. Questioning was neither her right nor her way. How does the Penelope—Odysseus pair fare with the second test which asks, Does the gender arrangement excite each partner sexually? Penelope emphatically places herself in the abundancy camp.

In the preceding dialogue we asked: What does Penelope do with sex, lust, and passion during the time of waiting? The ancient world's answer would be, She does not assign high priority to sex and passion. Is this the case, then, for modern women who "choose" the traditional gender arrangement? Or does this arrangement neccessarily create conditions of neglect, attrition, and frustration in the sexual realm?

To go by my own studies of nonclinical couples and families, the answer is decidedly "no." Many of these "satisfied" couples seem to sustain their sexual interest despite the psychologically absent mate because that interest is embedded in those same institutionalized roles and relations. "What appeals to me," they say along with Penelope, "is the very idea of being with a man who is out there exploring the world." The traditional gender arrangement does not necessarily create conditions of sexual neglect, frustration, and attrition. Indeed, the hero's absence and his very journey may lead to a bristling sexual anticipation and a flowering sexual readiness.

The third test of adequacy is, unlike the other two, externally imposed. For the *sense of abundance* to hold up over time, the relationship must also have depth, which is most richly acquired if both the man and the woman embark on an independent spiritual quest—if each takes the hero's journey, if each succeeds in the search for self-realization, if each has the blessings of the other during the journey, and if, in coming back, each not only transcends self but difference as well. The compassion for otherness that develops overcomes the strain put on commitment and mutuality when the man's and the woman's trajectories pull in different directions. If all this happens, the time of waiting, for all its uncertainties and strains, will serve to strengthen rather than weaken the sense of mutuality and autonomy that defines a successful quest for intimacy.

At bedrock, choice determines the nature of the culture of waiting. With regard to the third test of adequacy—whether neither, one, or both partners undertake a hero's search—most feminist activists would belittle Penelope's search, because it appears to take place without visible or viable alternatives. *Choice* to them implies the right or privilege of choosing freely between alternatives. The ancient Penelope did not have this option. Power to choose between alternatives rested exclusively in patriarchy, and men did not grant such choice to women. Nevertheless, Penelope claimed to choose freely; that is, she not only cooperated in these politics of choice, she appeared guided in this judgment by psychological preference. Modern Penelopes (e.g., Penelope 2) do, of course, have the right to choose between alternatives, and some choose as Penelope did, free of political resistance or psychological conflict. Modern Penelopes, as was the case with Homer's Penelope, if they pass all three tests of adequacy, can establish the possibility that a period of waiting will be accompanied by a sense of abundance.

The Culture of Adequacy

Whereas Homer's Penelope willingly and uncomplainingly muted her own sexual drive while waiting for Odysseus' return, Penelope 2 did not. Whereas the original Penelope remained faithful, Penelope 2 had a brief passionate affair, which she then voluntarily gave up. Reading between the lines, Penelope 2 had no trouble separating her tender and sensual feelings for her husband from her purely lustful feelings for a lover.

Fortunately for Penelope 2, the Ulyssean man she married had not split off tenderness and affection from sensuality and passion. Modern Penelopean types tend to have trouble with men in whom this split prevails. Sexually, Penelope 2 wanted it all: tenderness, sensuality, and passion. Her mythic gender ideal might have been a man like Hector and her husband's a replica of Hector's tender, feminine wife Andromache, an accomplished beauty like Athena. Thus, this couple's gender arrangement satisfied two of the three tests of adequacy which determine the nature of waiting: They had matched gender ideals and the images associated with these ideals helped to sustain a high degree of sexual interest during the period of waiting.

With regard to the third test (who embarks on a hero's journey), Penelope 2's career compromise ruins the couple's overall score. Splitting herself between work and family inevitably muddled Penelope 2's commitment to self and other. Perhaps this is a modern woman's journey: to solve the perplexing riddle of discovering how to do both. Because Penelopes often have "two natures," their spiritual journeys can either tear them in two or immobilize them. Consequently, some delay or never embark on a heroic journey. Their satisfaction with the sexual arrangement may erode away as a result. What saves a Penelope's interest is her remarkable compassion for others—if anything, she has too much compassion—a great sign of love. Nevertheless, her dilemma over what to do while waiting and the way she resolves it, defines her situation as a culture of adequacy.

The Culture of Deprivation

Rebecca's plain-rimmed glasses and don't-look-at-me makeup and hairstyle draw attention to her repressed sexuality. During therapy, Carlton, her fiftyish, balding, and boyish-looking husband sits gawkishly spread-eagled in the defiantly unattractive chinos and satin athletic-club jackets usually worn by working-class teenagers. As a fully tenured professor at a local university, he acknowledges having taken "more than" one step down from illustrious Harvard, where he started his promising academic career 25 years ago.

"We don't fuck enough, that's our problem. And when we do, the path I'm asked to take is so dangerously mined with 'Don't do that,' 'That's wrong for me,' 'That hurts' that it feels god-damned lousy," he whines like a teenager. And then, in contrast, he says, "Her inconsolable complexity is what continues to draw me to her most." This is said with the twang of the in-charge professor. Then about his mother he says, "I knew she liked being 'out there' where she was powerful enough to attract a lover who had worldwide fame, that she merely 'played at' being a good mother and good wife. She was neither."

"He can make love two or three times a day," Rebecca intones sadly, "but I get the feeling that I am invisible. It makes me sad enough to cry." (*And she does cry, each time she says this.*) "That's one of the reasons we don't make love." Eight years ago, Rebecca had "lost" her orgasm and with that she gave up all sexual interest in Carlton. Carlton's and Rebecca's gender ideals for self and other were provocatively mismatched. Nevertheless, it took couples therapy, after 25 years of marriage, to reveal the deadly effects which that previously unexamined mismatch had wrought on their sexual relations. In moving revelations, Carlton and Rebecca shared their ideals:

CARLTON: In the Cambridge years, I was full of myself, and saw myself as the original Renaissance Man—art, literature, architecture . . . nothing was outside the grasp of my hungry intellect. Though it was not the kind of thing I shared with you, each day I awoke to the blossom of my pride, and nothing would suit me better than to make love with you in its sweet fragrance. What I wanted from you . . . ? (*Because he'd never thought to ask, I fed him the line: a Penelope of sorts to your intellectually adventuring Ulyssean–Renaissance Man.*) "Not quite Penelope, because I wanted her with me . . . (*Imposing my mythic tools a bit too strongly: Athena, perhaps? She was herself accomplished in all the arts of life. She directed and encouraged all mental activity.*) Well, Athena more than Penelope. It sounds selfish to me now, but I just wanted you to be there and to have you with me. But you resisted, so I took in everything Cambridge/Harvard had to offer.

REBECCA: By yourself, because I hated Cambridge. I hated every moment I spent there; I hated every moment you spent there. But that doesn't mean I wasn't proud of your accomplishments; I just wanted you home more.

(*Rebecca revealed gender ideals similar to Penelope 2's but without the split between family and work. I think Rebecca would have wanted to play an Andromache to Carlton's Hector. Like Andromache, Rebecca is a gentle, modest, and affectionate woman. When she married, she was sure she'd realized the dream of joining her devotion to husband and family with his ability to participate nobly in the world while seeking his real happiness in a "well-founded house."*)

Although claiming that, through therapy, they had become more intimate, Carlton and Rebecca's intimacy level was low when they began couples therapy. And their sexual interest was meeting its death.

Carlton found their gender arrangement quite adequate, but not because of shared gender ideals. He had not searched and found Rebecca's ideal mythic choice for *herself* to be to his liking; rather he was, as he himself said, so full of himself (e.g., the Renaissance Man) that he never questioned or engaged Rebecca's deeper images at all.

Rebecca, for her part, never consciously challenged the gender mismatch or considered what it meant to her. During the first year or so of marriage, she seemed the more sexually liberated of the two. If he was the more aggressive (his compulsive sexual interest exceeded her apparently normal interest during that early period), she was the more inventive (to his delight, for example, she'd daringly hold his penis, not his hand, in a darkened theatre). Soon, however, the mythic gender arrangement began to lose its original appeal. Rebecca began to feel frustrated with Carlton's happy absorption in career and work. Restless with her increasing loneliness, she felt that her personal depths remained untapped and stagnant. On petty grounds, she fought his unavailability, but by continuing to make love on his schedule, she at once misled him and accelerated the centrally important *process of disappointment*. The process of disappointment gained momentum when Rebecca no longer saw Carlton as sexually appealing.

With regard to the third criterion, this couple again scored low: Rebecca evidenced no involvement in a hero's journey beyond her deep investment in family and place. This became painfully clear when Rebecca spoke in the melancholy tones of loss about how she had deeply and desperately longed for a place in the country. To her, country life was the essence of "family" and "the intimate life." Carlton had refused outright: "It clashed with my image of the Renaissance Man," he said. "Being in the country was totally antithetical to my image." Carlton believed he would have to give up part or all of his journey, and was unwilling to do so to support Rebecca's search. "I had no place and needed one," Rebecca said wistfully. Carlton countered: "I needed no place to fulfill *my* identity." Such "tragedies of love" can propel the environment of waiting into a culture of deprivation.

Rebecca's yearning for place; her commitment to family; and her fierce wish for a partner who wanted to share both place and family with her indicate that early on she might have intended to embark on a search of her own. But she lost heart and direction, in part because she wasn't conscious of her options until too late and because Carlton offered little cooperation or compassion for her desires. One would have to conclude that Rebecca's and Carlton's gender arrangement did not grant her the liberty to conduct such a search.

Carlton, on the other hand, may have started out on one; there is some small evidence that he was aware of having been on a journey he never completed. But at that point, he claimed the image of the Renaissance Man is all but gone. My career has reached a plateau lower than I dreamed. But if you asked me today to give up what's left of it, I would do it for the sake of our relationship."

Disappointment

Gender contracts unavoidably lead to some disillusionment. How each couple creates and manages this disillusionment ultimately determines whether each will experience the environment of waiting as a culture of abundance, adequacy, or deprivation. When disappointment persists and is unrelieved, gender contracts get broken. Thus it is one of the pivotal forces in sexual withdrawal. Rebecca and Carlton failed on all three of the tests of adequacy. Thus, sexual disappointment, which every couple faces as a possible consequence of the quest for intimacy, became a reality for them.

From Rebecca, and men and women like her, I learned that while waiting we resurrect childhood experiences of grief, loss, and sacrifice during the spiritual disasters of adult relationships. When these sentiments of grief, loss, and sacrifice become dominant themes in an adult intimate relationship, they drive a wedge in the relationship and its mythic gender ideals—reality disturbs the couple's professed ideals for the relationship. The couple experiences this disturbance as a profound disillusionment; its disappointment hits them with the impact of a spiritual disaster.

Rebecca experienced this disaster as she saw her environment of waiting change, by degrees, from a garden of promising hope to a field of dense disappointment. She recounted a process typical of what other women (and men) report in therapy: "It was like participating in the building of your own house of horror and not being able to put the tools of destruction down." Although the impacts of disillusionment are cumulative, they are recalled as singularly shocking moments. Tracking the three that Rebecca singled out will help us to see how her gender myths were dismantled while "her house of horror" was being built.

A Stranger in My Bed

Because Rebecca was not herself involved in a hero's journey in the world of work, it was logical that she should want to explore her own resources in the private world of emotional intimacy. Carlton was a lustful lover, but he knew little, she felt, of the tender and sensual side of things. Important as lust was, more crucial was the gathering sense of powerlessness she felt while postponing her own sexual impulses. In unknowing innocence, Carlton believed, during this period, that Rebecca was taking vicarious pride in his academic accomplishments. He remained unaware that she had emotional demands and sexual rhythms of her own.

After years of denying that something was seriously wrong, her illusion that he was her ideal lover began to dissolve. In an attempt to undo her frightened grief, she sought out situations that intensified her own pleasure-giving, wish-granting needs, and tried in this way to retrieve some part of the lost delight of fulfilling sex. This compensation did not work for long; soon the disturbing sense of loss returned, especially during those times when she reached out in hope of company, and he didn't notice.

One morning, awaking to his familiar sexual arousal, and unable to respond because of feelings of loss, she reached the conclusion that there was a stranger in her bed. The patterning for sexual disappointment and the eventual breaking of the gender contract had begun.

The Absence of the Loving, Smiling Hector

The second shock of disillusionment occurred later, when Rebecca's first born, Ted, was 14 years old and beginning to show signs of emotional difficulty:

> I was responsible for everything. For shoes and teeth, of course, but I expected that. But for loving and disciplining; I did not expect that. Ted was becoming a tyrant—soiling or spoiling everything he touched. He had no friends, other kids avoided him, even Rex (his younger brother by 2 years) was embarrassed by his antics. At 15, Ted was a full-blown iconoclast—a

destroyer of images and institutions. He hated school, friendships, and family. I was staggered by the irony—I who loved family so much.

I had all I could do not to hate him, to pay him back for his hating. But he was in trouble and I needed your company, your attendance, your council, and your participation in a growing mess. I could not get you to turn around and look, much less comfort me in my growing confusion.

I was alone in all this. Until our trip to Paris, that is, when you had no choice. When Ted caused that embarrassing stir in Customs and disappeared for 2 hours, your abuse was for me, not him, and you had no compassion for either of us. Somehow you turned everything around—comaraderie between you and the boys, exclusion and isolation for me. In that episode, I recognized a pattern that continues to this day. Your bond with them is through a hatred of women. They hate family. They hate marriage. They are confused about women—ridiculing and sneering at women's issues. When they act this way, it brings them closer to you. When they ignore me and direct all their conversation at you as if I do not exist, they think they are making up for the dreadful things I do to you.

Rebecca's dreams of a loving, tightly knit family unit with a home in the country, guided by the gentle and affectionate hand of a woman and supported by a tender and attentive spouse, became a horrible and frightening nightmare of loss, grief, and excruciating disappointment.

The Brave Hero Shrinks

The third shock of disillusionment over gender ideals came 2 years after the Paris episode, when Rebecca and the children spent a year abroad in an exotic Third World country. With the assistance of a group of younger colleagues, Carlton was doing a joint project with one of the best-known authorities in his field while on sabbatical. Until this time, Rebecca had merely avoided facing her animosity toward the world of Carlton's work. Now, however, she could not escape. Every evening after the day's work, there was a ritual gathering of the researchers and their respective spouses and children in a predinner social hour.

Rebecca was aghast at what she saw. Although second only to his older superior in official status, Carlton did not act the part. The "social hour" turned out to be an opportunity for the senior sage to hold forth and show his intellectual prowess. It was also an opportunity for the others to show their mastery. Although the younger colleagues took up the sage's challenge, Carlton did not. He sat, in what Rebecca saw as obsequious silence, at the sage's feet, while the younger men jousted daringly, "on their feet" intellectually.

Carlton lost credibility: He was not the brave warrior and noble patriot who, in anguish over Andromache's plea to avoid a battle certain to make a widow of her, said: "I do take thought of all these things, my wife, but I have very sure shame of the Trojans . . . if, like a coward, I shrink from battle." Despite Andromache's tragic fate, Rebecca might have preferred it to her own tragedy. Noble hero and warrior, loving father, and tender spouse were all attributes of Hector that Rebecca mythically idealized and sought in Carlton. During Carlton's sabbatical, this final mythic illusion was shattered.

When they returned home, Rebecca began to notice these same "weaknesses" in Carlton on occasion after occasion. He was finally judged guilty for committing gender crimes. Rebecca's body carried out the sexual sentence—her sexual interest waned.

An Afterword

In therapy, Carlton redeemed himself. He did not attack Rebecca, nor defend himself, nor even offer "other explanations" unless Rebecca asked for them. He was more than ever committed to the marriage, he said. The hungry scholar of his youth, still within him, wanted to know everything—most of all, how Rebecca's loss of sexual interest had come about. He learned, and is continuing to learn, much about his own aborted hero's journey and about his own sexuality.

The most valuable insight Carlton gained regarding his own sexuality occurred when for a time he lost his own sexual interest. Starting to pay more attention to his own sexual frustration, Carlton became more tender. He discovered that he had never had a clear mythic ideal for his wife. When he considered the consequences of this failed opportunity, he understood what it was to experience loss, disappointment, and withdrawal of sexual interest. For Carlton, this loss of sexual interest moved him a step forward in his construction and choice of a female mythic ideal, a process he should have begun before his marriage to Rebecca.

REFERENCES

Bellow, S. (1984). *Seize the Day*. New York: Penguin.

Bolen, J. S. (1985). *Goddesses in everywoman: A new psychology of woman*. New York: Harper & Row.

Campbell, J. (1949). *The hero with a thousand faces*. Princeton, NJ: Princeton University Press.

Campbell, J. (1968). *The masks of god.* New York: Penguin.

Campbell, J. (1972). *Myths to live by.* New York: Bantam.

Klaven, A. (May 24, 1988). Joseph Campbell, myth master. *The Village Voice,* pp. 57–64.

Kunitz, S. (February 22, 1987). The quest for the father. *New York Times Book Review,* pp. 1, 36–38.

Lifton, R. J. (1987). *The future of immortality and other essays for a nuclear age.* New York: Basic Books.

Perry, W. C. (1898). *The women of Homer.* New York: Dodd, Mead.

Sartre, J. P. (1964). *The words.* New York: Braziller.

Stoller, R. J. (1979). *Sexual excitement.* New York: Pantheon.

11

THE SEXUAL GENOGRAM: ASSESSING FAMILY-OF-ORIGIN FACTORS IN THE TREATMENT OF SEXUAL DYSFUNCTION

Larry Hof and Ellen M. Berman

The field of family therapy has had considerable difficulty acknowledging sexuality as an organizing force in family life. In breaking from the Freudian position, with its central focus on oedipal struggles and sexual drive states, to focus on system and context, family therapy has chosen a neutral—indeed, avoidant—attitude toward sexuality in general.

Sexuality is a central binding and organizing force in the life of a couple, enabling them to break from their family of origin to form a dyad. In addition, gender-based sex-role behavior contributes greatly to the structure of life within the new dyad. However, a search of three classic texts in the family therapy field (Boszormenyi-Nagy & Spark, 1973; Framo, 1982; Minuchin, 1974), as a representative sample, reveals a total of about four pages devoted to sexuality, most in case examples with no accompanying theoretical discussion. Boszormenyi-Nagy and Spark (1973) did briefly describe a case of sexual dysfunction related to unresolved guilt over disloyalty to parents.

For the authors cited, the lack of a specific focus on sexual issues was primarily because they were interested in developing other salient aspects

Larry Hof. Marriage Council of Philadelphia, Philadelphia, Pennsylvania; Department of Psychiatry, University of Pennsylvania, Philadelphia, Pennsylvania.

Ellen M. Berman. Department of Psychiatry, University of Pennsylvania Medical School, Philadelphia, Pennsylvania.

of their new theories. In addition, sexual dysfunction was viewed, in these texts at least, as part of a larger, systemic problem. It is notable, and rather discomforting, that, as the years progressed, the important issues relating to sexuality as a specific dimension of family functioning were left almost exclusively to the sex therapists.

Sexuality and sex-role development are also certainly major concerns in the life of the developing child. The literature on human sex education and child development is extensive, but it is organized around traditional models of Freudian, cognitive, and behaviorally learned responses. There has also been much work on cross-cultural sexual attitudes and behaviors. Although it is obvious from this work that much sexual learning is from direct interaction between parents and children, the models presented and discussed are basically nonsystemic in nature. There is little sense of how specific patterned behaviors and attitudes are carried from generation to generation, or how different children in a family can embody different aspects of their parents' sexuality.

The concept of sexual scripting as presented by Gagnon (1977) is one apparent exception to this general trend in the human sexuality education literature. Although he primarily emphasizes the concept of cultural scripts, he at least devotes some attention to the interactive nature of scripts between partners and, very minimally, discusses scripts developed and transmitted between familial generations.

It is interesting to note that writers strongly influenced by the Transactional Analysis school of therapy (e.g., James & Jongeward, 1971; Steiner, 1974), on the other hand, strongly emphasize the interactive nature of scripts between partners and scripts developed and transmitted between familial generations (usually limited to two generations). These writers, however, generally fail to develop the sexual aspects of such scripting processes. The one notable exception is Wyckoff's (1974) work, which focuses on sex-role scripting in men and women but does not address the issue of sexual dysfunction at all.

In some ways, Wyckoff's (1974) work was representative of the beginning attempts to link sociocultural aspects of human sexuality with intergenerational (two-generation) messages and/or scripts and the consequent effects on male–female interactions. Since Transactional Analysis developed from more dynamically oriented roots, the rich potential for further development of Wyckoff's (and others') ideas through interaction with the family therapy schools was not fulfilled because at that early date there was simply too much myopic parochialism on all sides to permit cooperative cross-fertilization of ideas and techniques.

In the sexuality education literature, there is also little reference made to family therapy and its possible relationship to sexuality issues in families or the lives of individuals. A review of four commonly used college texts in human sexuality (Doyle, 1985; Gagnon, 1977; Gagnon & Greenblatt, 1978; Victor, 1980) reveals a total of three pages devoted to family therapy, and even then it is not described in the context of sexual problems. Further, Framo (1982), Minuchin (1974), and Boszormenyi-Nagy and Spark (1973) are each cited only once.

Sexual problems and/or dysfunctions are also family-related issues, and they are not minor problems in the general population or in couples requesting therapy. Several studies have suggested that over 50% of couples have at least some complaints about their sex life, or a specific sexual dysfunction. Yet, family therapists, including those who work primarily with couples, have been so uneasy with this topic, and/or so preoccupied with other issues, that an entire subspecialty, sex therapy, has been developed to fill this void. While practitioners of this subspecialty have done great service in integrating physiological information about sexuality with basic issues of education, learning theory, and dynamic psychiatry, a negative effect has been further fragmentation of the field. To some extent, simple sex therapy techniques have been rendered with an aura of mystery, which has made it even harder to incorporate them into usual family therapy approaches. Sex therapists, on the other hand, seldom use three-generation considerations in their work. Kaplan (1974, 1979, 1983), for example, makes extensive use of dynamic material but utilizes few concepts from Bowen, Framo, and so forth.

We believe that family therapy theory has much to offer in the treatment of sexual issues and dysfunctions, and that sex therapy has much to offer to family therapy in terms of both theory and treatment. It is the thesis of this chapter that sexuality is best understood within the context of family theory, particularly those theories involved with family structure and three-generation transmission of loyalties and myths, as well as the more familiar dyadic issues of power, intimacy, and sex-role learning. This chapter reviews salient issues in the field, as part of a beginning integration of sexuality into family theory. As an example of clinical integration, we offer a method of exploring a person's three-generation sexual history that links their sexual issues to wider issues of family structure and loyalty. The specific technique described, the sexual genogram (Hof & Berman, 1986) and family journey—which builds on the work of Bowen, Framo, and others—has been found particularly useful in the treatment of a wide variety of sexual dysfunctions, as well as enables a deeper understanding of the couple's issues of intimacy and gender.

THEORETICAL ISSUES REGARDING SEX AND THE FAMILY

Sexuality is a biological given whose function in humans includes not only reproduction but affectional bonding, which offers additional biological advantages for the species. Because all biologically based behaviors in people became elaborated in complex symbolic ways, sex becomes transformed as well into a set of ideas about self and others. Sexuality is particularly confusing in this culture because it links so intimately and obviously our most basic biology with our highest and most complicated feelings and ideals, such as love, and our deepest sense of self, which is as much sexual as otherwise. This section examines the ways in which the affectional bonding produced by sexuality affects the family and the ways in which the transmission of ideas about sex by the family affect subsequent bonding.

Sex and Family Structure

The need for appropriate boundaries and a functioning hierarchy has been a major concern of family therapists, especially those of the structural school (Minuchin, 1974). Well-functioning, intact families maintain relationships with previous generations, with clear, appropriate, flexible boundaries and a clear hierarchy between grandparents, parents, and children. So-called single-parent families, where there may be a wide variety of part-time or alternate-generation caretakers, must establish their own system of maintaining boundaries and hierarchy. What is seldom mentioned is that sexuality plays a major part in the maintenance of such a hierarchy.

Parents' sexual behavior, a private activity that is known about (an open secret) but is neither witnessed nor for the most part discussed with the children, is proof of the parents' separateness and the inability of the children to take the place of an adult partner. The parents' closed door, a major symbol of the separation of generations in this culture, is most likely to be enforced not by a parental wish for privacy while reading, but for privacy while being intimate and especially sexual. The parents' ability to have a sexual relationship serves as a generational marker, proving their adulthood both to their own parents and to their children. Their willingness and ability to impart sexual information and values to their children, while helping them to delay expressions of some aspects of sexuality until developmentally appropriate, is a necessary part of parenting and both expresses and maintains appropriate family structure.

A lack of effective sexual expression or the presence of sexual dysfunction between the members of the dyad renders the couple more open to cross-generational coalition. Conversely, cross-generational coalition and the forces that produce it may render a couple more vulnerable to sexual dysfunction. Such coalitions, traditionally between the parent who experiences himself as more helpless and a "helpless" child, may often have a strong sexual component that will powerfully affect the internal life of the next generation.

> *Case 1.* Ben, a man in his thirties, entered therapy for marital issues related to being "too close to his mother." He also reported lack of sexual desire, although not impotence. History revealed that his parents had been unhappily married and that his mother had poured her energy into Ben, who was breast fed for 4 years and was permitted to sleep between his parents at will. His father had essentially "abandoned the field" and spent little time with his son. In therapy, Ben's fear of being disloyal to his mother, and possibly contributing to a divorce if he abandoned her, emerged with great turmoil.

A family structure of cross-generational and cross-sex coalition, such as just described, encourages the development of internal conflicts in the child at what is traditionally called the oedipal stage. The family model emphasizes the part of all three members in the development of these issues in the child. In addition, such a structure will later produce severe loyalty conflicts in the child, which continue into adulthood.

Couples in the process of divorce may have major structural problems around intimacy and sexuality. During the extremely stressful period of separation and the early postdivorce period, a parent may lean inordinately on one or all of the children. It is common to find that, during a separation or divorce, one child begins to sleep with one of the parents. This behavior is stressful and confusing for both child and parent, and indeed is doubly stressful because eventually the parent will choose to return to adult sexuality and attempt to remove the child from the bed.

> *Case 2.* Debbie, the 9-year-old eldest child of divorcing parents, said she wanted to "sleep with Daddy, so he won't be so lonely." Besides, she said, "I'm afraid to be alone at night." Her father experienced conflict regarding the request, but nevertheless permitted his daughter to sleep with him for 5 months on weekend visits. When he started to date again, Debbie was enraged and refused to stay with him on weekends. She expressed strong resentment toward "Daddy's girlfriend" and felt "more lonely than ever." With insight beyond her years, she mused, "I guess little girls can never win."

Following a divorce, both parents must negotiate issues around dating and forming other sexual relationships. Arguments over hierarchy may be remarkably worsened when a teenage child just beginning to explore her own sexuality is living with a single parent who is just beginning to date again. These tremendous concerns about parent and child sexuality are often hidden beneath arguments over minor matters of dating such as curfews, thus avoiding the very real issue of what it means to both child and parent to be exploring their sexuality at different points in the life cycle, where one is still responsible for the other.

> *Case 3.* Anne and Bobby, two siblings, aged 14 and 16, had been sexually active with their respective boyfriend and girlfriend. When the two were confronted by their recently divorced parents, they replied, "Why shouldn't we be allowed to have sex before we're married? You two are sleeping with your lovers, and you're not even married." The parents' reply was, "We're adults, and you are simply too young." Needless to say, the children were not satisfied with the reply, and the subsequent argument led to some much-needed family therapy for this "divorced family" of four.

The most serious markers of dysfunction involving sex and family structure include cases of actual incest, which have been treated in the literature with considerable detail, and sexual intrusiveness, which has been less well described. Sexual intrusiveness is here defined as the activity of a parent who becomes excessively involved in the child's sexual development to the point of, for example, bathing a 12-year-old child, giving frequent enemas, or demanding gynecological examinations in order to "find out the truth" about the child's sex life.

> *Case 4.* Martha, a 37-year-old female, told of having to give her mother a "blow-by-blow" account of every date when she was a teenager, even being pushed to divulge details regarding "how far" they went. In her marriage, Martha felt sexually inhibited with her husband, and it was having a serious impact upon their sexual enjoyment. In therapy, the lack of privacy when she was growing up and her mother's intrusiveness were identified as the sources of an ever present "brake" on Martha's spontaneity in the sexual area. The brake enabled her to avoid embarrassment, punishment, or rejection, and to protect her own sense of self and power as a teenager. When she was helped to identify how her relationship with her mother was present in her mind in her current sex life, she was able to set more effective boundaries with her mother in other areas of her life, contributing greatly to the resolution of the sexual problem.

The therapist working with an adult couple must be able to reestablish the structure in the family of origin, by taking a client history or interviewing other family members. In this regard, the genogram techniques described later in this chapter are particularly helpful. The therapist working with cases in which the therapy includes adolescents or children must focus primarily on the family's structure, but within that one must also consider the effects of sexual issues on the structure and consider the sex itself as a substantive content issue. A therapist's willingness to deal directly with the sexual issues, rather than with the peripheral issues of curfew, room cleaning, disobedience, and so forth, is extremely important, since both parents and children tend to be reluctant to deal with sexual issues directly, even when these are uppermost in their thoughts. The therapist's ability to discuss sexuality directly opens the possibility for parents and children to have more appropriate communication.

Sex and the Family Life Cycle

If sex within the dyad is a strong binding force, allowing a new family to develop out of the two families of origin, the developing sexuality of the children may be considered "subversive," albeit developmentally necessary. That is, the child's sexual urges move his life, both in fantasy and reality, away from that of his parents and into his own. The preschool child who learns to masturbate in private and who develops nonspecific but nevertheless sensually related feelings about other children is learning that it is possible for her to be a private and separate person with boundaries that her parents cannot breach. In the teen years, the crucial marker of adolescence and movement into adulthood is the sex hormone related physical development, and the subsequent intense erotic/intimate impulses allow the teenager to move the emotional focus out of the home and begin to attach elsewhere. This normal developmental event can be impacted in many ways by parents, who may have their own unresolved sexual issues and be overly fascinated or frightened by the child's development. In the face of this tremendous concern in both the teenager and parents, it is all the more remarkable how seldom these issues are discussed in therapy unless the child is specifically acting out sexually.

Obviously, sexual issues can be hidden by other issues that appear to be unrelated power struggles. In addition, sexual developmental issues can mask or affect other problems.

> *Case 5.* Connie, a 39-year-old single woman, presented with a case of long-standing depression. Psychopharmacological intervention impacted greatly

upon the depression, but the client was still left with a sense of a vague yet pervasive cloud hanging over her that would not go away. A discussion of the nature of the cloud led to a sense that "it doesn't all belong to me," which led to an in-depth exploration of her mother's pervasive and untreated depression, which had lasted throughout Connie's life. Each of the five children in the family was expected to do nothing to "upset" mother, but Connie was specifically chosen to "make Mom happy." The criterion for her selection was her lack of physical development at puberty. The other children, one older and three younger, were all perceived to be appropriately developed, but Connie's lack of breast development led to protectiveness by her mother and father, which was expressed in statements such as, "Maybe you should wait before you date, because you might be embarrassed. After all, guys make fun of flat-chested girls, and the nice boys won't even look at you." The added comment, "Besides, your mother will welcome the extra company," betrayed a hidden agenda designed to protect the mother and the marital dyad from having to deal with the consequences of the mother's real depression. Connie concluded that the onset of her own depression was at puberty, "or at least it became worse then." She connected it with the heavy responsibility associated with "making Mom happy," with her sense of repressed and suppressed anger at being "the chosen one while the others got off the hook," and with her guilt over not being able to accomplish the assigned task.

The Transmission of Sexual Loyalties, Values, and Concerns

Boszormenyi-Nagy and Spark (1973), Framo (1970), and others have eloquently discussed the transmission of family values from one generation to the next. Among the binding forces on each family member is the acceptance of at least some portion of the family's belief system and traditions. This is part of "being loyal" as a family group member. Among the belief systems that are most central to family life are those of gender, intimacy, and sexuality. These are indeed matters of great interest to the culture at large, and each family interprets these in their own way. Beliefs about gender-based behavior in the family—such as that men are powerful and women are passive—go hand in hand with beliefs and attitudes regarding intimacy and specific sexual behavior. It is not unusual, for example, to find that several generations of men in a given family (or only the youngest, oldest, or "special" child for several generations) have had a specific type of sexual dysfunction or a specific pattern of getting married and divorced. Sometimes a particular child in a single generation will be singled out to redress a long-standing family imbalance by becoming "mom's child" or "the boy my mother never had" and may be programmed for a specific set of sexual attitudes and behaviors in this way.

This information is seldom transmitted directly, especially about sexuality, but is usually conveyed through stories about other people whose behavior was acceptable to the family, or stories about family members who have been cut off. These feelings and attitudes may be held very strongly and will certainly directly affect the sexual life of each generation.

> *Case 6.* A 21-year-old man, Sam, entered therapy complaining of problems with his girfriend which included a sense of personal passivity, inhibited desire, and frequent premature ejaculation. He was seen with his girlfriend, who was indeed the more extroverted and controlling of the two. Sam was then seen with his parents in a family session, in which his depressed and controlling mother complained about his passive and quiet father and hinted strongly at sexual problems. Sam's father stated that his dad (Sam's grandfather) had had similar marital dynamics and, to his knowledge, so had his grandfather. Sam, who was overtly allied with his mother, was able to recognize that his behavior was, in part, a covert way of being loyal to his father, as well as a set of well-learned behaviors.

Specific events in a family's life in one generation may dramatically alter the shape of the next. For example, a woman reported a family secret that her aunt had had a child out of wedlock. This had terrified her mother, who proceeded to raise the client with rigid strictures against sexual expression, which the client was now passing down to her own daughters. In families where strictures such as these become too binding, members of the next generation may rebel by acting out sexually and becoming pregnant. This will, of course, confirm the mother's worst fears.

It is not only patterns that are transferred. Older generations may directly intervene in the lives of the nuclear family, responding to their own concerns.

> *Case 7.* A 3-year-old child, Gabrielle, was brought into the clinic after a minor episode of sexual touching by an adolescent stranger. This molestation was stopped in a couple of minutes and never repeated, and the child was not injured. Nevertheless, a year later, the parents were still bringing Gabrielle into therapy, and the clinic therapist was the third expert to be consulted in trying to find out if she was all right. The parents had been treating Gabrielle somewhat like a wounded princess, interpreting any evidence of upset as related to her "trauma." The parents themselves were having some conflicts, and it appeared that some of these were being detoured through the child. However, a brief review of the three-generation system revealed that the maternal grandmother had a sister who had been raped when she was 14. This had been extremely upsetting to the grandmother. It was she, in fact,

who had been pushing the mother to take Gabrielle to therapy, repeating over and over that she was concerned about the child's mental health. A strong message was given to the parents that their daughter was now "well" and that continued focus on the event would produce more problems. This enabled the mother, who had been feeling this way already, to reassure the grandmother with more conviction. She reported relief at all levels of the system.

It is probably fair to generalize that, in the majority of American families, sexual "traditions" include insecurity around sexuality, inaccurate information, and silence within the family around sexual issues. A highly sexually focused culture, combined with a ban on sharing information and feelings about sex, produces great confusion in young people and leads to increased sexual dysfunction. The specific ways a family copes with this cultural confusion are crucial to understanding sexual issues. Because sex therapy has focused either on intrapsychic conflicts or on the dyad, less attention has been paid to multigeneration transmission of both sexual attitudes and handling of problematic sexual issues. However, as many of the preceding case studies have indicated, intergenerational messages, loyalty issues, and family patterns are frequently core aspects of a sexual problem or dysfunction.

Object Relations Theory and the Transmission of Sexual Loyalties, Values, and Concerns

Each of us develops and evolves our own unique sexual script, based upon our emerging sense of self-image, our sexual experience, role modeling by our parents, relationships with our peers, and a host of other cultural aspects. That script is molded and shaped throughout our lives by a variety of forces and events. There can be little argument, however, with the statement that the foundation of a person's sexual script is laid early in life. The quality of attachment and bonding with those significant others who give us our primary care, be they members of our family of origin or not, greatly affects our ability to give and receive, make commitments, love, trust, and be intimate with ourselves and others. The quality of that early care thus sets the tone for the emerging sexual script.

As theorists and therapists have endeavored to understand the growth and development of sexual scripts, there has been a gradual movement away from the more traditional dynamic theories that emphasized instinctual sexual and aggressive forces toward a more interpersonal model.

Many people have settled upon an "object relations" perspective, which focuses on the desire for, and the quality of, those primary intimate relationships, and the possible positive and negative effects upon the individual and subsequent relationships when that quality is high or low. Issues of attachment, separation, and loss; internalized objects; positive and negative introjects; and projective identification are all part of such a perspective. These are important concepts which enable us to understand key aspects of an individual's sexual and relationship script.

The emphasis with this approach is upon how *internalized* objects or images impact us in such a profound way that they block our ability to see current reality, or they color that reality. When this occurs, the ability to separate the inner reality of the past from the real attributes of a significant other in the present is difficult, at best. Furthermore, when two partners in a relationship are both engaged in the process of projective identification—that is, projecting attributes onto each other and identifying with each other's projections—the possibility for significant relationship dysfunction, including sexual dysfunction, is extremely high.

Our experience has been that, for many clinicians moving into family therapy from an individual psychodynamically oriented framework, object relations theory becomes a convenient stopping place, which the therapist uses to focus only on internalized objects without really looking at the family's wider realities. This is reinforced by some of the writers in this area (e.g., Scharff & Scharff, 1987), whose work is focused almost entirely on the internalized issues, even while acknowledging the interplay between fantasy and reality.

The question could be raised, why does it matter if the messages were real, partially real, or not real at all? Our answer would be that clarity in this area facilitates shared meaning in the family, increases intimacy, increases assumption of self-responsibility, diminishes one-sided interpretations of reality, increases the possibility of forgiveness and reconciliation within the family, and increases the ability of the individuals and family to change what can be changed and accept the realities and limitations of what cannot be changed. Perhaps this is particularly true in the area of sexuality, where so little is talked about and so much is implied nonverbally.

To illustrate, I (L.H.) had polio when I was 2 years of age. For 2 months, I was placed in a contagious-disease ward of a local hospital, isolated from parental and familial contact, with the exception of visual contact through a glass partition. The nurses told my parents that I cried "continuously" for almost 30 days, then abruptly stopped. I did not have a "deep" cry again until, as an adult, I dealt with the suppressed and repressed pain regarding that experience. In retrospect, it is clear that, in order to survive emotionally and handle the narcissistic vulnerability caused by that experience, as a young child I made several conclusions, utilizing projective identification as an ego defense: (1) The world is all bad for doing this to me; (2) I must be bad for the world to do this to me; and (3) Mommy and Daddy are bad for doing this to me. But, if all the world, and Mommy and Daddy were bad, I could not survive, so a gentle but passive and somewhat absent father was cast in the role of "all bad" and a more active and present mother was cast in the role of "okay," although I was still leery of her.

When, as a young adult, I saw an old family picture of my father holding an infant child above his head and beaming with joy and love, I felt tremendous anxiety. My "world-view" was called into question and effectively shattered. Subsequent conversations with both parents (and a helpful therapist) helped to modify the "inventions" of my mind so that I could experience my family and parents in a new, more balanced and loving way.

Those family discussions also paved the way for self-disclosure on my parents' part of some rather significant issues. For example, in the 1940s, one approach to parenting was not to "spoil" children by picking them up when they cried. In fact, my mother told of an experience when she started to pick me up when I cried in the doctor's office and was sternly repri-manded by the physician. Her desire to be a "good mother" and not "spoil" me conflicted with her internal sense of appropriate nurturance. My sense of having received ambivalent messages regarding touch in general and physi-cal and emotional support and nurturance in particular were confirmed by these and other family stories and by the expression by my parents of their long-withheld pain and guilt regarding not trusting their own instincts to touch me more. Yet, both of them came from nonemotional Germanic origins in which affectional touch was severely limited.

Out of such discussions came an increased sense of reality versus internalized object or image, a sense of mutual struggle and having done the best I could, an assumption and expression of self-responsibility by all parties, a more balanced view of reality, and increased closeness and intimacy from sharing, empathically hearing each other, understanding each other's motivations, and forgiving each other when needed.

For some people, family-of-origin interviews yield the inescapable conclusion that some parents, due to their own "craziness," family pat-terns, or personality flaws, are incapable of loving their children or of perceiving them as good people. In such cases, the psychological task of clients is quite different. Instead of learning that early fantasies are flawed and that connection and shared adulthood are possible, these clients must accept their own worth and the possibility of love elsewhere. With this task comes a different kind of disengagement and a goal of giving up a hopeless struggle in order to move on to other relationships.

An understanding of multigenerational family patterns allows for a deeper understanding of the parents as people with pasts and problems of their own. This understanding is often critical to becoming one's own person. At the least, one can gain the freedom of knowing as much as is possible, what is "me" and what is "them," what is "invention" and what is "reality," what can possibly be changed and what cannot or will not. Having done the best that one can do in the present with the "there and then" and the "here and now" realities and inventions, one can become free to work toward genuine acceptance of the possibilities and limitations of one's self and family.

The sexual genogram process discussed later in this chapter helps the client and therapist to get a broad yet specific overview of the family of origin and its potential impact upon the presenting problem. It also helps clients to sort out reality from internalized object or image. The utilization of such a process can lead to a greater variety of treatment approaches than is generally common in sex therapy.

Sex therapists who rely primarily upon intrapsychic and brief behavioral sex therapy approaches may miss many of the interpersonal dimensions of a specific sexual dysfunction case. Those who focus primarily on object relations may miss many of the very real intergenerational issues that can contribute to a sexual dysfunction. On the other hand, those who rely primarily on intergenerational approaches, like many Contextual family therapists, may miss other significant dimensions.

Intergenerational messages are an important part of any systemic overview of clients with sexual dysfunctions, and they are an important focus for sex therapy, but they are not the only or necessarily predominant focus. What is needed is the renunciation of parochial approaches and the practice of genuine integration of sex, marital, and family therapy, with the therapist using the best from all of the theoretical schools, so that each piece of the systemic puzzle can be identified and utilized. It is the therapist's task to help the client(s) to identify the salient forces impacting upon the relationship or sexual dysfunction, so that appropriate, insight-oriented, family-of-origin, or behavioral interventions can be devised to resolve the issues. Our clients are entitled to and deserve no less from us than this.

SEX THERAPY AND THE FAMILY THERAPIST

It is probably correct, if somewhat oversimplified, to suggest that family therapists doing clinical work have two main responses to patients' sexuality. One is basically to ignore it. If a sexual problem arises, these therapists refer the case immediately to a sex therapist, believing that they are not knowledgeable enough to handle the problem. The second response is the assumption that the sexual problems are simply one more symptomatic response to the general family malaise, whether this be framed as lack of differentiation, problems with family structure, or poor communication techniques. Therapists who hold this view believe it is not necessary to discuss sexuality directly, assuming that if they solve the basic problem, the sexual dysfunction will go away. A few family therapists do insist that they discuss sexuality with great frequency and comfort, although some of these have had no specific training in techniques of sexual diagnosis and therapy.

Two really fascinating questions are why family therapists have not eagerly adopted this clinical knowledge as well as why they have contributed so little to the literature on sex therapy. Given the fact that most people would agree that sexuality is an important and binding force in maintaining a dyad and, by implication, a family, why has there not been an explosion of literature on the subject? Sex therapists have presented a number of possible reasons.

1. *Sex therapy is "too medical" and nonsystemic.* It is certainly true that a reasonable percentage of sexual dysfunctions have a medical cause. For this reason, before treating a sexual dysfunction, it is necessary to make a diagnosis, and an individual diagnosis at that. This presents two problems. One is that there is truly a separate body of knowledge on sexuality to be learned, and this takes time. It is also uncomfortable material for people who have not been trained medically. (It is interesting, however, that therapists who are afraid of the medical aspects of sexuality have not hesitated to deal with other illnesses that have equal medical—and, in fact, more life threatening—components, such as anorexia and asthma.)

The second problem is that this has to be an individual diagnosis as well as a couple diagnosis. This often leaves therapists experiencing it as "nonsystemic" and therefore not within their area of expertise. Family therapists, in general, have been trained to make only relational statements about what is going on between people, and the idea of a formal diagnostic evaluation of one or both members of the couple often makes them uncomfortable and gives them a sense of cognitive dissonance.

2. Sexual issues are totally systemic. Although sexual dysfunctions may require medical diagnosis, sexual symptoms and issues are often part of the larger couple dysfunction. Therefore, in a fair number of cases, it is possible to treat the sexual symptoms without dealing with them directly. It should be said, however, that a good many couples find that marital and family therapists refuse to bring up the topic at all and look acutely uncomfortable when the couple brings it up. In this way, the therapist never really knows whether or not there is a problem. These couples often report that the relationship is better in general but the sexual relationship or problem has not changed. This has been a surprisingly frequent complaint in couples referred to us.

3. Sex therapy is an educational process and therefore not very interesting. Because, particularly in the early days of sex therapy, ignorance was one of the principal problems couples brought into therapy, a great deal of early sex therapy was done in the form of education, followed by behaviorally focused exercises. Masters and Johnson's program initially came out of a medically focused institution, and their writing was not systemic in a larger sense. In addition, because their program was based on behavioral desensitization, most marriage and family therapists did not observe (or discounted) the large relational component that was built into the exercises. It was a long time before therapists realized that these exercises could serve a number of functions in allowing access to the couple's systemic issues and difficulties. Many early systemic therapists were specifically against educational processes, believing that, once the system was functioning, people would find out information by themselves. (We believe that these writers frequently failed to reckon with the couple's societally scripted discomfort at dealing with sexual material, which decreased their ability to obtain or remember information.)

The fact that certain sexual dysfunctions, particularly premature ejaculation, impotence, and primary orgasmic dysfunction, must be dealt with directly by using the sensate focus exercises is particularly distressing to those therapists who prefer to work with brief therapy in an indirect manner. Because of the physiological processes involved, these indirect methods seldom work with those dysfunctions, while a direct approach involving education about the person's body and the techniques necessary for stimulation frequently works quickly and completely. Of course, with other sexual issues and certain desire-phase disorders, indirect methods are often more likely to work.

4. Sex is a low-priority item. Early work in family therapy was done with the entire family, and extremely dysfunctional and rigid families at that. In families in which the presenting problem was a life-threatening illness on the part of one of the members (e.g., suicide, violence, anorexia), the sexuality of the couple assumed a very low priority. In many of these rigid families, where issues in the child arose because of the couple's fierce insistence on detouring their conflict through the children, the couples were highly resistant to any specifically oriented couples' work and frequently totally refused to discuss sexual issues. Therefore, much early literature ignored sexuality in favor of problems that seemed to be more serious.

5. *Therapists are personally uncomfortable.* Although all of the preceding reasons are important, we believe that they are not as important as therapists' personal discomfort with the area of human sexuality. In all studies, family therapists have been shown to be like other people of their social class. They have the same value system, the same marriage and divorce rate, and the same comforts and discomforts, including a sharp discomfort with sexuality. In a society that is basically sexually repressed, virtually every individual experiences some degree of sexual traumatization, sexual secretiveness, and sexual ignorance. This has been demonstrated frequently in human sexuality programs.

At the Marriage Council of Philadelphia, all incoming marital and family trainees—usually experienced therapists—are required to take a sexual enrichment program and a course in human sexuality. Most of the trainees report that they have gained greatly from this exposure and that it has drastically changed the way they have worked with couples. In therapy situations involving family therapists who have not had specific training with treating sexual dysfunction and who have not had a chance to deal with their own sexual issues, the therapists' anxiety, coupled with their clients' anxiety in dealing with sexuality, has allowed all members of the triad (or family unit) to avoid the subject. This continuing discomfort may make therapists unwilling to acquire the expert knowledge needed to treat couples effectively, let alone to consider what family therapy might have to offer the treatment of sexual dysfunction, or to write a paper about it.

Since comfort, knowledge, and expertise are all positively correlated, it is important that marital and family therapists deal with their sexual issues and increase their comfort and knowledge levels with sexual issues. As these increase, therapeutic expertise with these issues will increase as well. Therapists will then be better able to assess the relationship of sexual issues or dysfunctions to the broader system and to treat or refer families or couples.

THE SEXUAL GENOGRAM AND FAMILY JOURNEY

Everything written so far in this chapter emphasizes one point: The sexual life of the adult client who arrives at the therapist's office is greatly impacted by family history and structure. The job of the therapist is to consider the effects of this upon the client. For example, if a person is sexually ignorant, is she emotionally free to take in new information? If a person becomes more directly sexual, will that be a betrayal of mother or father? If he becomes intimate, will he break a family tradition of distancing? Access to this material is best obtained by transforming some traditional tools of family therapy in order to gain some new information. We use the term *sexual genogram* (Hof & Berman, 1986) to describe a process designed to facilitate the gathering of that information.

The sexual genogram uses a traditional family therapy tool to explore issues of sexuality in the structure and belief system of the client's family of origin. The genogram itself, as developed by Murray Bowen (1978) and enlarged on by Guerin and Pendagast (1976) and Wachtel (1982), has traditionally been used to obtain an "aerial view" of the larger system.

The genogram is a three-generational diagram or map of the people who make up one's family. It can include whatever data the therapist wishes. At the minimum, births, deaths, marriages, and divorces should be included. However, feelings, myths, and stories about significant events can also be included. Its advantages over a standard narrative history is that it casts a wider net: By including everyone, not only those the clients see as important, it is more apt to reveal emotional cut-offs, secrets, and previously unnoticed alliances. The process of drawing the genogram gives a sense of organization and distance to the material, thus facilitating objectivity and rationality; and it offers the possibility of increasing or decreasing affect as the history progresses. The family contacts that are usually initiated as a way of gathering history often contribute to basic shifts in family dynamics.

We have adapted the genogram to pinpoint sexual issues. By providing a gentle, careful overview of sexual issues across generations, the sexual genogram enables the client to explore previously hidden affects and study family patterns of interaction around sexual issues. This, in turn, provides information helpful in resolving immediate sexual problems and often produces shifts in the basic quality of the couple's relatedness.

The Sexual Genogram Process

A sexual genogram is most appropriately utilized after the initial evaluation has been completed. The exploration of sexual issues is best done when a climate exists in which therapeutic trust and rapport have been established, there is no acute marital crisis (e.g., violence, one partner is planning to leave the relationship, etc.), and the couple has agreed to explore their sexual issues and problems.

The process involves five parts: introduction; creation and exploration of a family genogram; creation and exploration of a sexual genogram; discussion of genogram issues with other family members; and a review of the total process and integration with the treatment plan.

Introduction to Genogram Concept

The process is facilitated by a cognitively oriented explanation of the concepts and goals. The roles of early learning, family structure, and intergenerational processes in the development of individual, couple, and family systems is explained. The concepts of *life script* and *family scripts*, as utilized by Transactional Analysis therapists (James & Jongeward, 1971), and of *family loyalties* (Boszormenyi-Nagy & Spark, 1973) have proven extremely helpful in presenting this idea to clients in a nonthreatening and interest-provoking way. Positive/facilitative and hurtful/destructive examples are drawn from the clients. Self-disclosure by the therapist may be used to model and emphasize the universal nature of these processes and normalize both positive and negative aspects for the clients. This can increase the likelihood of further exploration in sensitive areas by the clients, which might be precluded if they believed that they were alone in their feelings, beliefs, or actions. As the concept is grasped and curiosity pricked, speculation as to how these concepts might relate to the presenting sexual problem is encouraged briefly. As the clients perceive the importance of considering the impact of their family of origin upon their development, relationships, and sexual problem, motivation usually increases to continue the process.

Creation and Exploration of a Family Genogram

A genogram is defined as a "diagram of extended family relationships including at least three generations" (Foley & Everett, 1984, p. 12). It graphically shows the names and ages of all family members; specific dates of significant life events such as births, deaths, marriages, separations, and divorces; and marginal notations regarding occupations, significant illnesses, and other important life events and transitions. We stress that, although facts are important, we are also very interested in the client's perceptions regarding the identified facts or events. In other words, what was the impact upon the client, other significant persons, and related systems?

Construction of the genogram can be done by the couple within the session, with the therapist and each partner in private sessions, or by the partners at home in private, with sharing done after the work has been completed. This is a matter of therapist preference, available time, and the clients' needs for either sharing or privacy.

Each client is instructed to use lines, symbols, and colors that might be personally relevant to show feelings, alliances, boundaries, coalitions, closeness, distance, emotional cut-offs, conflicts, connectedness, and so forth. Personal creativity is encouraged, to make the process a lively one for the clients, tapping memories of things past and present. They are encouraged to look at family pictures and albums. Gaps where information is missing are noted, for these are often the domain of a living secret that still impacts upon the system. Feelings, thoughts, and dreams experienced by the client as the genogram is being created are to be noted. If there is permission within the family system to talk openly regarding the "family tree," clients are free to do so in order to gather information. However, if such a discussion would threaten the client or disrupt the broader family system, we advise waiting until later in the therapy process.

It is evident that we are describing a graphic device that combines the data-gathering approaches of a variety of writers, including the history-gathering aspects of Guerin and Pendagast (1976); the relationship/family "mapping" features of Minuchin (1974); the impact, internal images, and "story" aspects of Duhl (1981) and Hof and Miller (1981); and the projective emphasis of Wachtel (1982). Development, family structure, and family loyalties may all be highlighted.

If the genograms have been done separately, which usually takes 1 or 2 weeks, the partners are encouraged to discuss their findings with one another. They frequently hear one another's stories from a new perspective and with increased sensitivity and empathy, as a result of adhering to this structured and reciprocal process. In addition, partners can frequently supply missing facts or remind one another of "forgotten" feelings, since they tend to be less emotionally involved in the other's family process.

In the therapeutic setting, the therapist can facilitate the exploration by asking what happened (identification of facts/events), what the impact was upon people and systems (analysis), and what generalizations can be made (specific learning) regarding the relationship of the "there-and-then" (one's living history) to the "here-and-now" issues that are the focus of therapy.

The therapist endeavors to help the client fill in gaps, make affective connections to nodal events, perceive overt and covert patterns, and remember positive images that may have lain dormant but have been helpful in bonding this person with other persons in this unique family. Verbal and nonverbal clues are carefully observed and, where it is deemed appropriate, explored to help create connections. The feelings, thoughts, and dreams experienced as the exercise was being completed are also examined.

Creation and Exploration of a Sexual Genogram

After the family genogram has been created and explored, each partner is asked to reconsider it during the following week, with a specific focus on the following questions:

- What are the overt and covert messages in this family regarding sexuality and intimacy? Regarding masculinity and femininity?
- Who said or did what? Who was conspicuously silent or absent in the area of sexuality and intimacy?
- Who was the most open sexually? Intimately? In what ways?
- How were sexuality and intimacy encouraged? Discouraged? Controlled? Within a generation? Between generations?
- What questions have you had regarding sexuality and intimacy in your "family tree" that you have been reluctant to ask? Who might have the answers? How could you discover the answers?
- What were the "secrets" in your family regarding sexuality and intimacy (e.g., incest, unwanted pregnancies, or extramarital affairs)?
- What do the other "players on the stage" have to say regarding these questions? How did these issues, events, and experiences impact upon them? Within a generation? Between generations? With whom have you talked about this? With whom would you like to talk about this? How could you do it?
- How does your partner perceive your family tree/genogram regarding the aforementioned issues? How do you perceive your partner's?
- How would you change this genogram (including who and what) to meet what you wish had occurred regarding messages and experiences of sexuality and intimacy?

Answers to the questions are to be written in a free-flowing manner, with the assurance that what is to be shared with one's partner or the therapist is under the total control of the writer. Feelings, thoughts, and dreams that are triggered as these questions are considered are to be noted. Sometimes lines, symbols, or colors on the original genogram are modified to express new realities discovered as these questions are considered. Partners are encouraged to share as much as possible and as much as they desire with each other prior to the next therapy session.

In the therapy session, meaning, insights, and ideas are explored using the processes of identification, analysis, and generalization/learning. When this has been shared between the therapist and both members of the couple, discussion focuses on deciding which issues could be, and/or need to be, explored directly and fruitfully with other family members. In some cases, this next step is not necessary, and we move directly to the fifth step in the process, the review of the process and integration with the treatment plan.

Discussion of Genogram Issues with Other Family Members

In most cases, the genogram is the first step in a family journey that leads to general goals of individuation and possible restructuring of family alliances in the present. Bowen (1978), Framo (1970, 1976), Paul and Grosser (1981), and Williamson (1981, 1982a, 1982b) have written extensively on various ways individuals can make contact with their families, with and without a therapist present, both for retrieving the past and for reconnecting and redefining family relationships in the here and now. Whatever the specifics of the approach, the goal is a slow, nonconfrontational connection, beginning with requests for information and clarification of family experiences. Respect for parents as well as children is crucial. Time for things to settle between contacts is always planned for. Confrontation or expression of painful feelings is done only when clients and family have been able to talk or share enough so that contact feels safe.

Before any contact is made, the client's fears and apprehensions are openly discussed, as is the potential impact upon other family members who are to be approached. The emphasis is placed upon enabling persons to tell and hear each others' stories, to gather information (facts, feelings, and impressions), to discover family scripts or legacies of an intergenerational nature, and to learn about one's family and use what is learned to facilitate understanding of current functioning and resolution of current problems.

With sexual material, this gradual and respectful attitude is even more critical. Clients are encouraged to make contact in a face-to-face manner if at all possible, by telephone or letter if not. This is done without the partner present, since the goal is to deal with relationships within the original family. Most clients find it easier and more productive to deal with one parent or sibling at a time, in a private place. Sexual material is approached after other historical issues are covered. The easiest questions to ask are those about values, such as, What were you taught about sexuality as a child? What did you want me to know about it? To think about it?

Parental ideas and feelings about sex are generally elicited far more easily than anxious adult children would believe. If the conversation becomes intimate, parents will often reveal sexual secrets, such as pregnancies, abuse, and so forth. It is seldom if ever necessary or desirable to obtain information about current sexual practices of parents, or for clients to share their own.

Clients are reminded that they should not expect, or even attempt, to cover everything in one meeting. If the client needs to discuss particularly painful material, such as sexual abuse by a parent, careful rehearsal and preparation is essential. Clients whose parents are dead, unavailable, or unwilling to talk should consider locating other family members. Siblings, aunts, uncles, and cousins usually are acutely aware of sexual feelings and attitudes of family members, and are often repositories of secrets as well.

When the contacts are made, partners are encouraged to keep each other apprised of what has occurred and what feelings and thoughts have been experienced. Specific supportive responses are modeled and encouraged. Throughout the process, the therapist should be available for phone consultations as needed and extended-family sessions where indicated.

After the contacts have been made, the conjoint therapy session is once again used to gather meaning, insights, and ideas from the exercise. The identification, analysis and generalization/learning processes previously utilized are once more used. This exploration leads naturally to the last component in the sexual genogram process.

Review of Process and Integration with Treatment Plan

The therapist and clients do a reflective review of the total process, emphasizing questions such as, What have you learned? and How can we use what you have learned to help resolve the sexual problem? As the insights, feelings, and legacies are discussed, a new perspective frequently emerges, with greater appreciation, empathy, and objectivity regarding what occurred in one's family and how it impacted upon all family members.

Insights regarding the etiology and maintenance of the sexual problem often lead to diminished blaming and a positive sense of reciprocity.

The learning and ideas of the clients and the therapist are then merged
with the more traditional behavioral components of a sex therapy treatment plan to resolve the presenting sexual problem.

Case Illustrations

The following two case illustrations give a sense of how a three-generational family model and the sexual genogram process itself can be of use in
the treatment of specific sexual problems and dysfunctions.

Betty and Bob

Betty and Bob, a well-bonded, married, middle-aged couple, presented
with multiple sexual dysfunctions. She had never experienced an orgasm,
and he experienced situational premature ejaculation. Both dysfunctions
were rather tenacious, resisting prior treatment efforts with a trained sex
and marital therapist, even when serious attention was paid to uncovering
unresolved intrapsychic issues. It was evident to all involved that "something" was blocking the resolution of the problems.

The sexual genogram process was employed. The questions that were
especially helpful to Bob were, What are the overt and covert messages in
this family regarding sexuality and intimacy? Regarding masculinity and
femininity? He discovered, through his family genogram, that the men
were scripted to be less powerful than the women in the family and were
not "allowed" to think "too highly" of themselves. Because he was a warm,
personable, dynamic individual and very successful in his own business,
the premature ejaculation served as a way of "keeping him in his place."
Discussions with other male family members gave him a clear sense that
his dysfunction enabled him to remain faithful to a nonhelpful family
script. An uncle, with whom he discussed some of the specific sexual
questions, confirmed how the "successful" men in the family were frequently the object of "good-natured" teasing about their sexuality. In Bob's
marriage, Betty played her part by teasing him and occasionally blaming
him and "his problem" for her inability to be orgasmic.

Betty, in discussing her family genogram, was struck by her drawing
of thin, red, "angry" lines (showing a negative impact) underlying green
"positive" lines, connecting her to her older brother, father, and grandfather (see Figure 11.1). The therapist was impressed by her frequent
references to "how close we were as a family." In the subsequent week, as
Betty wrote the answers to the sexual genogram questions, two had
particular significance for her: What were the "secrets" in your family

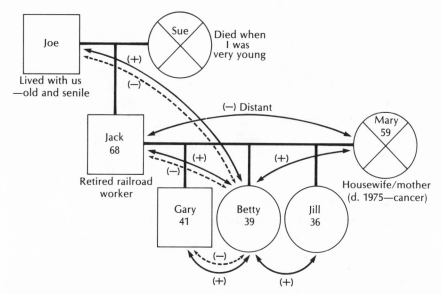

FIGURE 11.1.   Selected Elements of Betty's Genogram. *Key:* Solid line between Jack and Mary = negative, "distant"; solid line between Betty and, respectively, Gary, Jack, and Joe = positive, "close;" dashed line between Betty and, respectively, Gary, Jack, and Joe = negative, "angry."

regarding sexuality and intimacy? and, What do other "players on the stage" have to say regarding these questions? What emerged was that Betty had kept hidden from her previous therapist and her husband a pattern of close sexual contact (fondling, but not intercourse) with her grandfather, father, and older brother.

At her own initiative, during the same week, but after she had written her answers, Betty approached her older brother, with whom she had a close and open relationship. She was seeking information from him regarding how he remembered those events and how the experiences impacted upon him. He responded, "Don't you remember how we both enjoyed it?" She was shocked at this, because she had "forgotten" the pleasurable aspects of the experience.

As Betty, Bob, and the therapist discussed the sexual genogram, what emerged even more clearly to her than ever before was her resentment at the loss of control she experienced when she had been approached by her grandfather (a senile man) and her father, and her anger at her mother for not believing her when she told her as a young child of the abuse. She began to see how her inability to have an orgasm enabled her to maintain control and at the same time block the remembrance of sexual pleasure that was experienced in a relationship with her brother that she had labeled "sick."

Betty believed that the sexual genogram process had enabled her to approach her secret in a very gentle way, with her being able to maintain complete control. In the discussion with the therapist, the collusive elements of the couple's relationship were also exposed: Bob helped protect Betty from remembrance of "sick" pleasure; Betty helped protect him from "thinking too highly of himself." When this material was explored, traditional sex therapy approaches to each of the sexual dysfunctions led to rapid resolution of the premature ejaculation and to somewhat slower, but no less certain, resolution of the pre-orgasmic condition.

In addition, Betty had several discussions with her father during the course of therapy which helped her to put the past behind her and to understand in a new way his relationship with her long-dead mother. At first she sought only information regarding several questions on the sexual genogram. She was instructed not to initiate a discussion of the overtly sexual aspects of their past relationship. Rather, she was to focus initially on her long-standing feelings at the "loss of control" in many aspects of her relationship with him. He surprised her by expressing remorse regarding several of the instances she noted, and by apologizing for his sexual intrusiveness and "taking advantage" of their close relationship. The genuine love between Betty and her parents thus became experienced in a deeper way, and, when her father died some 6 months later, Betty had a sense that the unfinished business of the past was fairly well resolved.

Janet and Dave

This second case illustration demonstrates how a family emotional legacy can be transmitted across the generations and impact upon a later generation in a sexual dysfunction.

Janet and Dave, married for 9 years, both aged 30, and college educated at the graduate level, presented with a case of long-standing inhibited sexual desire on Janet's part and with both describing the marriage as being "in serious trouble." The sexual genogram process enabled both of them to see how the "abandonment" by their respective fathers (his at age 8 via divorce and hers at age 12 via death) and the way it was handled or not handled in the family led to a significant amount of unresolved grief, as well as a mutual-protection society between them, with each endeavoring to help the other avoid pain of any sort. Contacts with their respective families enabled the grief work to be completed for each of them and for the extended family to address the long-avoided pain.

Janet and Dave were able to identify how they colluded in "not growing up," in avoiding death and adult responsibilities. In addition, both were invested in not increasing sexual intimacy, so that love would not get too deep and the pain then would not be so great when the "inevitable" loss finally came again.

Janet also realized through this process that her maternal grandfather had literally abandoned her grandmother, mother, and her siblings, when Janet's mother was 6 years old. This fact had never been disclosed, the grandfather always being referred to as the one who "died." Discussion of the genogram with a paternal uncle (the designated family historian) revealed this fact and led to a significant meeting with Janet's mother in which her long-denied grief was exposed in a helpful manner.

When she asked her mother how the abandonment experience had impacted upon her, her mother replied that she "determined then and there never to get close to a man again—no one would do that to me!" In the therapy session, Janet's comment was, "No wonder it's been so difficult; I've had to carry my grief and hers for over 20 years!" This was significant both in its truth as well as in its power to enable her to feel free to move closer to Dave sexually. In this case, specific sex therapy interventions were not needed to overcome the sexual dysfunction. As marital therapy continued, the sexual desire was kindled.

Indications and Contraindications

A brief and less detailed sexual genogram is appropriate as a part of any routine sexual history, as a way of pinpointing potential problem areas. The length of time it takes to gather the information and the amount of detail desired vary with the therapist. A clinician who takes a primarily fact-oriented genogram in the office can accomplish a great deal in a short period of time. We see no contraindications to this type of information gathering, provided that the couple is not in an acute crisis and is at an appropriate point to start discussing sexual issues. For therapists using a brief behaviorally focused treatment model, the sexual genogram in its more detailed and elaborated form should probably be used only when an impasse has been reached.

The family journey is a more complex issue. Although there are probably no absolute contraindications other than active psychosis in one of the parents, timing and planning are critical. A person in the midst of a major, hostile struggle with parents needs to work through those issues with a therapist well trained in family-of-origin work, before sexual themes are dealt with.

We have been using the sexual genogram method informally for several years and in a formal manner for the last year, involving some 20 couples. In addition, 35 students in the Marriage Council of Philadelphia's family therapy and human development courses have done family geno-grams and journeys in which some sexual material was elicited. We have not personally encountered serious problems, although some experiences were more helpful than others. This does not mean, however, that an unprepared client could not have a most unpleasant experience.

CONCLUSION

Family therapy theory adds much to the conceptualization of sexuality and its problems in dyads. Sexuality plays an integral part in organizing family structure along generational lines. Family-of-origin patterns, beliefs, and loyalties affect later sexual functioning in the family of procreation. The sexual genogram is a data-gathering and assessment process that enables people to explore multigenerational issues in a rapid, effective way. It may also represent the first stage of a treatment process that involves family exploration and family journey, or it may simply facilitate more traditional insight-oriented therapy. It may be used in combination with a variety of other therapy modalities and represent an addition to the usual sex and family therapy armamentarium.

PERSONAL RESPONSES: LARRY HOF

Ever since I began teaching a course in sexual function and dysfunction at the Marriage Council of Philadelphia, I have been interested in the impact of family-of-origin factors and issues in the treatment of sexual dysfunc-tions. Part of that interest came from the realization that such forces were frequently downplayed or even relatively ignored by many sex therapists. To be sure, early social learning was emphasized as an important factor in the etiology of sexual dysfunction; however, little was done to identify and utilize gender and generational socialization issues fully in the treatment of sexual dysfunctions.

I also realized that an early experience with polio, as well as being raised in a family that gave ambivalent messages regarding touch in general and physical and emotional support and nuturance in particular, impacted greatly upon my own view of the world, my family, each parent, and myself, as well as my initial ability and capacity for interpersonal intimacy, self-disclosure, trust, and vulnerability (discussed in the body of the chapter). The "working through" of those issues involved not only dealing with the "inventions" or internalized objects of a child's mind (from an object relations perspective), but actually dealing with the realities of the family and parents in a face-to-face manner.

Out of that intergenerational process came a sense of healing and mutual struggle, a sense of understanding and mutual responsibility, a sense of reality and increased closeness and intimacy. If such forces could be so powerful for me, I believed that they must have a central place in the treatment of sexual dysfunctions, in which such intimacy, gender, and generational socialization issues frequently emerge. It was for this reason that I developed the sexual genogram process and have made it a core aspect of my approach to the treatment of sexual dysfunctions.

This chapter emphasizes the need for serious, in-depth consideration of intergenerational messages as part of any systemic assessment of clients with sexual dysfunctions, and as part of the treatment process as well. The addition of such an emphasis to the more traditional behavioral, object relations, and interpersonal/marital emphases can lead to a truly systemic integration of sex, marital, and family therapy. Such an approach is necessary if our clients are to be enabled to identify and resolve the salient issues impacting upon their relationship or sexual problems. Such an approach is also needed if sex, marital, and family therapy trainees are to avoid the parochialism that has for too long infused too many of the training programs in the field.

REFERENCES

Boszormenyi-Nagy, I., & Spark, G. (1973). *Invisible loyalties*. New York: Harper & Row.

Bowen, M. (1978). *Family therapy in clinical practice*. New York: Jason Aronson.

Doyle, J. (1985). *Sex and gender*. Dubuque, IA: Brown.

Duhl, F. J. (1981). The use of the chronological chart in general systems family therapy. *Journal of Marital and Family Therapy*, 7, 361–373.

Foley, V. D., & Everett, C. A. (1984). *Family therapy glossary*. Washington, DC: American Association for Marriage and Family Therapy.

Framo, J. (1970). Symptoms from a family transactional viewpoint. In N. Ackerman, J. Lieb, & J. Pearce (Eds.), *Family therapy in transition* (pp. 125–171). Boston: Little, Brown.

Framo, J. (1976). Family of origin as a therapeutic resource for adults in marital therapy: You can and should go home again. *Family Process*, 15, 193–210.

Framo, J. (1982). *Explorations in marital and family therapy.* New York: Springer.

Gagnon, J. (1977). *Human sexualities.* Glenview, IL: Scott, Foresman.

Gagnon, J., & Greenblatt, C. (1978). *Life designs.* Glenview, IL: Scott, Foresman.

Guerin, P. J., & Pendagast, M. A. (1976). Evaluation of family system and genogram. In P. J. Guerin, Jr. (Ed.), *Family therapy: Theory and practice* (pp. 450-464). New York: Gardner Press.

Hof, L., & Berman, E. M. (1986). The sexual genogram. *Journal of Marital and Family Therapy, 12,* 39-47.

Hof, L., & Miller, W. R. (1981). *Marriage in Richmond: Philosophy, process and program.* Bowie, MA: Brady Co.

James, M., & Jongeward, D. (1971). *Born to win.* Reading, MA: Addison-Wesley.

Kaplan, H. (1974). *The new sex therapy.* New York: Brunner/Mazel.

Kaplan, H. (1979). *Disorders of sexual desire.* New York: Brunner/Mazel.

Kaplan, H. (1983). *The evaluation of sexual disorders.* New York: Brunner/Mazel.

Minuchin, S. (1974). *Families and family therapy.* Cambridge, MA: Harvard University Press.

Paul, N. L., & Grosser, G. H. (1981). Operational mourning and its role in conjoint family therapy. In R. J. Green & J. L. Framo (Eds.), *Family therapy* (pp. 377-391). New York: International Universities Press.

Scharff, D. E., & Scharff, J. S. (1987). *Object relations family therapy.* New York: Jason Aronson.

Steiner, C. M. (1974). *Scripts people live.* New York: Grove Press.

Victor, J. (1980). *Human sexuality: A social psychological approach.* Englewood Cliffs, NJ: Prentice-Hall.

Wachtel, E. F. (1982). The family psyche over three generations: The genogram revisited. *Journal of Marital and Family Therapy, 8,* 335-343.

Williamson, D. S. (1981). Personal authority via termination of the intergenerational hierarchical boundary: A "new" stage in the family life cycle. *Journal of Marital and Family Therapy, 7,* 441-452.

Williamson, D. S. (1982a). Personal authority via termination of the intergenerational hierarchical boundary: Part II. The consultation process and the therapeutic method. *Journal of Marital and Family Therapy, 8,* 23-37.

Williamson, D. S. (1982b). Personal authority in family experience via termination of the intergenerational hierarchical boundary: Part III. Personal authority defined, and the power of play in the change process. *Journal of Marital and Family Therapy, 8,* 309-322.

Wyckoff, H. (1974). Sex role scripting in men and women. In C. M. Steiner (Ed.), *Scripts people live* (pp. 196-209). New York: Grove Press.

12

SEXUALITY IN MAY-DECEMBER MARRIAGES

Florence Kaslow

May-December marriages of younger women to older men are certainly not a new phenomenon. There have been well-known celebrity age-discrepant couples like Pablo and Pauline Picasso, Marta Montanez and Pablo Casals, Charlie Chaplin and Oona O'Neill, and John and Bo Derek. Over the years, such marriages have been the subject of books and films and have evoked various emotional reactions ranging from curiosity to empathy to derision.

Age-discrepant or May-December marriages, as the terms are utilized in this chapter, are those in which the husband is a minimum of 10 years older than the wife (Magdoff-Singer, 1988). This chapter will not deal with comparable age-discrepant relationships where the wife is the older partner (known as December-May marriages), as the dynamics are believed to be different enough to warrant separate attention.

LITERATURE REVIEW

The literature on May-December marriages, even including work that is tangentially relevant, is relatively scant. Cowan (1984) conducted a study of the perceptions of two different age groups of subjects, regarding age-discrepant relationships. One group of subjects was composed of adult males and females (mean age of 28 years), while the other was made up of male and female high school students. Subjects were randomly assigned to read one of five different resumés about couples of various ages, as

Florence Kaslow. Florida Couples and Family Institute, West Palm Beach, Florida.

follows: male and female same age, male 7 years older than female, female 7 years older than male, male 18 years older than female, female 18 years older than male. Participants read the short resumés and were asked to rate these relationships.

The adult as well as the adolescent subjects viewed highly age-discrepant relationships (in which there was an 18-year difference) more negatively than moderately age-discrepant ones (age difference of 7 years). All subjects reported more suspicion of and discomfort with fe-male-older relationships than male-older relationships. Adult males, similar to the adolescents, viewed the female-older relationships with 18-year discrepancies quite negatively. Generally, Cowan (1984) found that relationships in which the female was older were thought to have less chance of success than those in which the male was older and that there was an acceptance of a "double standard" by both adolescents and adults, which approves relationships between older males and younger females, but not the reverse.

Research on the effects of the double standard upon people's perceptions of age-discrepant couples was also conducted by Hartnett, Rosen, and Shumate (1981). One interesting finding was that the wealthy older person was perceived more positively than the older person of average income, regardless of sex. The younger woman in age-discrepant relationships was seen more favorably than the younger man by female subjects; the reverse was true for male student responders.

Presser (1975) reported on age differences in marriage and how they reflect on the status of women, based on a review of census data and the literature. She asserted that many young women marry older men to improve their social status. They select an intelligent, high-achieving man who will immediately provide them with a higher standard of living. (This is clearly borne out in the two cases presented later in this chapter.) Presser highlights the irony in these choices. Frequently, these women actually delimit their own achievable status by foregoing their personal, educational, or career goals when they marry. She asserted that there will continue to be status differences between men and women as long as there are (large) age differences in marriages and women are thought to be solely responsible for child rearing. (Perhaps data collected in 1988 might reveal different patterns, given the greater involvement of fathers in child rearing in the past decade.)

In an interesting study, Foster, Klinger-Vertabedian, and Wispe (1984) explored the effects of age differences upon male longevity. They found that 50- to 79-year-old men who were married to younger women tended to outlive their contemporaries who were married to older women.

They suggest caution in interpreting these findings and speculate about the meaning of them. These researchers hypothesize that premarital selection factors and the couple's interaction pattern during marriage may also be contributory factors to this increased longevity. Nonetheless, they concluded that there is a relationship between age difference and longevity and recommended further study.

Magdoff-Singer (1988) uses an object relations perspective in her analysis of 25 age-discrepant couples—some May–December and some December–May pairings. She focuses on the frequency with which she observed the mechanisms of "projective identification" and "splitting" in the treatment of these couples, stating, "They were couples who were locked in a collusive process which was built upon mutual projective identifications." She utilizes the concepts of splitting and projective identification in the same way these were delineated by Klein (1948), that is, that the perceived "bad" parts of the self are "split off" from the ego-syntonic "good" parts and then discarded by being projected onto another person, who is usually a very significant other.

In addition, Magdoff-Singer (1988) takes Kernberg's (1980) elaborations regarding the defensive maneuvers of splitting and projective identification and applies them to the dyadic interaction of age-disparate married couples. Denial, assertion of omnipotence, and devaluation are other mechanisms of defense utilized in conjunction with splitting and projective identification. She concludes that these deeply ingrained patterns are deleterious to the relationship and need to be brought to the level of conscious awareness and resolved in therapy, if the marital relationship is to improve and endure.

According to Slipp (1984), in order for projective identification to occur, there must be relatively permeable ego boundaries. This fluidity permits one partner to place pressure on the other to think, feel, or act in a way that is congruent with the projector's internalized self or object. For this to happen, a close, continuing relationship between the projector and the object is essential so that there can be a reinternalization through identification with the precipitated behavior of the object.

In my search of the literature, I found no in-depth analysis of various important sexual themes in age-disparate marriages. In clinical discussions of this topic, however, there is often mention made of the fact that the woman who enters such a union is living out her oedipal fantasies in the choice of a partner who is old enough to be her father. Also, her rapid attainment of social status or financial security sometimes contributes to an eroticized sense of excitement toward the husband who provides a glamorous, affluent lifestyle, at least in the early years. There is sometimes little direct connection made between what she attains and her dispensing occasional sexual treats, a "trade-off" that we have found to be implicitly assumed in many of the age-discrepant couples we treat. For example, as one angry and disappointed 60-year-old male patient told me when his 33-year-old wife of 3 years sued for divorce, "She was so delightful and cuddly with me, I thought she really loved me. I didn't believe my friends when they warned that it was my estate she was in love with. I didn't realize it until my will and estate planning became the daily thrust of her conversation and each sexual encounter had a price tag attached to it."

FOCUS

This chapter attempts to explore these sexual themes based on clinical observation and analysis, in order to expand our knowledge base of the sexual dynamics and patterns of May–December couples. Two cases will be used illustratively to trace the evolution of such relationships, the *essence* of the mutual attraction, and the nature of the sexuality and sensuosity experienced, in order to help clinicians glean a fuller understanding of such couples so that their interventions can become more effective. Given the high divorce rate and the longer life-span now extant, there is a great likelihood that there will be an increasing number of remarried couples in the May–December bracket, many of whom will seek help from therapists in unraveling the complex problems they confront. Perhaps it is from this sociocultural context that this topic derives its significance.

The two cases presented here are representative of 20 such cases I have seen in my Florida-based practice in the past 7 years. The population being discussed is white and upper middle and upper class. Patients in this group have been almost exclusively Protestant or Jewish, therefore one case illustration is taken from each of these religious groups. They are drawn from a multiplicity of ethnic backgrounds and countries, although members of the 20-couple sample being discussed here are all at least second-generation Americans and many come from families that have been in the United States since the 19th century. Such marriages are not particularly atypical in Southeast Florida, an area people relocate to in order to fulfill their dreams.

Age-discrepant couples differ from other couples in several dramatic ways. First, the two partners are at very different places in their individual life cycle development, with many accompanying implications. These include the fact that they generally were raised in different generations and often like different music styles, clothing, sports, and so forth; there is a wide variation in energy levels, including libidinal energy and energy for beginning a new family; and they respond to the parent generation differently, in that frequently the husband is a contemporary of the wife's parents, so that generational boundaries become confused. A second major category of difference is that the attraction and interaction pattern is more often one of complimentarity, rather than symmetry, with the husband better educated, wealthier, more power oriented, and more dominant than the wife. With couples closer in age, there is likely to be greater egalitarianism, especially since the advent of the feminist movement.

This chapter is written from a diaclectic, integrative, theoretical framework (Kaslow, 1981). It incorporates psychodynamic and object relations postulates about intrapsychic and interpersonal functioning, as well as structural and systemic theoretical formulations about complementarity and symmetry in dyadic relationships (Bateson, 1958). Such defense mechanisms as denial, splitting, and projective identification, alluded to earlier (Kernberg, 1980; Klein, 1948; Magdoff-Singer, 1988; Slipp, 1984), were manifested quite frequently by the couples in the sample. High complementarity characterized most of the couples when they got married; as the wives became more assertive and autonomous and sought greater equality, many of the marriages became more turbulent, partly because the wives were chosen for their docility and dependence and the husbands resented giving up power and control.

FACTORS CONDUCIVE TO AGE-DISCREPANT DYADS

Various psychosocial, medical, and cultural factors seem to have converged in recent decades to produce what appears to be an upsurge in the number of May–December marriages. These variables include but may not be limited to:

- Men and women marrying at an older age.
- Greater longevity in the life-span of the male (Riley, 1983).
- Heavy emphasis on staying young and having fun.
- The relative ease of obtaining a divorce and remarrying.
- The preference of many men for a woman with a firm, trim, young body; a lovely, unlined face; and a fairly unformed or amorphous sense of self.

- The preference of many older men for a woman who can bear children and who isn't embittered yet by life.
- The pursuit of security, social status, and material wealth by some women who wish to acquire it easily.

Each of these factors will be briefly explored in two intertwined combinations that form a composite.

Marriage Occurring at a Later Age

The trend, visible in earlier decades of the 20th century, of young women marrying as soon as they finished high school, in order to have a legitimate way to move out of their parents' home and to "have sex," has diminished in the past 20 years, particularly in upper-middle and upper-class socioeconomic groups. As a result of the women's liberation and feminist movements, many young women now move out of their parents' homes to go away to college and never really return "home" again to live there full time, even if they are still single after graduation. Others move out when they become financially and emotionally ready to do so. Many young women, like their male counterparts, want to be well established in their careers and want to have achieved a good sense of self and a high level of overall independence before making a commitment to the kind of permanent relationship marriage entails. With the greater sexual freedom afforded to women in the 1960s and 1970s, attributable to more permissive attitudes toward sexual expressiveness and the easy accessibility of various means of birth control and legal abortions, many women ceased to feel pressured to get married in order to be sexually active.

The 1980s has seen some curtailment of uninhibited sexual expressiveness because of the increasing number of cases of venereal disease including herpes and AIDS. Responsible singles have become concerned about "safe sex" and prefer longer-term involvements. Nonetheless, a return to the stringent doctrine of no premarital sex is unlikely with members of nonfundamentalist or nonorthodox religious groups. Rather, it appears that sexual involvements are being entered into more slowly and selectively and less frequently, since what may be at stake if one makes a "wrong choice" of a sexual partner is nothing less than one's life.

As women marry later—in their twenties and early thirties—and desire to continue pursuing the careers they have worked so diligently to establish, some decide not to have children. They believe it will impede their freedom and their continued ability to invest a major portion of their time and energy in their work-a-day world. Whereas men in their own age bracket may now be eager to start a family and want a partner who views full- or part-time mothering as important, a man in his late forties or fifties may already have raised his family and be delighted at the prospect of a young, vital, attractive, interesting, and ambitious career women/wife with whom he won't be tied down by a second family. He finds her interest in him ego gratifying, as it enables him to feel younger and more virile. She respects his achievements and finds his cosmopolitan view of the world—acquired through years of experience—appealing. Initially they are highly compatible. He finds her still young and well-toned body more sexually enticing than that of the softer, more mature body of a woman closer to his own age. The younger woman, consciously attracted by his knowledge, status, *savoir-faire*, and wealth, may not be too concerned about his middle-aged pulchritude—especially if he jogs, works out at a spa, or is an avid participating sportsman and has remained reasonably fit. Initially, concern over his greater age is more than compensated for by his numerous attributes.

Greater Male Longevity

As more and more men have a life expectancy into their seventies, some appear to crave a second (or third) partner after they have raised their first family and become disenchanted with and/or bored by their first wife (Ahrons & Rodgers, 1987; Kaslow & Schwartz, 1987), whom they perceive as dowdy or no longer interesting, sexually appealing, or stimulating. There may be no novelty, intrigue, or "turn-on" left. Conversely, his wife of many years may reject him for being dull, stodgy, too passive, or too domineering, or because she believes she has outgrown him or can no longer tolerate his alcoholism, spouse abuse, selfishness, or TV addiction. If she has achieved a successful career and has a strong sense of her own identity, she may be ready to venture forth on her own, unwilling to be stifled.

With 40% to 50% of all marriages ending in divorce in the United States in the 1970s and 1980s (National Center for Health Statistics, 1985), the stigma attached to divorce prior to the 1970s has decreased markedly. Also, since the number of awards of permanent alimony has decreased, being replaced in many jurisdictions by none (Texas) or temporary rehabilitation alimony (Florida), men whose children are grown no longer face the financial burden of having to pay spousal support until their own or their ex-partner's demise. When there is no, very low, or temporary alimony awarded, economically the woman fares poorly after a divorce (Weitzman, 1985). The man, however, may emerge into the single world in good to excellent financial shape. Money has its own sex appeal to many, which may make him a sought-after partner by women. As indicated earlier, his solvency may make him particularly attractive to a younger woman; she, in turn, helps him to feel rejuvenated and holds out the promise of a "second chance" for marital fulfillment, sexual arousal, and gratification.

With the emphasis on youth in our culture, the man, in order to enhance his opportunities to meet the younger women he perceives to be the most desirable, may create a new, younger image for himself. These efforts may include a combination of exercise to tone up his body, plastic surgery for a sagging face and/or body, more stylish clothing, and the like. Nonetheless, no matter how much he tightens and tones, attempts to deceive others and/or himself, he cannot "turn back the hands of time." The biological/physiological time clock ticks steadily away, and his real age and the disparity between his age and his new wife's may well surface to haunt them a decade or more later. His sexual prowess often diminishes whereas his wife's is ascending, creating frustration for both because their life rhythms may be so out of sync. If his normal, gradual biological slowing down is accelerated and complicated by his need to take medication for such conditions as hypertension or diabetes, or if years of heavy drinking have contributed to sexual dysfunction, his occasional inability to achieve or maintain an erection may turn into frequent impotency. If her reaction is anger or derisiveness, their interactive difficulties will be heightened. This sexual manifestation of the age disparity may be the harbinger of a more serious and eventually irreparable rift in the marriage, unless the couple seek and receive expert marital and sex therapy (Kaplan, 1974, 1979).

CASE HISTORIES

Let us consider two cases, both first marriages for young women in their early twenties. In the first case, the husband was 16 years older and never married. In the second, he was twice divorced and 20 years her senior. The cases are summarized, highlighting the underlying personality dynamics, interactions and transactions, unconscious and conscious bases of attraction, and sexual themes. Both cases are drawn from my recent clinical files and have been carefully disguised to protect the identity and privacy of the people involved. As indicated earlier, in our West Palm Beach, Florida practice, my associates and I see numerous patients who exhibit attitudes, ideas, and characteristics similar to those described here.

Case 1

Mrs. Germaine (Judy) originally came to see me in 1984. At that time, she was a lithe, petite woman of 58 years, 4'11" tall and weighing 100 pounds. She always came in well groomed, often in a golf outfit, and slightly breathless from rushing after a game. Her pretty blue eyes fit her sweet face, and it was easy to understand why friends still found her "adorable and cuddly."

In telling her story over the first few sessions, she relayed that she had been raised by strict parents and felt that her mother had been withholding of affection and very critical. Judy had developed little self-confidence and no real skills. She had learned to be soft-spoken, compliant, and ingratiating. Her two older brothers doted on her, and she became accustomed to expecting men to take care of her, emotionally and financially, in return for her being cute, appreciative, and pleasant to have around. She had learned well how to play up to boys and, later, men, with wide-eyed looks and verbal flattery. With coy innocence, she remained a virgin until she was married, conforming to the behavior expected of a "nice girl" in the 1940s.

When she met Mr. Germaine (Rich), shortly after she finished high school, she was working as a receptionist in a large firm. Her salary was much too meager to allow her to buy a car or rent her own apartment; besides, her parents shared the attitude of many others of their generation almost 40 years ago: "No daughter of ours will move out until she gets married. 'Nice girls' simply don't do that, and no good Jewish parent would permit it."

Rich was a well-established, young corporate executive 35 years of age. He was captivated by the sweetness, gentleness, and attractiveness of his firm's new receptionist. First he brought flowers for her desk and often stopped by to chat. A few months later, when he extended a gracious invitation to her for dinner at one of Boston's fine restaurants, Judy was delighted and highly complimented. Rich was completely ready to get married, and he wanted a docile wife whom he could pamper. Judy adored his kindness and attentiveness. A whirlwind courtship ensued. Her parents encouraged the relationship, as they respected Rich and his increasing affluence. They intuitively sensed he'd be a good caretaker for their daughter. He respected and valued her moral values and did not pressure her for premarital sexual intercourse. Rather, he wanted to keep her "purity" intact until after the wedding ceremony.

Nine months after their first meeting, Judy and Rich were married. They easily agreed that it was inappropriate for Judy to work. She spent her time shopping and developing impeccable and expensive taste in clothing and home furnishings. She also observed carefully and read avidly in order to become a gracious and skilled hostess and a popular guest. When Rich was promoted, they joined a country club, built a home in a wealthy suburb, and had two children. Judy grew to "worship" her indulgent, adoring, successful husband, and he delighted in his charming though somewhat histrionic and overly sensitive wife. She had full-time domestic help while her sons were growing up, so that her time and energies were free to devote to them. She did this gladly and blossomed in her role as an adoring mom who loved to play with her sons and participate in their activities. They treated their mom as they saw their father and uncles treat her—as a lovely, fragile doll.

Judy spoke wistfully of the first 33 years of her marriage. They sounded almost idyllic—secure, uncomplicated, full of love and closeness. Rich possessed all of the warm attributes her parents lacked, and she felt nurtured and valued. Their physical relationship had been tender, affectionate, considerate, and cuddly, but never passionate, intense, or erotic. Judy assumed that she would continue to live a relatively charmed life and garnered no experience in coping with adversity.

Her first real disillusionment came when her oldest son, Don, a 30-year-old physician, got married. Judy's new daughter-in-law lacked the gentility and refinement she was accustomed to and did not fit into the family's harmonious mold. She was assertive, outspoken to the point of vulgarity, and eager to move far away from the tight, tight world of Don's family. Judy, who had eagerly anticipated welcoming a daughter into the fold, was crushed by her daughter-in-law's open rejection and dislike. It was apparent that Don's wife viewed her mother-in-law as a helpless, parasitic ornament and as a competitor for Don's affection. She cleverly pressured him into accepting an offer to join a practice in Michigan rather than in Boston, and told him it was time to "escape" from his tightly knit Jewish family.

The year after Don's marriage, when Judy was 53 and Rich was 69, Rich had a mild coronary and decided it was time to retire. He no longer could tolerate the brisk New England winters and thought it was advisable to relocate in South Florida. The couple's younger son, who had a good job as an engineer in Boston, chose to remain in their hometown. Judy did not adjust well to the disruption and relocation. She longed for the familiar, secure world of her past. In the 4 years subsequent to their move to Florida, Rich's health slowly deteriorated.

When Judy began therapy, she was in an agitated, mild depression. She asked, "How could he do this to me? How could he get so old so fast?"

She rapped her fist on my desk and in a restrained shout said, "It isn't fair! I'm too young to sit around all day and play companion/nurse to an old, tired man."

When I queried Judy about her realization of the significance of their 16-year age disparity, she said it had only registered with her when Rich became 60 years old. In the early years, it was wonderful having a well-established, older man as a husband, as she didn't have to make any decisions or worry about anything. He did it all for her. But now it seemed like a vast difference. She was still young, energetic, and very much alive. She still wanted to have an active social life, go out dancing, and play golf and tennis. She also had come to realize, from discussions with friends, television, and reading, that she had never experienced a truly passionate, grand love affair and that Rich had been more of a husband/father than a husband/lover. She felt deprived and deeply resented it.

Rich, then 73, was quite sedentary due to his heart condition (he had had a second coronary) and arthritis. He was impotent and lacked any strong desire for sexual play. His expectations, alluded to in the few joint sessions he was willing and able to participate in, were that, since he now needed the attention and nurturance, Judy would take care of him as he had taken care of her for so long. He lightly indicated that part of the reason he had selected a much younger woman was to insure that she'd be alive and well enough to take care of him if and when he became infirm. He hinted at the fact that he had more than earned this as a loyalty debt repayment (Boszormenyi-Nagy & Spark, 1973/1984), and he conveyed his expectation that, of course, Judy would want to "be there for him." This was much less of an established fact for Judy than for her husband, but she was unwilling to relate to him how "trapped" she felt or that the main reasons she planned to remain with him were her fear of loneliness and fear of independent functioning—not gratitude, love, or unending devotion.

It became apparent that Judy had remained an infantile and dependent personality. She longed for her parents' approval and had always wanted affection from her dad to offset her mother's cold strictness. She was unable to express overtly and therefore to resolve her oedipal strivings. Instead, she displaced them onto her brothers and became proficient at being charming, ingratiating, subtly manipulative through her helplessness, and sweetly seductive, only at a level of coy flirtation. In a sense, this was her vocational training—to learn how to please a man so he would support her and protect her from the stresses of the external world.

Her choice of someone like Rich was multiply determined. She craved a father figure who would treat her as his darling daughter. In a somewhat disastrous way, she lived out her oedipal wishes, with Rich as the father substitute. The meager satisfaction was that, materially and in some ways emotionally, she triumphed over her mother in that Rich became much more affluent than her biological father had been. Her mother's critical statements that "you can't do anything right" ceased when Judy married Rich, as he was a fine choice by her mother's criteria. It is also possible that her mother, who repeatedly held sex in disdain as something "a woman only did when her husband wouldn't take no for an answer anymore," at some unconscious or perhaps even conscious level knew that sex across generations is surrounded by taboos. Perhaps, because of her philosophy of marriage, Judy's mother wanted to spare Judy becoming the recipient of excessive sexual demands. Or, perhaps less kindly motivated, she did not want Judy to experience greater sexual pleasures than she had known.

Whatever her mother's intentions, Judy never fully blossomed into a sensuous woman with Rich, as throughout her marriage she responded to him more as a daughter than as a full partner, wife, and lover. It was only after several decades of marriage that Judy realized, from talking to other women, reading sexy novels, and watching television, that some "nice" women enjoyed feeling lustful, and that they initiated sexual play and were passionate and uninhibited with their partners. At that point, she wanted to experiment and experience much more, but Rich was already too old and set in his ways. She was angry over her sense of deprivation and at him for not introducing her to the world of sexuality beyond infrequent lovemaking, limited to intercourse in the missionary position. The fantasies in which she eventually indulged about massage, tactile pleasuring, and oral stimulation inevitably had partners other than Rich as the love object. He simply did not and could not fit her image of a passionate lover.

He, in turn, apparently had a low level of libidinal energy. From the outset, he was paternal, affectionate, and considerate but never "hot blooded." In his cool, methodical, well-planned manner, he selected a compliant, attractive "people pleaser" person for a wife, which left him in total control and with a built-in caretaker for his later years. He wanted a daughter and found one. She was more of a sibling to her sons than a mother. He articulated, and I believe sincerely meant, that Judy had always been the perfect wife for him. He sensed her sexual naïveté and that she would not assertively place sexual demands on him that he would find onerous. This conservatism and inhibition never changed.

In his less-than-golden older years, he really wanted her to stay home and take care of him. She planned to do so, but more as a daughter than as a mature wife who had experienced the rich fullness of a sexually active and fulfilling marriage. At the time that she entered therapy, she was depressed because she felt that life had passed her by and she would never know the joys of full sexuality. She resented his low sexual desire and impotency. Neither could allow themselves to consider a penile implant. Despite her resentment, the idea of pursuing an extramarital affair was unthinkable given her code of fidelity and her fear of high-risk behavior. Her frustration was overwhelming.

Judy did not know how she would manage alone when Rich died, nor could she fathom how she could cope much longer, feeling trapped by him, even though she continued to laud "how wonderful" he then was and always had been. This kindly and considerate "gentleman" had enabled and perpetuated Judy's dependency because this kind of *Doll House* marriage (Ibsen, 1979) suited him extremely well. He had told her never to worry her "pretty little head" about money, thereby keeping her in luxurious bondage. Further, their sons were named his executors, and funds for Judy were placed in a trust so she would never need—or be able—to become independent. Dependence and sexual fulfillment with a person upon whom one is dependent may well be incongruous.

This scenario appears often in May–December marriages, where the reciprocal and interlocking reasons that the choice occurs often become the taboos and impediments to healthy sexuality within the marriage.

Case 2

Several years ago, Dr. Flier (Greg), a psychiatrist who resides and practices several cities away from the Palm Beaches, called to arrange for marital therapy. Because of his prominence in his local and neighboring communities, he decided it was worth traveling some distance to insure privacy and confidentiality. He had specifically and carefully selected me, ostensibly because (1) he felt that both he and his young wife, Bonnie, would relate better to a female therapist; (2) he was familiar with my writings and respected the quality of my work; and (3) we had met briefly at a professional conference where I had made a presentation, and he had "liked my warmth and candor." None of this struck me as atypical, since these reasons are similar to those given by many therapists when they seek treatment (Fay & Lazarus, 1984; Kaslow, 1984, 1986).

During the first interview, the following history unfolded: This was Greg's third marriage. He had a daughter, Colette, aged 21, and a son, Phillippe, aged 19. By now Colette was a senior in college and lived with them on vacations and during the summer. She had always been Daddy's girl. Although her biological mother, Greg's first wife, had originally been granted primary custody at the time of their divorce some 10 years earlier, 2 years later, when Colette was 13 years of age, she had convinced everyone involved that life would be better if she went to live with Dad, who was still "single." For Greg and Colette, all was "comfy-cozy" until Dad remarried briefly, for a year, when his daughter was 16. She apparently attempted to punish him by spending larger blocks of time at her mother's or with friends, and by "hanging out with a druggy crowd and cutting school." Greg came to think that his second wife was too strict and not appreciative of his daughter and had driven her away, and that he had betrayed Colette by marrying again when she was at the vulnerable age of 16 years. His second divorce ensued rapidly, and Colette came home to cuddle with her adoring "papa."

His son, Phillippe, 2 years Colette's junior, was ostensibly handsome and perplexing, as he had a neurologically based learning disability that caused great academic difficulties and lack of acceptance from peers because of his poor ability at sports. His mother never found him to be an appealing child, so he had remained in his protective and competent father's custody (Adamson & Adamson, 1979).

Two years before coming to me for therapy, when Colette was a college sophomore at 19 years of age and Phillippe was a 17-year-old high school sophomore, Greg, then 44 years old, saw and immediately gravitated toward Bonnie at a party. He was attracted by her slim yet sexy build, her dark and sensuous complexion, and her vivacious appearance and actions. Bonnie was flattered by the obvious attentiveness of the tall, good-looking doctor with the sparkling green eyes. Both described how rapidly the sparks were ignited and how strong the chemistry was that they felt for each other. Bonnie, then 24 years old, was literally and figuratively swept off her feet, into Greg's romantic arms and out onto the dance floor. Bonnie had majored in drama at college and was an aspiring actress, working wherever she could find a role in a play. Her theatrical flair made her stand out in a crowd and whetted all of Greg's appetites.

A whirlwind and passionate courtship ensued. Greg fell "madly in love" with his young flame and not only wined and dined her but paid for drama, dance, and vocal lessons. Bonnie had a generous and affectionate nature and was very kind to Phillippe, who responded well to her interest and attention. Greg was ecstatic, as he felt happier and more fulfilled with Bonnie than he had in many years. Despite his training and experience as a clinical psychiatrist and the warning of his long-time male and female friends that Bonnie was truly young enough to be his daughter (she was only 3 years older than Colette, and there was enough of a physical resemblance that they could have been sisters), he was so blinded by his passion and sense of good fortune in meeting and captivating Bonnie that he was able to deny to himself that any incestuous longings were being fulfilled in the relationship or that his needs to be all-powerful and financially indulgent were now being expressed with yet another person.

Bonnie had been an "only, lonely child" of a struggling, blue-collar family. Through charm, determination, hard work, and talent, she had obtained a scholarship and put herself through college. She had an artistic flair and an observant eye. In her expanded, heady college world, she learned how to make the most of her good looks, high cheekbones, and 5'6" amply bosomed body. She had modeled, gone to dance classes and practiced faithfully, and had acquired endearing interpersonal skills. She found Greg's interest both baffling and flattering. How wonderful to have a wealthy, prominent, handsome, and successful psychiatrist so much in love with her!

During the next few sessions, both volunteered further information about their early history as a couple and family quite easily. As the story went, Bonnie willingly moved in with Greg and his son. They had a wonderful few months of a prewedding honeymoon period. Bonnie alternated between her theater classes, rehearsals, and doing some drama therapy in a psychiatric facility. Phillippe responded well to her, and Greg was "on a prolonged high." Colette, similar to other Protestant girls from "good families," was spending her junior year abroad and was too absorbed in her life in Paris to express any opposition; besides, she apparently thought Bonnie would be another of "Daddy's passing fancies."

Greg and Bonnie decided to get married and had a relatively modern and open marriage, in terms of pursuing individual interests while maintaining sexual exclusivity (O'Neill & O'Neill, 1972). Bonnie had made it clear that she wanted to have at least two children, and Greg had consented.

About 2 months after the wedding, Colette returned from France and spent the summer between her junior and senior year "in residence" with her dad and new stepmother. She competed for her dad's affection and treated Bonnie as a hated rival. She used every opportunity she could to turn her father against Bonnie and was cunning and beguiling in her maneuvers (Sager, et al., 1983). She treated Bonnie as a contemporary, not respecting her ascribed and inherited parental role (Visher & Visher, 1979). Bonnie didn't particularly want to be in a parental relationship with a young and sassy woman only 3 years her junior. She was closer in her own life cycle development, interests, and behaviors to her stepdaughter than to her husband (Carter & McGoldrick, 1980). When young men in their late twenties and early thirties came to the house to see Colette, they found Bonnie enticing and mysterious. She was unconsciously drawn to their vibrations of high sexual energy and began to perceive Greg as a much older man.

The heretofore ignored 20-year difference in age then became prominent. Having Colette home also stirred up the incestuous aspects of Greg's and Bonnie's mutual attraction, as it was mirrored in Greg's interactions with his daughter.

Bonnie, who had initially been so patient with Phillippe, became disenchanted with him and "all of his problems" when she began to take over more and more of the daily responsibility for supervising his school-work and at-home activities. She found him to be whiny, spoiled, and demanding. Greg totally indulged him, not only because it was the easiest way to bypass a temper outburst, but because he felt guilty about having contributed to his son's problems. There was a history of minimal brain damage in Greg's family, but not in his first wife's, and he had "broken up" his first family of procreation by initiating the divorce. He was assuaging his guilt and overcompensating by not setting any guidelines or rules for behavior. Phillippe had truly become a tyrannical despot (Abrams & Kaslow, 1979; Kaslow & Cooper, 1978), as many learning-disabled children are inclined to do if given unbridled freedom from their parents.

Bonnie had no desire to spend inordinate amounts of time supervising and entertaining Phillippe. This was not part and parcel of her ideal marriage. By the time they began therapy with me in 1985, after 2 years of marriage, she was "totally fed up" with Phillippe and Colette and with her husband's unwillingness to see his children's excessive demands for attention and their lack of consideration and respect for their stepmother. Greg sided with his children and decried Bonnie's unanticipated "hardheartedness and lack of empathy." He was still "madly in love with her," but they were at an impasse. Since Colette's return from France and her spending of more time in her father's home during her college year, Greg's and Bonnie's ardor had cooled and they rarely made love, unless both children were away from the house at the same time, an infrequent occurrence (Kaslow, 1988). When Greg was in his protective parenting role, he was much less seductive and amorous.

With the children home, it became evident that Bonnie was more of a sibling who was competing for attention, understanding, and money than she was a wife/mistress. She felt manipulated and short-changed. Bonnie's accurate perception of her husband's deliberate manipulativeness was validated when, in the first session, she said, "I can't imagine how Greg found a therapist he didn't know; he knows and intimidates everyone. I'm so glad he heard about you and followed through, as our marriage is really in trouble." Ethically, I thought it incumbent upon me to have Greg clarify that we had had a previous brief contact. It also seemed to be therapeutically essential to win the "battle for structure" (Napier & Whitaker, 1978) and let him know that I would not enter into a collusive and deceptive alliance with him. He was not pleased, but he recognized and came to respect my commitment to ethical practice.

Within the second month of treatment (sessions were held weekly), Bonnie indicated that she wanted to start her family. She was now well into her mid twenties and eager to be a mother. Greg wanted to renege on this part of their premarital contract (Sager, 1976). He felt that they had their hands more than full with Phillippe and Colette and that this was a sufficient family. He didn't want to be going to PTA meetings and Little League games at 50-plus years of age, when he would look like a grandfather compared to the other younger fathers. He was looking forward to an "empty nest" so he and Bonnie could resume their fun times alone together. He was eager for his active parenting years to draw to a close.

Conversely, Bonnie wanted to have her own children and admitted to having chosen Greg partly because she knew he "made beautiful babies" and could immediately supply a financially secure environment for them. She resisted his vague postponement suggestions, realizing these contradicted his newly stated wish for an empty nest. She was also concerned that he would certainly be much older than most other fathers of newborns, and she had come to think that time was of the essence. She was irate and resentful of his changed position regarding wanting children.

Bonnie delivered an ultimatum: Either Greg would express his full commitment to her and their marriage by limiting his children's intrusiveness and demands and participating in "helping me become pregnant," or she would take time out to go to New York, try out for a Broadway play, and see what her life would be like without him. Although Greg said that he didn't want her to leave, his behavior was a reflection of the fact that he was father first and husband/lover second. He had become the good father he himself had always longed for, different from his powerful and competitive surgeon father.

Within 6 months, Bonnie landed a part in an off-Broadway show, found a 33-year-old actor boyfriend, and let Greg know she was filing for divorce. She told him he really was "too old" for her and that his best, productive years were behind him, while her most productive years—professionally, financially, and maternally—were ahead of her. Greg was shattered, but, as could have been predicted, Colette came to the rescue.

Greg resisted looking at the incest and age-related themes and at his inability to set limits with his children lovingly. He blamed Bonnie for all of their problems, splitting off the "bad," adventuresome part of himself. He also reified his daughter, seeing her, like himself, as "all good." His psychiatric background further enabled him to rationalize and intellectualize about what had occurred. Even when presented with fairly confrontative interpretations in therapy, he was never willing to come to grips with the core dynamic that led to his selection of Bonnie, namely, his displaced desire to be sexually involved with Colette.

When therapy terminated, Bonnie felt wonderfully liberated and Greg gloried in his martyrdom and constructed a reality (Reiss, 1981) in which he could get continuing satisfaction from his overprotective and overpossessive, seductive father role.

Clinical Findings from Case Histories

There emerge from these two cases, which are quite representative of the 20 May–December pairs I've seen clinically in the past 7 years, numerous important clinical findings that highlight the typical issues in these relationships:

- Oedipal sexual wishes are often part of the latent substrata of the attraction.
- The husband's already-realized financial success enables him to be generous to his wife and provide her with a very comfortable lifestyle; he rapidly becomes perceived as the potential "good daddy" she always wanted.
- The man's wealth was a definite plus factor in both of these cases and in almost all of the others in my clinical sample. This is congruent with the finding reported earlier by Hartnett, Rosen, and Shumate (1981) that society sanctions age-discrepant marriages of a younger woman to an older man, when he is wealthy.
- Initially, the man is flattered and rejuvenated by the attention of the much younger woman; later, he resents her desire for a larger variety of pleasures, which may include frequent and experimental sex, children, athletic activity, and travel. He's done much of this and is ready to be more settled and sedentary.
- These much younger wives, whether the first or second spouses of their older husbands, evolve or "inherit" a sibling rivalry with their children and stepchildren.
- Frequently, at the beginning, the woman is a dependent and somewhat submissive person and the man is seemingly independent and

dominant. The relationship has a great deal of complementarity (Bateson, 1958), which is mutually satisfying. However, if and when the woman becomes more assertive and autonomous, as Bonnie did, most of these husbands are not able to accept a shift to a more egalitarian, symmetrical marital system. They cannot tolerate the perceived loss of power and control entailed in a more equal relationship.

• Often the man perceives the woman as flighty, charmingly inadequate or lightweight, and somewhat lacking in depth. He simultaneously criticizes yet enjoys these traits and her dependency, because of his own ambivalence about his child/wife. She is confused by his contradictory messages.

• Ultimately, the woman comes to see their husband as "too old for me" and realizes that, chronologically and emotionally, he is in her parents' generation and not her own. When it is a second marriage for him and a first for her, she is often truly an age peer with his children. The couple are at vastly different stages in their personal life cycles.

• Because of the frequency and intensity of cross-generational themes (Minuchin, 1974; Minuchin & Fishman, 1981) and transactions in the relationship, the incest taboo is periodically activated and inhibits the full flowering of a rich and continuous, sensuous, sexual relationship. To the extent that true intimacy only flourishes between relatively equal and mutually respectful partners of the same generation, these May-December marriages seem to have a low potential for long-term sexual gratification, emotional closeness and understanding, and physical intimacy. In fact, the specific and multidetermined choice of partner may well be a manifestation of a primitive protective defense against intimacy.

• Eventually, and sometimes all too soon, the partner's sexual appetites and interests are out of rhythm. Not infrequently, as the woman becomes less inhibited and feels a sense of heightened sensuosity and sexuality in her thirties and forties, he is experiencing a decline in his sexual desire and/or prowess. He may have increasing difficult having and/or sustaining an erection, or he may become a premature ejaculator (Kaplan, 1974, 1979). The causes may be psychologically and/or physiologically based, as in the Germaine case. The vastly different levels of libidinal energy and sexual desire can contribute to an exacerbation of any existing schism and incompatibility and be one of the trigger factors that precipitates the move toward divorce.

This study confirms what Magdoff-Singer (1988) reported, which is that women in May-December relationships generally "appear to have had critical, demanding mothers and remote or unpredictable fathers. The older men they married had fathers who were highly competitive and presented a strong macho image; their mothers were narcissistic and dependent" (p. 140). Basically, the women were overwhelmed by the tasks of individuating and achieving a high level of autonomy. They were unconsciously quite competitive with their mothers and were attracted to men with rescue fantasies. Most seemed to transfer their "symbiotic attachment from their mothers to older, protective, potentially nurturant" (p. 140), yet often dictatorial men. As daughters growing up, the large majority of these women received the message that it was not particularly advantageous to be independent, that it was better to "have a man who will take care of you and look after you" (pp. 140–141).

In effect, they were reared to be beautiful and dependent, as a way of ultimately earning a living (being supported). We also found, as did Magdoff-Singer (1988), that some of the "December" males could easily be categorized as very special in that they were very wealthy or very famous. Although most appeared to be competent and able, they were not "exceptionally talented" by external standards. Nevertheless, the women in our sample reported that their husbands exceeded their expectations, at least in the early years, and they viewed themselves as fortunate.

In order that therapy be a curative experience for May-December couples, the therapist should discern whether the basis of the attraction and continual involvement is an attempt, conscious or unconscious, to rectify missed aspects of close relationships from their childhood or a more pathological interactive sequence. To the extent that the younger woman has transferred her dependency needs from her parents to her husband, the therapist should attempt to help her achieve sufficient self-confidence, competence, and assertiveness to end her symbiotic attachments to parent(s) and spouse. Concurrently, in conjoint sessions, the husband's need for power, control, and dominance must be addressed so that he can come to accept his wife's burgeoning selfhood and maturity.

Ultimately, the mechanisms of splitting and projective identification must be interpreted and contained so that each partner can be perceived as his or her "real self," not as the idealized or hated personification of the good or bad imagoes. Each partner must be helped to tolerate ambivalence and accept it as a fact of daily existence, if they are to be able to integrate the good and bad aspects of self and others and establish a solid and realistic sense of self as a whole and separate person.

Helping them to assess honestly their past intentions and current needs and desires is essential. As indicated earlier, for true intimacy to be possible, the spouses must become "equals," transcending the generational difference so that they can become real partners. Only then can their sexuality flourish in a healthy, mutually gratifying, adult-to-adult relationship.

PERSONAL RESPONSES

Influence of Gender and Generational Socialization. As a woman who saw realization of her own career aspirations as an important and legitimate goal before the groundswell of the feminist movement occurred, autonomy and self-sufficiency were and remain key components of my personal value system. Although I consciously believe in the hackneyed phrase "options for women," the "best" option in a male–female love relationship, where emotional and physical intimacy are sought, seems to me to be a reciprocal one where each utilizes and expands his or her assets in a healthy, egalitarian dyadic system (Kaslow, 1982). This entails, but is not limited to, joint problem-solving efforts; mutual respect and consideration; space for individuality as well as togetherness, and for separate as well as shared activities; having fun together; and being basically in agreement regarding values and lifestyle. These beliefs may also reflect the socialization pattern in my family, in which one was raised to marry for love, to make a permanent commitment, to treasure and be loyal to one's mate, and to expect the same in return. My mom was a bubbly, assertive, energetic dynamo; she always felt equal to the task and able to meet the many challenges that arose in the life of a first-generation, poor, immigrant family. During the Depression and for many years thereafter, my dad worked 7 days a week from 7:00 A.M. to 10:00 P.M. to "make ends meet" during my childhood and adolescence. Initiative, hard work, and shouldering responsibility, side by side in a family unit, were ideals that became deeply ingrained. The family believed in and lived "all for one and one for all."

It may well be that seeing women who are socialized to be and remain helpless and dependent, and who then choose to stay in this position rather than make a personal contribution to the world, as did Judy Germaine, is an anathema to me. They seem to lose out on enjoying the self-enhancement that accrues from pursuing one's own productive efforts. To the extent that women like this want to become more autonomous, I believe I can be a very valuable ally, through therapy. I can usually empathize with the level of stress their husbands feel, since I have much respect for people who have achieved a great deal through their own activities. Many are over functioners and can be helped to begin to relinquish some of their desire and need for total responsibility and control. They are then enabled to move toward a healthier, more balanced relationship (Lewis, Beavers, Gossett, & Phillips, 1976; Walsh, 1982), rather than a system in which the husband is superior because of greater age, education, and wealth, and the wife is inferior due to being a dependent personality, younger, less educated, and from a lower socioeconomic class.

I was raised in a lower-middle-class, hard-working, Jewish family of very conservative morality. The extended families of origin on both sides were striving for survival. My dad's family in particular placed a high premium on education, intelligence, social justice, and freedom for all, which they saw as essential elements in the Jewish tradition and as compatible with the pursuit of the American Dream, which was the reason they had emigrated to America from Eastern Europe. My mom was openly affectionate to my older sister and me; my dad was emotionally cool and reserved. They would hug one another and were very devoted to each other, but there were never any sexually seductive behaviors exhibited, nor was there ever any child abuse, spouse abuse, alcoholism, or drug addiction. Arguing was virtually nonexistent. Struggles were with the harsh realities of the economic and political world, not the inner private world of the family. Although we were a close and rather cohesive nuclear family, sexuality was not an issue to be addressed. It was probably considered insignificant. As I reflect back, I believe both parents were shy and inhibited. Our sex education consisted of occasional admonitions to "never let a boy touch you," to "be a virgin when you get married," and to "always be a lady." On the rare occasions when I dared to wear a dress with a decolleté neckline or a tight-fitting sweater and short skirt, Dad would send me upstairs to change into something less revealing and much more proper. His few words and disparaging look had the force of strict family rules in them.

Influence of Personal Intimacy and Sexual Experiences. Given what I was to realize was my own passionate and highly sensuous nature, I sought out a marital relationship with a warm, affectionate, devoted, considerate, intelligent, and ethical man. It was intended to provide the cocoon in which I could express and fulfill my own vivid sexual fantasies and longings and in which, I hoped, he could also. Fortunately, we met while we were both in college and dated off and on for many years. Sol respected, fully accepted, and admired my high energy, career ambitions, need for autonomy, and the (displaced) physicality that was expressed in many forms of dance. When we married 7 years after we first met, he said he knew exactly what he was getting and it was what he wanted. Thirty-plus years later, we share a continually deepening physical and emotional intimacy in the frame of a basically egalitarian marriage. Many of our long-time friends, who consider their marriages to be essentially satisfying after 25-plus years together, also seem to have a similar respect for each other's individuality, integrity, honesty, and fidelity and welcome growth and change. They started out on a relatively equal footing and share a history of dreams they have fulfilled together, particularly of having mastered the vicissitudes of adult life together and of respecting each other's contributions to their nuclear and extended families and their personal ecosystems.

Conversely, the May–December couples in our clinical population often start out on an unequal footing and the inequalities are perpetuated, often by mutual tacit agreement. As indicated earlier, when the wife attempts to redress this inequality, the "doll's house" crumbles. It may be that my own gratifying experience of intimacy in a peer friendship/love relationship stands out in sharp contrast to what is usually achieved in age-disparate, cross-generational relationships.

Implications for Family Therapy Training and Practice. Despite the fact that I agree with core training for family therapy practice that emphasizes systems thinking and interventions to interrupt dysfunctional relational patterns, I believe there must also be some focus on the intrapsychic world of the individuals who make up the couple and family, on sexual themes in family life, and on different types of pairs, including the kind delineated in this chapter. Although part of training should be generic, clinical practice is specific to each patient or patient unit. Clinicians should have a grasp of the dynamics of various dyadic systems and their *raison d'être*, the kinds of problems they enounter, and the range of strategies for coping with these. Would that I had had at least some exposure in graduate school to sexual dysfunctions and sexual themes in marriage and family therapy. They weren't taught then and are still generally underemphasized, so that individuals must fill in the gaps through reading and attending institutes and workshops. There is always so much more to do; trial and error, both sexual and clinical, are still excellent modalities for learning and are often more enticing than the classroom or library. Yet, here, too, balance is essential. Formal training in taking and understanding a sexual history, in the importance of prescribing a complete medical work-up when there is a sexual dysfunction, and in appropriate interventions should, in my opinion, be part of any graduate or professional school or institute training program.

REFERENCES

Abrams, J. & Kaslow, F. W. (1976). Learning disability and family dynamics: A mutual interaction. *Journal of Clinical Child Psychology*, (1), 35–40.

Adamson, W., & Adamson, K. (1979). *A handbook of specific learning disabilities*. New York: Gardner Press.

Ahrons, C. R., & Rodgers, R. H. (1987). *Divorced families: A multidisciplinary development view*. New York: W. W. Norton.

Bateson, G. (1958). *Naven* (2nd ed.). Stanford, CA: Stanford University Press.

Boszormenyi-Nagy, I., & Spark, G. (1984). *Invisible loyalities*. New York: Brunner/Mazel. (Original work published 1973)

Carter, E., & McGoldrick, M. (Eds.). (1980). *The family life cycle*. New York: Gardner Press.

Cowan, G. (1984). The double-standard in age discrepant relationships. *Sex Roles, 11*, 17–23.

Fay, A., & Lazarus, A. A. (1984). The therapist in behavioral and multi-modal therapy. In F. W. Kaslow (Ed.), *Psychotherapy with psychotherapists* (pp. 1–8). New York: Haworth Press.

Foster, D., Klinger-Vertabedian, L., & Wispe, L. (1984). Male longevity and age differences between spouses. *Journal of Gerontology, 39*(1), 117–120.

Hartnett, J., Rosen, F., & Shumate, M. (1981). Attribution of age discrepant couples. *Perceptual and Motor Skills, 52*, 355–358.

Ibsen, H. J. (1979). *The doll house*. Morton Grove, IL: Coach House Press. (Original work published 1879)

Kaplan, H. S. (1974). *The new sex therapy*. New York: Brunner/Mazel.

Kaplan, H. S. (1979). *Disorders of sexual desire*. New York: Brunner/Mazel.

Kaslow, F. W. (1981). A diaclectic approach to family therapy and practice: Selectivity and synthesis. *Journal of Marital and Family Therapy, 7*, 345–351.

Kaslow, F. W. (1982). Portrait of a healthy couple. *Psychiatric Clinics of North America, 5*(3), 519–527.

Kaslow, F. W. (1984). *Psychotherapy with psychotherapists*. New York: Haworth Press.

Kaslow, F. W. (1986). Therapy with distressed psychotherapists: Special problems and challenges. In R. R. Kilburg, P. E. Nathan, & R. W. Thoreson (Eds.), *Professionals in distress: Issues, syndromes and solutions in psychology* (pp. 187–210). Washington, DC: American Psychological Association.

Kaslow, F. W. (1988). Remarried couples: The architects of stepfamilies. In F. W. Kaslow (Ed.), *Couples therapy in a family context: Perspective and retrospective* (pp. 33–48). Rockville, MD: Aspen.

Kaslow, F. W., & Cooper, B. (1978). Family therapy with the learning disabled child and his/her family. *Journal of Marriage and Family Counseling, 3*(1), 41–49.

Kaslow, F. W., & Schwartz, L. L. (1987). *Dynamics of divorce: A life cycle perspective*. New York: Brunner/Mazel.

Kernberg, O. (1980). *Internal world and external reality*. New York: Jason Aronson.

Klein, M. (1948). *The psychoanalysis of children*. London: Hogarth Press.

Lewis, J., Beaners, W. R., Gossett, J. T., & Phillips, V. A. (1976). *No single thread: Psychological health and the family system*. New York: Brunner/Mazel.

Magdoff-Singer, L. (1988). May/December marriages. In F. W. Kaslow (Ed.), *Couples therapy in a family context: Perspective and retrospective* (pp. 133–146). Rockville, MD: Aspen.

Minuchin, S. (1974). *Families and family therapy.* Cambridge, MA: Harvard University Press.

Minuchin, S., & Fishman, H. C. (1981). *Family therapy techniques.* Cambridge, MA: Harvard University Press.

Napier, A. Y., & Whitaker, C. A. (1978). *The family crucible.* New York: Harper & Row.

National Center for Health Statistics (December 26, 1985). Advance report of final divorce statistics, 1983. *Monthly vital statistics report, 34*(Suppl 9), 86–120.

O'Neill, G., & O'Neill, N. (1972). *Open marriage: A new life style for couples.* New York: M. Evans.

Presser, H. B. (1975). Age differences between spouses. *American Behavioral Scientist, 19,* 190–205.

Riess, D. (1981). *The family's construction of reality.* Cambridge, MA: Harvard University Press.

Riley, M. W. (1983). The family in an aging society. *Journal of Family Issues, 4*(3), 439–454.

Sager, C. J. (1976). *Marriage contracts and couple therapy: Hidden forces in intimate relations.* New York: Brunner/Mazel.

Slipp, S. (1984). *Object relations: A dynamic bridge between individual and family treatment.* New York: Jason Aronson.

Visher, E. B., & Visher, J. S. (1979). *Stepfamilies: A guide to working with stepparents and stepchildren.* New York: Brunner/Mazel.

Walsh, F. (1982). *Normal family processes.* New York: Guilford Press.

Weitzman, L. J. (1985). *The divorce revolution: The unexpected social and economic consequences for women and children in America.* New York: Free Press.

13

A CYBERNETIC–SYSTEMIC APPROACH TO PROBLEMS IN SEXUAL FUNCTIONING

Gary Sanders and Karl Tomm

There are few human activities that occur so frequently and yet are so shrouded in privacy, misunderstanding, and myth, as sexual activity. The privacy fosters misunderstanding and myth making, and the mythologies in turn foster further misunderstanding and privacy. Despite the recent increase in the amount of public information about sexuality that is available in books, popular magazines, and newspapers, person-to-person exchange of information about sexual experience tends to be stereotyped, surreptitious, or altogether absent. Consequently, sexual ideas, values, expectations, and activities vary enormously from one individual to another, from one couple to another, from one religious community to another, and from one culture to another. Add to this the variety of purposes and meanings associated with human sexuality—such as reproduction, physical attraction, attachment, sexual identity, sexual orientation, sexual preferences, the politics of male–female relations, morality, and spirituality—and the subject becomes extremely complex. In other words, sexual activity at any one moment may fulfill a variety of personally felt physical, psychological, social, and/or cultural expectations. These could include experiencing intense physical and psychological arousal, expressing interpersonal intimacy and uniqueness, fostering interpersonal bonding, producing offspring, seeking self-affirmation, seeking personal power, or fulfilling conjugal duty and commitment. With such complex

Gary Sanders and Karl Tomm. Family Therapy Program, Department of Psychiatry, The University of Calgary, Calgary, Alberta, Canada.

demands being made of one's sexuality, it is not surpising that adolescents and adults often seem heavily preoccupied with issues of sexuality. At the same time, however, because so many individuals remain constrained by the shroud of privacy and by family and social sexual taboos, it is also not surprising that they develop concerns about and symptoms of sexual dysfunction.

Increasing numbers of these people are now seeking help for their sexual concerns. In North America many of these couples seek such help from marital and family therapists, particularly when specialized sex therapists are not available. The issues brought to family therapy are mostly related to sexual functioning and less so to issues of sexual development or identity. Concerns about partner fidelity, sexual abuse, and the sexual activities of children or adolescents are also commonly presented but will not be addressed here. We will limit our discussion to therapeutic responses to problematic experiences of persons in a sexual relationship, that is, to problems of sexual functioning. Within this domain, clients are usually concerned about how they *should* be performing sexually. They compare their current performance to a past time, or to their performance with another partner, or to the performance of others (as imagined or as seen in print and movies), and regard themselves as falling short.

The majority of these complaints and symptoms may be mapped onto the five phases of the sexual response cycle: sexual desire, arousal and excitement, orgasm, resolution, and evaluation/pleasure. For instance, one partner may complain that the other is insufficiently desirous of intercourse. Others may report lack of physiological arousal, despite a strong desire. Still others may complain of early ejaculation or inability to achieve orgasm.

From our point of view, what is more important than the specific nature of the symptoms is the experience of and concern about these symptoms. These concerns could be quantitative, such as worries about the frequency of sexual activity or intercourse, or they could be qualitative, such as complaints about lack of sufficient intimacy for adequate arousal before coitus. These types of concerns are, of course, often interrelated in that one partner may complain about lack of frequency of sexual contact while the other may complain of lack of sensitivity to his or her feelings. The partners' respective experiences and consequent problem-solving efforts often form a feedback system that tends to maintain or aggravate their problems, with increasing dissatisfaction for both. It is this interpersonal pattern of complementary experiencing, meaning giving, and responding that interests us the most in organizing our efforts to facilitate therapeutic change. In other words, our focus is on patterns in the here and now. This does not mean that we are not interested in our clients' past sexual experiences. We are, but only insofar as that past is active and having effects in the present. In our view, an in-depth interview about past sexual experiences and events can be more pathologizing than healing. As therapists, we prefer to orient ourselves in therapy toward fostering a future-oriented self-healing process rather than a past-oriented analytic process. Because of this preference and our recognition of the applicability of cybernetic and systemic thinking toward this end, the primary focus of our chapter will be on the use of systemic* therapeutic principles in dealing with concerns about sexual functioning.

A PRAGMATIC DEFINITION OF SEX

Whenever possible we try to maintain a view of sex and sexuality as centering around persons' perceived experiences within a dyadic relationship. Sex is not merely regarded as the physical encounter of sexual organs or any particular sequence of actions; it is regarded as a uniquely sensuous experience in an intimate relationship. The terms *sex, sexual,* and *sexuality* will refer to those conditions, both personal and interpersonal, that permit the creation of the experience of an interpersonal state of sensuous mutuality. Thus, the term *sex* will not be used to refer primarily to anatomy, physiology, or those actions necessary to reproduce the species. Instead, we conceptualize sex as mutual sexuality.

The decision to focus on the experiential and relational aspects of sex rather than on the physical and reproductive is based on two factors. One is the nature of our clientele. The clients that present to us with sexual problems describe concerns about sexual functioning that takes place in the context of intimate personal relationships. Clients with genuine physiological sexual problems seldom present themselves to us for treatment. Furthermore, in contemporary North American culture, the vast majority of the population who engage in sexual activity take active measures to limit or obviate their reproductive possibilities. These measures may

---

*The use of the term *systemic* throughout this chapter refers to those ideas and theories alternatively referred to as Batesonian, Milan, ecosystemic, or cybernetic. The common thread among these views is a focus on circular patterns of interaction triggered by "differences." This is in contrast to the physicalistic view of systems associated with general systems theory, where interaction is based on mass, energy, and power. For a more detailed discussion of these differing systems views, the reader is referred to Bradford Keeney's book, *The Aesthetics of Change* (1983).

include anything from the rhythm method, condoms, diaphragms and the pill, to surgical sterilization. The second reason for defining sex as mutual sexuality is that it orients us as clinicians in a more therapeutic direction. If we were to focus on and to attend to primarily the physical and physiological aspects of sexuality in our treatment efforts, our clients would be invited to do the same. Doing so would be to contribute to a process of objectifying, mechanizing, and perhaps even trivializing a unique human event that has the potential to be experienced as holistic, aesthetic, and spiritual. Shifting one's view from sex as a physical act to sex as a relationship process opens more possibilities for the latter potential to be actualized.

Our circumscribed definition of mutual sexuality includes four major criteria:

1. Each person in a dyadic relationship experiencing self as having desire (with or without physical arousal) to be sexual with the other person
2. Each person in the relationship perceiving the other as also experiencing sexual desire and/or arousal
3. Each person actively choosing to participate in whatever intimate interaction takes place and not being coerced to do so
4. Each person experiencing this mutual desire, arousal, and/or activity in a context of emotional and physical vulnerability, with trust that one will not be taken advantage of by the other

Please note that our definition of mutual sexuality does not *necessarily* include intercourse. Although coitus may be entailed in an episode of mutual sexuality, it is not considered a key criterion for a gratifying sexual experience. On the other hand, anything that does not fulfull the four conditions is considered something other than mutual sexuality. For instance, if one person is sexually desirous and/or aroused while the partner is not, but the latter participates willingly for social reasons, we might regard the activity as "sexual obligation" or as "sexual duty," but not as mutual sexuality. If one partner is aroused while the other is not interested or willing, but the former tries to impose his or her desires upon the latter, we regard the activity as "sexual assault" or "sexual harassment," depending on whether physical force is employed or not. If sexual activity is taking place between an adult and child, we consider the activity "sexual abuse," whether the child is interested and aroused or not. This follows from our cultural point of view that the adult is seen as not respecting the child's best developmental interests.

In evaluating different forms of sexual interaction from our particular sociocultural perspective, we have found it useful to make two basic distinctions. The interaction could be distinguished as socially responsible or socially irresponsible, and it could be distinguished as violent or nonviolent. It is important to note that for the purposes of this discussion we are using Humberto Maturana's (personal communication, 1986) rather broad definition of violence as *any attempt to impose one's will upon another,** whether by physical, chemical, psychological, or social means. The reason for using such a broad definition is that it invites us to recognize the violence being perpetrated in certain situations that we otherwise might not consider violent. At the same time, however, it invites us to evaluate whether this "violence" is socially responsible or not. In other words, Maturana's definition leaves space for some violence to be accepted as socially responsible, such as appropriate discipline of children, confrontation of adults who persist in problematic patterns, enforcement of social legislation, and control of criminal behavior. However, the fact that violence may be involved in some situations not ordinarily considered violent stimulates us and our clients to try to think of alternative patterns of interaction that are not violent.

Given these two distinctions, it is possible to categorize a variety of sexual interaction patterns and contrast them with the sexual mutuality we strive to facilitate. Sexual harassment, sexual assault, and most sexual abuse are regarded as both violent and socially irresponsible. Sexual abuse of children may in some circumstances be seductive and not violent, but in our opinion it remains socially irresponsible because of the socially generated developmental view that the adult has failed to respect and protect the future of that child. Similarly, voluntary prostitution and other forms of sexual exploitation may not be violent, but they can be readily distinguished by many as socially irresponsible in that someone is being taken advantage of and/or the sacredness of sex is being trivialized. On the other hand, a sexual encounter based on obligation (as for instance, when one person concedes to the sexual requests or demands of another, not because he or she is desirous or interested, but because of prior commitments or other social circumstances) may be socially responsible, but it

---

*I (G.S.) generally use a more expanded version of Maturana's definition of violence. It is *The holding of a view by one person or group to be true so that another person's or group's view is untrue and must change.* It is the belief that others' views *must change* rather than the difference of views that creates the interpersonal "mind set" that Maturana says all violence stems from.

would be considered violent insofar as the second is imposing his or her desires upon the first. Likewise, some forms of sexual refusal following intentional invitations to sexual activity may also be regarded as violent. Based on our two basic distinctions, these and other kinds of sexual interaction are tentatively categorized in Figure 13.1.

What is interesting to note is that the sexual activity entailed in "marital duty," that is, one spouse (usually the wife) responding to the sexual demands of the other spouse, not because she or he wants to, but because they happen to be married, may be socially responsible but, given our framework, it still would be considered violent. Thus, many "normal" couples may be seen to be living a relationship of sexual violence (with episodes of sexual duty and/or sexual refusal) rather than a relationship of mutual sexuality. Unfortunately, much of this type of violence is considered socially responsible and hence tends to be perpetuated rather than presented for therapeutic intervention. Nevertheless, such relationship patterns usually become a chronic source of stress for both partners. The form of sexual activity that we consider mutual sexuality is nonviolent, in that both persons are genuinely interested and desirous; and it is socially responsible, in that neither participant is being taken advantage of by the other.

	Violent	Non-Violent

Socially Irresponsible	- sexual harassment
	- coercive sexual abuse
	- sexual assault
	  (including "rape")
	- coercive prostitution
		- sexual exploitation
		- voluntary prostitution
		- pornography depicting
		  violence or degradation
		- non-coercive sexual
		  abuse

Socially Responsible	- sexual obligation or
	  "marital duty"
	- sexual refusal after
	  intentionally
	  fostering expectations
		- sexual and reproductive
		  education
		- declining unwanted
		  sexual invitations
		- mutual sexuality

FIGURE 13.1.   Violence and social responsibility in sexual relations.

EARLIER APPROACHES TO SEXUAL DYSFUNCTION

During the last century there have been two major therapeutic approaches to concerns about sexual functioning. The use of "folk medicine" remedies is the oldest and the most established. For instance, men with rapid ejaculation have often been told to entertain anti-erotic thoughts during sexual intercourse, to provide distraction. Having an affair has sometimes been prescribed for men with erectile dysfunction, while testosterone has been administered to others. For female arousal and orgasmic dysfunctions, "common-sense" suggestions have included using lubricating gels, faking orgasm, and passively taking care of the husband's sexual needs no matter what the woman's state of arousal.

The second major approach has been psychoanalytically oriented psychotherapy, to which most professionals practicing in the mental health field have been exposed. This approach is based on the theoretical assumption that the failure to accomplish the childhood developmental tasks associated with an appropriate resolution of the Oedipus complex results in arrested, delayed, or distorted psychosexual development. Treatment usually consists of reenacting the oedipal situation in the transference relationship with a therapist and thereby completing those developmental tasks that were seen as not accomplished in childhood (Heiman, LoPiccolo, & LoPiccolo 1981). Partly as a result of the failure of the analytic approach to deal effectively and efficiently with sexual problems, the first approach of "common-sense remedies" once again became more prevalent.

In the last 20 years, more modern methods of dealing with couples' sexual concerns have been developed. A major milestone was Masters and Johnson's (1970) pioneering work. Soon after it was published, behavioral treatment strategies became widespread. They involved the therapist in educating clients about normal sexual functioning, in restructuring maladaptive behavior patterns and cognitions, and in using anxiolytic and skill-training techniques. The work of Masters and Johnson filled in many of the gaps about the physiological and anatomical basis to sexual activity. Other researchers (Hoon, Hoon, & Wincze, 1976, 1977; LoPiccolo, 1980) have carried on their work, and many changes have occurred in the understanding and treatment of sexual problems, particularly in the last 15 years. Several behavioral treatment methods have been extended and elaborated.

Today, however, there are comparatively few people who practice strictly behavioral approaches. Instead, most sex therapies involve quasi-behavioral techniques. For instance, Kaplan (1974, 1979) in her "New Sex Therapy" uses many behavioral techniques, such as systematic desensitization, the construction of successive client successes, and so forth, but her work is combined with the psychodynamic analysis of the individual. The work of Price and colleagues (Price, Heinrich, & Golden, 1980; Price, Reynolds, Cohen, Anderson, & Schochet, 1981) is also based on behavioral principles but tends to be more interactional in its application. These therapists pioneered the use of group treatment strategies for sexual concerns. All of these approaches had the following in common: attempts to reduce performance anxiety, use of sex education, skill training, communication in sexual technique, and the use of a variety of attitude change procedures.

The elaboration of systemic therapy methods by the Milan team (Selvini Palazzoli, 1978, 1980) and others (Hoffman, 1981; Tomm 1984a, 1984b) opened the door for another useful clinical tool to be applied to the treatment of sexual problems. Both of us (especially G.S.) have been involved in applying Milan concepts to sexual difficulties since 1980 (Sander, 1986). The use of these systemic principles has been extremely gratifying in some cases. Nevertheless, we continue to use some of the quasi-behavioral treatment principles as well, remaining mindful of the systemic context in which they are being applied. Indeed, one of the things we have found is that applying quasibehavioral techniques in the context of systemic understanding potentiates their effectiveness.

MULTIPLE DOMAINS OF EXPLANATION AND INTERVENTION

Despite our preferred focus on the experiential relationship aspects of sexuality, we acknowledge the fundamental importance of our clients' biological status, knowledge base, and behavioral repertoire. At least some assessment of these aspects is required, in addition to an evaluation of the meaning our clients give to their sexual activity and to their interpersonal relationship. For this reason, an approach that uses a model with multiple domains of assessment and intervention will be described and elaborated.

At any particular point in therapy, inquiries and/or interventions may be directed toward the biological domain of physiology, the informational domain of facts about sex, the behavioral domain of sexual actions, or the experiential/relational domain of meaning. We tend to organize ourselves by thinking of these domains as reflecting nonhierarchical levels of increasing comprehensiveness which are interconnected (by us as observers) in a circular fashion (see Figure 13.2). The model is nonhierarchical in the sense that we assume bidirectional, rather than unidirectional,

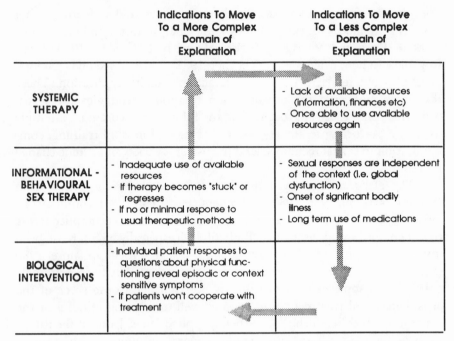

	Indications To Move To a More Complex Domain of Explanation	Indications To Move To a Less Complex Domain of Explanation
SYSTEMIC THERAPY		- Lack of available resources (information, finances etc) - Once able to use available resources again
INFORMATIONAL - BEHAVIOURAL SEX THERAPY	- Inadequate use of available resources - If therapy becomes "stuck" or regresses - If no or minimal response to usual therapeutic methods	- Sexual responses are independent of the context (i.e. global dysfunction) - Onset of significant bodily illness - Long term use of medications
BIOLOGICAL INTERVENTIONS	- Individual patient responses to questions about physical functioning reveal episodic or context sensitive symptoms - If patients won't cooperate with treatment	

FIGURE 13.2.   Nonhierarchical model of multiple domains of intervention.

patterns of influence among the several domains. A basic feature of the model is the implied flexibility to move from one domain to another whenever this seems appropriate. By moving from one level of conceptual abstraction "up" to more comprehensive levels and back "down" again to simpler levels recurrently, therapists should be able to change the nature of their explanations as needed to guide their interventions. Whenever possible, however, therapists remain mindful of the experiential/relational effects of any assessment or treatment initiatives while working at the biological, informational, and behavioral levels. For instance, if inquiring about certain aspects of biological functioning, about a person's sexual knowledge, or about specific sexual behaviors were likely to be experienced as humiliating (and not just embarrassing) in the presence of the partner, the therapist would refrain from asking in the conjoint context. Thus, the systemic relational view still provides the overall umbrella that contextualizes explorations in the other domains.

With a complete assessment, movement in the model might proceed in a stepwise fashion up from a biological focus, through an informational and behavioral focus, on to an interactional and experiential one. At the same time, however, the model suggests that there are times when it might be appropriate to move back down to lower levels of complexity, to generate more appropriate interventions. Implicit in this model is the invitation for therapists to recognize that it might be useful to move from one domain of understanding (and concomitantly from one domain of intervention) to another in certain circumstances. Before proceeding to focus our discussion on the emotional/experiential domain, which we are most interested in, we will provide some comments about the other domains and our movement from one to another.

At some point in the assessment it is important to inquire about the biological capabilities of each partner. Numerous prescribed drugs, some nonprescription drugs including alcohol and tobacco, and a large number of medical illnesses can severely affect the physiological capability for sexual functioning. Although many marital and family therapists may not feel that they have the expertise to evaluate the biological aspects of sexuality, there is a series of simple questions that can be used to rule out any significant biological dysfunction. These questions can be organized around the five phases of the sexual response cycle.

1. Desire phase
   Are there ever occasions when you feel sexually desirous, whether or not you act on those desires? In other words, have there been times when you experienced a desire to be involved with someone sexually, even though you may not have done so?
2. Excitement/arousal phase
   On an occasion when you do feel sexually desirous and you choose to act sexually, whether with yourself or another person, are you able to increase your arousal through the sexual actions you engage in?
   (*for males*) Do you have physical changes such as an erection, testicles swollen and pulled up against the body, and the like, that accompany arousal?
   (*for females*) Do you have physical changes such as a feeling of pelvic fullness, vaginal wetness, and so forth, that accompany arousal?
   What about arousal associated with dreams in the night or on waking in the morning?
   Are you able to maintain your arousal for whatever sexual purposes you desire?

3. Orgasm phase

Do you get to a point where you feel the urge to release your arousal through a rapid rhythmic release usually called orgasm?

(*for females*) Are you usually able to be orgasmic when you want to be?

(*for males*) Are you able to influence the timing of your ejaculation?

4. Resolution phase

About how long does it take for your body to return to normal after you have been sexually active—seconds, minutes, hours, or days?

(*for females*) Do you have feelings of pelvic fullness, aching, or pain afterward?

(*for males*) Have you had the experience of prolonged aching of the testicles or an erection failing to subside?

5. Evaluation phase

Do you reflect upon the sexual experience you have had and evaluate and/or discuss it?

Do you find the sexual activity to be as pleasurable as you would want it to be?

Any responses to these questions that are unusual should invite the therapist to explore further and could become a basis for requesting a complete physical examination. In particular, negative responses to the questions concerning the excitement/arousal phase in the presence of sexual desire could suggest some underlying medical problem, particularly if no drugs, alcohol, or medication can be implicated. On the other hand, if the clients' answers to these questions suggest that their physiological capabilities are intact, it would be more appropriate to move on to explore the informational, behavioral, and experiential levels before proceeding further with physical investigations, even if a client has predominantly biological concerns. The reason for this is that the client's preoccupation with biology may be limiting her capacity to become aware of relevant factors in the other domains and the therapist's continued focus on biological functioning may inadvertently foster rather than ameliorate the client's misdirected concerns.

Until the more recent interest in medical management (Morales, Surridge, & Marshall, 1981; Morales, Surridge, Marshall, & Fenmore, 1982), specific sexuality oriented biological interventions have focused almost exclusively on surgical methods. These have consisted of the implantation of erectile prostheses or the creation of artificial vaginas.

Although these interventions are beyond the professional scope of most therapists working with sexual concerns, the assessment of the need for biological intervention is not.

If there appear to be no biological problems—that is, the "dysfunction" appears context dependent—the therapist would move up a level and ask a series of questions about the clients' knowledge about sex and their specific sexual behaviors, to give the therapist some benchmark with respect to their sexual understanding and behavioral repertoire. One of us (G.S.) uses a modified version of the Derrogatis Sexual Functioning Inventory as a questionnaire in the form of a handout. A client's lack of adequate information may quickly become apparent in his responses on the questionnaire. Sometimes the judicious use of specific information or behavioral suggestions as to how a couple could enhance the quality of their sexual interaction is all that is required in treatment. In other words, some sexual problems have simple solutions. For instance, setting time aside for a sexual encounter and/or creating the conditions for intimacy, such as being alone together after dinner or an evening out, may seem obvious to most of us but may not be arranged because of the assumption that to do so deliberately would interfere with sexual spontaneity. Occasionally basic information is required to correct misunderstandings. For example, physiological arousal in females is not as obvious as it is in males and may take more time, especially when the male takes the initiative. Thus, if the male proceeds with penetration without realizing his partner is not yet ready, he is unknowingly risking inflicting physical and emotional pain. On other occasions, simply receiving "permission" from an authority figure to perform certain valued behaviors while being sexual is enough to liberate some clients from constraining myths. Some clients feel attracted to oral-genital contact but think it is abnormal. A clear statement that such behaviors are perfectly common and usual and are not unhealthy (provided both parties agree) may be all that is required.

The therapist could also evaluate and monitor client access to sexual information. Although there have been notable changes in the media during the recent years of increasing sexual openness, our community is still relatively secretive and closed regarding information about sexual behavior and experience, compared to other meaningful aspects of life. Because of these restrictive societal values, very few of our clients feel as free to search out useful information about sexual issues as they would about parenting, adolescence, marriage, old age, and similar events. Bibliotherapy, the prescribed reading and reviewing of specified information or use of audiovisual materials, may be helpful in situations in which clients need basic information or gradual desensitization.

Other clients appear to have the opposite problem. They have seen too many sexual movies and/or have read too many sexual novels or manuals. Consequently, they have given themselves so much "permission to perform" that they are unable to keep up to the level of their misguided or unrealistic expectations. For instance, many couples who present with clinical concerns assume their sexual behaviors and feelings should be goal directed, that they should achieve a particular end, such as a "spectacular simultaneous orgasm." Their focus is on achievement. By directing their attention toward the goal of performance or of pleasuring the mate and away from self-directed sensual feelings, these clients miss or lose what they could experience as a quality sexual exchange. The preferred focus in mutual sexuality is one's own experience of heightened *personal* sensual awareness while perceiving the other as also intensely aware of her own experience. What one shares with the mate is not so much one's own sensual feelings but, rather, the interpersonal context. When this context consists of mutual physical and emotional disclosure, vulnerability, and trust, at the same time as one experiences enjoyment and physiological sexual arousal, we think of the event as sexually intimate. If, however, the interpersonal context has evolved to become one of purposeful striving, such as toward some self-imposed performance standards for oneself or one's mate, the couple could benefit from some redirection. Some directive behavioral techniques such as sensate focus exercises and self-stimulation for orgasmic experience may be useful. Depending on how it is implemented, the squeeze technique for early ejaculation could also fall into this domain. If it seems apparent that the couple has an adequate behavioral repertoire, it would be appropriate to move on to focus more squarely on the experiential meaning level. Continuing to focus on specific sexual behaviors could inadvertently promote further performance anxiety.

One positive indication for the need to move to a more complex or comprehensive level of understanding would be the therapist's perception of apparent "resistance" to the interventions based on an explanation at a lower level of conceptualization. For instance, when certain sexual problems that normally respond well to information or behavioral prescriptions are not changing in the direction of resolution, these more usual approaches appear to be resisted. Such situations could benefit from an understanding of the so-called "resistance," thereby enabling the therapy to continue. A useful view of resistance is that held by Steve de Shazer (1982), who suggests it is a property of the client–therapist relationship and not of the client or couple. He uses the therapist's felt experience of client resistance as an indication that the therapist has, as yet, to understand fully enough the couple's symptoms and the system of interaction.

Indeed, as therapists, we prefer to take the pragmatic view that *client resistance does not exist, but therapist resistance does.* Adopting this orientation helps us in using the experience of client resistance to evaluate our own position and recapture an inquisitive stance, which may then enable an exploration of something other than "more of the same wrong solution" (see Luckhurst, 1985, p. 4). On the other hand, when the clients comply appropriately with therapist suggestions and directives, this suggests that further trials of informational or behavioral interventions may be fruitful. In other words, if therapy appears to be progressing well, there is no need to change levels of explanation and intervention. It is such feedback in the therapeutic system, that becomes the cybernetic "steersman" guiding the course of therapy.

An indication for movement downward in the hierarchical model could be any perception on the part of the therapist of the absence (or a deficit) of some important resource, be it financial, physical, physiological, behavioral, informational, emotional, or contextual. If a therapist, working within the relational/experiential domain, perceives a lack of behavioral capabilities, she might be well advised to return to that level of explanation. If, while working at the behavioral level, she notes insufficient knowledge about sexual behavior, a move back to informational input would be appropriate. Likewise, if lack of physiological responsiveness became apparent, further exploration at the biological level would be indicated. The therapist must continually monitor the clients' actual and experiential *access to basic resources* for adequate sexual functioning and try to open space for these resources to be obtained, if they are not readily available. On the other hand, if *inadequate use of available resources* is perceived, it is usually best to move on up to a more complex framework of understanding in which the nature and effects of such inadequate use may be understood and challenged. Thus, one impetus for moment-to-moment changes in the nature of the interventions used is movement between domains of therapist understanding, which is triggered by the clients' responses to the therapist's actions.

THEORETICAL BASIS OF A CYBERNETIC-SYSTEMIC APPROACH

As noted earlier, some sexual problems remain unresponsive to treatment, even when adequate physiological, informational, and behavioral resources are available. It seems as if some clients have a motivational problem of mobilizing and applying these resources to deal effectively with their sexual difficulties. When the usual sex therapy techniques are inadequate, some therapists rely on psychoanalytic methods to treat the "resistance" they distinguish. In a sense, the locus of treatment moves "inside the head." When we encounter this kind of difficulty, however, we prefer to remain "outside the head" as much as possible and continue to explore the couple's human relationship systems, including our relationship with them. Indeed, we are currently often more inclined to explore relationship interventions, even before trying behavioral methods. Desire disorders, for instance, are often too complex to treat effectively and efficiently with the usual methods. Furthermore, we have sometimes observed that, once one problem like vaginismus is resolved, the partner often develops another problem, such as erectile dysfunction. Thus, in these situations we find it more efficacious to use interpersonal systemic interventions from the outset.

There are two levels of complexity involved in applying an interpersonal systems approach. One may be regarded as based on first-order cybernetics—the cybernetics of *observed* systems. The other is based on second-order cybernetics—the cybernetics of *observing* systems. The first entails the identification and description of reciprocal patterns of interaction between mates that generate, maintain, or aggravate, problems. In other words, the focus is on identifying pathologizing patterns of interaction between the members of a couple that are recurrent or circular. These problematic patterns may be classified as negative feedback patterns, positive feedback patterns, or disruptive or extreme oscillations from one pattern to another. Negative feedback in cybernetics entails a difference-minimizing loop. For instance, a male with erectile dysfunction experiencing sexual insecurity might express sexual interest in a partner who responds by evaluating the size and firmness of his penis and, thus, inadvertently raises performance expectations, which undermines his sexual arousal and maintains the insecurity. Such interaction minimizes the possibility of a change or a difference in the symptoms: The man continues to have erectile dysfunction, which continues to invite a focus of interest and concern for the partner. In contrast, positive feedback in cybernetics involves a difference-maximizing loop. For instance, when one person with low sexual interest is pursued incessantly by another with high interest, the sexual appetite of the first is blocked even further, while that of the other is intensified out of frustration. The third type of cybernetic pathology, excessive oscillation from one pattern to another, may be manifest by periods of excessive sexual demands alternating with long periods of complete avoidance of physical contact.

Therapeutic interventions based on these kinds of assessments are oriented toward interrupting the pathologizing pattern. Because the pattern is interactional and circular, the focus of the intervention can be on any link in the chain, that is, on the behavior of the symptomatic person, on the behavior of the partner, on both, or on their sequence in the interaction. Alternatively, the focus of intervention could be on the pattern as a whole, that is, on the meaning systems that organize the whole interactional process. Whenever possible we prefer to focus on the whole pattern by using a more comprehensive intervention, which may be modeled after the Milan systemic methods of offering a paradoxical opinion (e.g., positively connoting the pattern of interaction in service of the relationship) or providing a ritual prescription (e.g., ceremoniously burning, freezing, or thawing a symbolic representation of the experienced restraints to change).

The cybernetics of observing systems entails a greater degree of complexity. It includes a *recursion*, which refers to the application of a process to the products of that same process. An example of second-order cybernetics is the process of distinguishing the nature of the distinctions being distinguished. In other words, within the cybernetics of observing systems, the observing system observes and acts upon its own products and/or habits of observing. Thus, a man with performance anxiety may become anxious when noticing his own performance anxiety. A woman with vaginismus may become tense by trying to relax her own muscular tension. Indeed, "doubled emotions," like fear of being afraid, guilt about feeling guilty, irritation about being irritated, being depressed about being depressed, can become especially malignant. There is a much larger degree of interaction with the "self" in these patterns.

This self, however, need not be thought of as "skin-bounded." Indeed, we find it more useful to think of the self as a socially defined unity that arises through, and is maintained and/or modified by, social interaction. In other words, the "autonomy" of the pathologizing patterns that entail self-observing may still be seen as a social process. Human beings see themselves through the eyes of other human beings. The interpersonal aspects of these second-order patterns may not be obvious at first glance, but they become more apparent when we reflect upon the distinctions we make about the distinctions others make of us, and the effects these distinctions have on our patterns of thought, feeling, and behavior. Take, for example, the ubiquitous blame-guilt cycle. If a woman distinguishes the man she is being intimate with as insensitive, and he distinguishes her as distinguishing him as such, he may concede and also see himself as insensitive and feel badly about himself, and/or he may distinguish her as too judgmental and blame her for being unfair. She, in turn, could take either or both responses as validations of her original distinction. If he tries to defend himself and blame her for being unfair or in error, she may feel obliged to bring forth more evidence to support her view. At the same time, however, she may also concede to his view of her and begin to feel badly about herself. If he then distinguishes his behavior as having triggered her into feeling badly, he may feel even worse and become more suspicious about his own sensitivity, seeing himself as preoccupied with himself, less sensitive, and more irritable with her, and so on. The "knot" of self-definition through mutual interaction begins to tighten. Talking about their views of one another becomes a process of blame inviting guilt and guilt inviting further blame, so that they see each other and themselves more and more negatively. Then, distinguishing themselves in a painful pattern of talking, they begin a new relationship of talking about their relationship, which also may become problematic with further blame-guilt cycles. In other words, sexual problems in couples often arise and are aggravated by their patterns of reacting to and/or talking about what they distinguish as a sexual problem.

However, inherent in this second-order cybernetic perspective is also the potential of autonomous self-healing. We are becoming increasingly interested in fostering this potential. If, for instance, the man referred to in the previous paragraph distinguished *his sensitivity* to his partner's criticisms of insensitivity (in relation to her), he could choose to redirect his emerging sensitivity to become a constructive resource for himself, that is, to help him become more aware of her experience. Thus, he could guide his own evolution in the direction of reducing the original insensitivity she distinguished. Similarly, if the wife of a man with erectile dysfunction noticed her own habits of noticing the turgor of his penis and noticed how her noticing invited him into feeling insecure, she could alter the focus of her noticing habits to attend to something that he felt more secure about, such as the texture of his skin or his gentleness. Likewise, if a man noticed that his own pattern of taking note of his level of sexual arousal (or of noticing his partner taking note of his arousal) raised his experience of performance anxiety, he could shift his focus of attention to something else, such as experiencing the affection and caring of his partner. Therapy toward such self-healing redirectiveness often entails a process of bringing forth descriptions (in the therapeutic conversation) of first-order patterns so that they subsequently can be distinguished and acted upon in a second-order manner by clients, on their own.

Psychodynamic therapists might regard this orientation as one of offering insight. We are not very comfortable with this notion because it is historically associated with intrapsychic phenomena and implies too much conscious awareness. The phenomenon we are interested in is more basic and general. It is a process of making new heuristic distinctions and perhaps new connections among them as a result of social interaction. Many of these distinctions take place in the coordination of therapeutic interaction and are not unconscious. Furthermore, we prefer to emphasize the interpersonal aspects of the process and would thus choose the term *outsight*, rather than *insight*. After all, the new recursive distinctions do arise in the interpersonal domain of therapeutic interaction. Our orientation toward outsight is consistent with our emphasis on the interpersonal contextual aspects of mutual sexuality; that is, rather than focusing on intercourse, we focus on "outercourse." Indeed, we regard the whole phenomenon of observing as fundamentally social. Even descriptions of the experience of self and of autonomy, depend on language that originally arises in the social domain.

When applied to the therapeutic system, this second-order perspective also enables the therapist and/or team to monitor its own behavior and to note whether it is actually guiding the session in a therapeutic direction or not. It enables therapists to distinguish their own resistance to considering alternative interventions when distinguishing the client as resistant. That is, the autonomous self-corrective potential of therapists is enhanced as well. If the therapist notes a lack of progress when working with a woman presenting with low sexual desire, the distinction of low desire as the problem could be distinguished as problematic. Perhaps both she and her mate are under the influence of excessive expectations for her. Perhaps her mate could be distinguished as having a problem of excessive desire. Or perhaps the discrepancy between them regarding sexual desire and the attempts of each partner to impose his or her preferences upon the other could be a more coherent distinction of the problem. The nature and consequences of these differing distinctions could be explored in the therapeutic conversation. Finally, the power politics entailed in determining which distinction should prevail could be brought forth for examination. The man or the woman may be operating from patriarchal assumptions in seeing the problem as her low desire. The woman might experience validation in distinguishing the problem as his excessive demands and control efforts. Both might be able to recognize the violence entailed in imposing each of their views upon the other. Consequently they might agree to accept a discrepancy distinction and proceed from there to a greater understanding of each other's experience and explore ways of escaping constraining assumptions. This process enhances the flexibility and autonomy of the therapeutic endeavor.

The major difference between a second-order cybernetic perspective of sexual problems and the more usual perspectives is one of epistemology, that is, the way in which we as therapists and clients know what we know about problems and solutions. The more traditional lineal views associated with biological, informational, behavioral, and causative-interactional understandings (and even a first-order cybernetic understanding) are based on the assumption of objectivity; that is, we assume that we know what we do about problems through lineal perceptual input from the world out there. This lineal epistemology works well for a large number of sexual concerns, but it may be rather limiting when dealing with the more complex or "resistant" concerns. With these, the second-order cybernetic epistemology may be particularly useful, since it temporarily abandons notions of objective truth and causation and looks more at the coordination of interaction that brings forth distinctions, the process of distinguishing rather than the distinctions alone, and the pattern rather than the content. The intent of therapy moves from one of achieving an outcome of specific behavioral change to one of increasing opportunities for alternative distinctions and behaviors. It is assumed that when people genuinely experience alternative behavioral options they will spontaneously select those that lead to more mutual pleasure and less pain. The goal of therapy becomes what has been dubbed *metachange*—a change in the couples' ability to change (Tomm, 1984b). From this perspective, change in a sexual relationship that occurs during the course of therapy is seen as a change in patterns of interaction attributed to the co-creation of new distinctions and meanings. The couple could make use of whatever biological, informational, and behavioral resources they have, in new ways that lead to their own experiential solutions.

CLINICAL ISSUES IN A CYBERNETIC–SYSTEMIC APPROACH

Therapist Style and Stance

The therapist's choice of interviewing manner and style may vary in its therapeutic quality. It may facilitate or impede the ease with which clients disclose and explore sexual matters. Obviously, it is incumbent upon the therapist to take leadership in establishing a pattern of interaction with clients that fosters healing. At the very least this implies developing an acute sensitivity to the personal vulnerabilities involved in talking about sexual experiences. Few of us are as carefully prepared for our sexual lives as we are for other human interactions such as meeting strangers, going to school, finding employment, parenting, and so forth. Our society generally prohibits preparing people for open and frank discussion of sexual experiences. At the same time, however, we tend to pick up a complex set of behavioral expectations pertaining to how we *should* feel and behave sexually. Clients enter the therapeutic context under the influence of these shoulds. They may feel that they should not even talk to an outsider about their sexual concerns and so may experience themselves as breaking implicit social rules in coming to therapy. If the therapist recognizes this, it is useful to comment on explicitly and express appreciation for their personal strength and courage in challenging these constraining assumptions by initiating treatment.

To acknowledge and accept the uniqueness of the client's experience enhances the possibility that the therapeutic context will, in fact, become healing. Often clients feel embarrassed or shy when sexually explicit material is talked about. Sometimes they even become mute and subsequently avoid sessions. Deliberately constructing a context of permission for embarrassment or shyness may alleviate the anxiety that could retard or prohibit the formation of a therapeutic relationship. This may be adequately conveyed with an accepting attitude, or it may require specific statements about the usualness of feeling anxious in such situations. For example, the following introductory statement could go a long way toward creating a therapeutic context of acceptance and openness while respecting the experience of the participants:

> Most people have limited opportunity to be as open and frank in discussing sexual issues compared to other important life issues such as finances, child rearing, and so forth. Usually, when we talk about sexuality, it is either about someone else's, as a joke, or with a detached air. If you feel some embarrassment or shyness as we talk today, that is perfectly usual and expectable. I would appreciate your being as frank as possible, since it helps my understanding of your situation and my ability to be helpful to you. And please feel free to use whatever words or terms you are used to. Now, what do each of you see as the major concerns that have brought you here today?

The covert cultural injunction that "one should not talk about sex" is challenged with this invitation to be frank and open and is further weakened by a coherent rationale for why disregarding it would be helpful.

Another series of "shoulds" that constrain the clients' ability to find solutions are moralistic injunctions that trigger guilt and blame. Clients are often quick to blame and berate one another, as the following examples show:

> HE: As a wife, she should be more affectionate with me. She hardly ever wants to have sex anymore.
>
> SHE: You shouldn't be so demanding!
>
> HE: If you were only more willing to have intercourse, I wouldn't have become so demanding.
>
> SHE: How do expect me to respond to you when you're bugging me all the time?

Or they blame themselves:

> HE: What is wrong with me that I can't control my ejaculation and give my wife an orgasm?
>
> SHE: I should be able to satisfy my husband; why can't I relax enough for him to make love to me?

In responding therapeutically to these shoulds, we have found it extremely useful to separate the moralistic expectations from the clients themselves. White's (1986) cybernetic methods in family therapy have been particularly helpful in this respect. The problematic expectations are attributed to cultural influences rather than to persons. In applying his method we ask questions about how certain expectations have influence over the clients and how these expectations "push" them into problematic patterns of behavior and experience. Then we ask questions about occasions when they might have been able to "escape the tyranny" of these expectations. When clients begin to experience the problematic expectations as something apart from themselves as persons, their guilt feelings and patterns of blame begin to abate. This externalized view of problems (in this case, the problematic sexual "shoulds" prescribed by our culture) is consistent with our orientation toward a social interactional basis for the mental phenomena with which we are dealing. What we try to introduce in the therapeutic conversation are increased possibilities for heuristic distinctions (e.g., between "self" and "not-self") and more space for choices in the direction of healing patterns of interaction.

To develop greater expertise in a cybernetic–systemic understanding that might cultivate more healing interviews, it is useful for therapists to work with colleagues in clinical teams and to practice adopting certain principles or conceptual postures in relation to clients. Our own evolution as therapists was significantly enhanced while employing the ritual five-part session of the Milan team (Selvini Palazzoli et al., 1978) for a few years and adopting their three guidelines for the conduct of the session:

hypothesizing, circularity, and neutrality (Selvini Palazzoli et al., 1980). One of us (K.T.) has summarized the Milan approach elsewhere (Tomm, 1984a, 1984b) and more recently has redefined the three guidelines as conceptual postures while adding a fourth: strategizing (Tomm, 1987a). The reader is invited to review these earlier publications for a more comprehensive description of the Milan approach; only certain aspects of the conceptual postures will be presented here, as they apply to sexual concerns.

Strategizing refers to the therapist's deliberate decision making in order to respond therapeutically to whatever emerges during the course of the interview. The therapist is continually making choices about what to attend to, what to do, what to say, and what *not* to do or say. The process of strategizing is organized by the overriding goal to have a constructive, healing influence. For instance, as previously suggested, a therapist may choose to attend to the clients' initial embarrassement, offer a normalizing explanation, and deliberately avoid any response that could be construed as judgmental or demeaning. When the clients' definition of a sexual problem seems to be pressuring the therapist into taking sides, the therapist may deliberately strive to maintain *neutrality*, which allows more space for spontaneous healing to take place. Skills in systemic *hypothesizing*, such as conceptualizing circular interaction patterns, are sometimes necessary to establish and maintain such a neutral stance. Thus, certain aspects of the conceptual postures of strategizing, neutrality, and hypothesizing are synergistic in enabling a therapeutic process. However, all of the activities involved in these postures are ultimately based on the *circularity* of recurrent interaction between therapist and client in the therapeutic system.

The circularity inherent in a therapeutic conversation (that is, in therapist questions triggering client answers, triggering questions, triggering answers, and so on) is easily taken for granted. Fortunately, one of the idiosyncratic features of a second-order cybernetic–systemic approach is to emphasize this circular process. Attention is drawn to the therapist's contributions to the distinctions being drawn by clients through the questions asked. It is not assumed that the clients' distinctions are offered spontaneously to the therapist, as if clients were in an unbiased vacuum. Certain kinds of questions invite certain kinds of reflections and responses. For instance, questions based on patriarchal assumptions (Does she respect your sexual needs as head of the household?) elicit different experiences and answers than questions based on feminist assumptions (Does she respect herself as fully equal in your sexual relationship?). Through their interaction in the clinical conversation, therapist and client tend to become coupled in their assumptions and patterns of drawing distinctions.

Indeed, they become coupled in an emotional domain as well as a linguistic one. The dynamics of emotional interaction between therapist and client in the therapeutic system makes an enormous difference in the quality of the relationship. The therapist who adopts a posture of *caring circularity* (interacting primarily on the basis of human affection) is more likely to offer clients an experience of empathic understanding than a therapist who adopts a posture of *obligatory circularity* (interacting primarily on the basis of the professional need to obtain information), who is more likely to give clients an experience of penetrating scrutiny. The latter can be especially problematic when exploring sexual concerns, which often include the experience of ones person being violated by another. The penetrating scrutiny of the interviewer may inadvertently aggravate the problems being presented.

There is probably more room for the therapist's own feelings of affection to emerge when working with couples oriented toward enhancing their mutual sexuality than in other kinds of therapy. Emotions are infectious, and the therapist's affection for his or her clients as persons can enhance a couple's affection for one another. However, in our opinion, there are *no* circumstances in which it would be appropriate or justified for a therapist to become sexually involved with a client. To do so violates our cultural understanding about the nature of therapy and would be socially irresponsible. A therapist taking advantage of clients for his or her own needs for intimacy or sexual gratification also would be contradicting the fourth criterion of mutual sexuality (as defined earlier). The best way in which a therapist's affection can be expressed is in the form of humor. To use humor effectively the therapist must continually listen to the clients' listening (to the therapist), so that he can be assured that they experience him as laughing with them, not at them. In other words, developing skills in the conceptual posture of caring circularity requires the ability to monitor the moment-to-moment effects of our behaviour on our clients, to compare these effects with what is intended, and to make changes accordingly.

The other conceptual posture that we have found extremely useful in guiding our interviewing style is neutrality. Adopting this posture implies accepting all persons as valued and equal and not taking the side of one person against another. Sometimes this is not easy, particularly when both members of a couple agree in their descriptions that only one of them is the problem, such as both confirming that one partner is very inhibited or "frigid." In these situations, externalizing the problem from the person (without projecting it onto another person) makes it much easier for a therapist, without jeopardizing neutrality, to agree that certain aspects of the situation are problematic. Useful questions include, How did these inhibitions get such a hold on you? In what circumstances do these childhood proscriptions take over? When they do, what happens to you? Have there been some moments when you have been able to escape them? These make it possible for the "identified patient" to experience the problem increasingly as separate from her as a person and alien to her personhood (which is affirmed and valued). Later the therapist could shift the focus to interactional elements, by asking her partner, When she is in the grips of her family view that "nice women are not sexual," what do you do to help her become a stronger person and free herself to make her own choices rather than caving in? What kinds of things do you do or say that might invite the inhibitions to take over her, without intending this? Similar queries can be addressed to the "identified patient": Have you noticed some things that your partner says or does that inadvertently feed the inhibitions and strengthen their power over you? In this manner, the woman as a person is separated from her inhibitions and her partner is invited to consider which of his or her own actions may support or challenge the pattern. Subsequently, the problematic contributions of the partner may also be externalized. This technique makes it easier for a therapist to remain more neutral with respect to persons but still take a strategic position against the continuation of problems.

We believe that the enactment of neutrality during the course of an interview has a general healing effect. It counters the ubiquitous tendency to blame the personhood of others when there are problems, and it opens space for clients to take a fresh look at one another as persons who mean well. Perhaps one of the most insidious enemies of neutrality is egocentrism, an orientation in which one is self-centered and in which one's views and oneself are collapsed to constitute a single entity. Thus, if someone were to challenge our views, we could experience them as challenging us as persons. Such an egocentric orientation leaves us extremely vulnerable to reacting to any difference from our preferred views as threatening to us. The typical response would be to protect ourselves by defending our views and to judge the other as incorrect or wrong. A commitment to neutrality helps us escape such egocentrism in ourselves and facilitates a similar orientation in our clients. To be neutral with respect to persons (including ourselves) when they manifest differing views and apparently differing contributions to problems, therefore, requires an ability to separate persons from their views and the consequent behaviors.

Neutrality is particularly important when dealing with sexual issues, because of the vulnerability of persons who hold idiosyncratic and/or stereotyped views that are maintained by the cultural shroud of secrecy over personal sexual experience. As already noted, sexual activities are not discussed as freely or as deeply as other significant life events. Because there is less open discussion, it is less obvious that our sexual views are derived from our social context; hence they are more likely to be directly associated with the self and tend to become egocentric. Furthermore, because of the shortage of explicit open discussion and modeling about sexual alternatives, we have fewer useful distinctions available to us to make comparisons and reevaluate our circumstances. One stereotypic belief, for instance, is that sexual activity and sexual intercourse are one and the same thing. On an experiential and even a physiological basis, there is much more to sex than the act of sexual intercourse, particularly for women, for whom it is often only a moderate physiological stimulant. Sexual intercourse is only one form of sexual activity, yet for many it is thought of as the "true" or ultimate—and therefore, only—form.

An egocentric perspective of sex entails the presupposition that what one as an individual understands to be most normal sexually (i.e., usual, reasonable, and acceptable) is, in fact, a true picture of sexual normality. Egocentric views have crippled the therapeutic impact of many professionals for years. For instance, psychoanalytic views of "normal" sex were based on the early-20th-century male view of sex as intercourse. Women who did not have "vaginal" orgasms (orgasm through vaginal containment of the penis) were considered psychosexually immature. These professionals, because of their egocentric orientation, tended to impose their views rather than look at what was, indeed, happening for people, let alone what was possible. We see similar but more subtle egocentrism today in the attempts to have clients' sexual lives conform to what the therapist considers appropriate. We are not neutral about this process. We are against such "therapeutic violence," that is, the imposition of the therapist's views upon the client. At the same time, however, we try to remain neutral with respect to the personhood of such therapists and see them as being under the influence of misguided patriarchal ideas or egocentrism. We also apply the same perspective to ourselves as we try to escape the lingering grip of patriarchy and egocentrism and the temptations to impose our views of mutual sexuality on our clients. We do, however, have our preferences. But, acknowledging our positions as preferences keeps us mindful that they are personal and that we do not have any right of "objective authority" to impose them on others. This guides us to try to remain open to discussion and to altering our views as we interact with clients and colleagues. In other words, neutrality helps us move away from potentially restrictive egocentrism within the therapy room and thereby helps us reduce the inadvertent negative impact of judgmental or moralistic attitudes of which we may be unaware.

It is useful to bear in mind that neutrality is not a static position that is attained, but rather is a conceptual posture that a therapist adopts to orient her behavioral responses in the interview. During the circular interaction of questions and answers, the therapist keeps moving his or her position in relation to answers, because of the tendency for persons to become identified with their views. Indeed, a conceptual posture of affirming neutrality potentiates the posture of caring circularity. By accepting persons more fully and separating them from the distinctions they make, the therapist can move closer and be more affectionate in relation to clients. At the same time, both neutrality and circularity depend on the ability of the therapist to operate as an observing system within the context of the therapeutic system. The therapist, by coupling with clients, contributes to their capacity also to operate more effectively as observing systems. The opportunity for clients to gain a new and more useful perspective of their sexual lives is enhanced when, holding a neutral stance in relation to the people whose lives are guided by beliefs, we remain intensely curious about their beliefs and the differential effects of holding one belief compared to another. The therapeutic impact is derived for helping the couple to take an observer position in relation to themselves as persons and thereby seeing the impact of their own observations, beliefs, and actions on themselves and others. The acceptance of neutrality can be useful in helping the couple examine the impact of stereotypic gender beliefs, beliefs about alternate sexual lifestyles, and other larger system issues that are often difficult to explore without a neutral perspective. The common pathology of "more of the same wrong solutions" is almost inevitably fed by judgments about what is believed to be sexually "normal" or "right." Unfortunately, beliefs about what is sexually normal tend to be ill-founded social myths.

The Therapeutic Use of Questions

We have already indicated how some questions may be used therapeutically in the course of an interview. This possibility has become a major focus of interest for us during the last few years. We also have become more sensitive to how some questions actually can be countertherapeutic. I (K.T.) have examined the issue of asking questions in clinical interviews in some depth and have devised a framework for classifying different kinds of questions that has proven useful in clinical work and teaching (see Figure 13.3). This framework has been published elsewhere (Tomm, 1988) but will be summarized briefly here, with a few examples of questions that might be asked in an interview approaching a sexual problem.

Figure 13.3 illustrates the two basic axes or dimensions used in the framework. The vertical dimension has to do with the therapist's *assumptions about mental process*, which underlie any particular question. At one extreme are lineal, cause-and-effect assumptions. At the other are circular, interactional assumptions. These assumptions may be either ontological, concerning what kinds of sexual problems or solutions exist, or epistemological, concerning how the client or therapist comes to know what they know about the problems or solutions that exist. The horizontal dimension has to do with the therapist's *intentionality* with respect to asking a particular question or asking it in a particular manner. At one extreme is the intent to ask a purely *orienting question*, that is, to obtain a response to orient the therapist. At the other is the intent to influence the client deliberately in some manner, through an *influencing question*. With the intersection of these two axes four quadrants arise with four different kinds of questions. *Lineal questions* are asked to elicit responses that

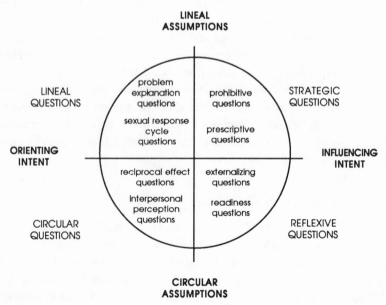

FIGURE 13.3.   A framework for distinguishing different kinds of questions.

orient the therapist to a lineal understanding of the situation. *Circular questions* are asked to elicit responses that orient the therapist to a circular understanding of the situation. The therapist's habits in the conceptual posture of hypothesizing will determine whether he or she will tend to ask predominantly circular or lineal questions to generate the information required to formulate explanations to guide her or his therapeutic efforts. *Strategic questions* are asked when the therapist intends to influence the client to think, feel, or behave in a specific manner that the therapist regards as most appropriate. In other words, the therapist assumes that he or she knows better than the client on a particular issue and, through the question, tries to direct the client toward the "correct" thought, feeling, or action, in a lineal manner. *Reflexive questions* are being asked when the therapist intends to influence the client in a general direction that the therapist considers therapeutic, while remaining respectful of the client's capacity and autonomy to choose to move in that direction or not. In other words, the therapist facilitates the client's own capacity to make appropriate choices for himself or herself.

In traditional sexual therapy, the therapist for the most part works with lineal, orienting questions. The primary intent is to attempt to get the "real picture" of what is going on. Much time is devoted to getting detailed behavioral descriptions of the sexual symptoms and dysfunction. The questions for obtaining information about the five phases of the sexual response cycle that were suggested in the early part of this chapter are examples of such lineal questions. Further lineal questioning could be devoted toward outlining the impact of earlier life events on the development of the symptoms. The therapist could be oriented toward becoming familiar with the sequence of sexual experiences and developments in the client's history. In addition, effort is expended in eliciting the clients' own explanations of the problem, which are almost always lineal. From the answers to these types of questions, the therapist typically arrives at a lineal, causal understanding of the problem. Consistent with this understanding, the therapist then gives a behavioral prescription, which the clients are expected to follow and report back upon. The whole process is based on lineal assumptions about the nature of problems and of treatment.

Cybernetic-systemic sex therapy may also begin with some lineal questions (to orient the therapist to the problem and to engage the clients in their lineal views), but circular questions soon enter the conversation. For instance, a series of *behavioral effect questions* may be used to clarify interaction patterns: When he approaches you for some sexual contact, what do you typically do? And when you try to put him off, what does he do? And when he gets irritable, what do you do? A series of *difference questions* may be used to clarify reciprocities: which of the two of you shows your disappointment about your sexual activities the most openly? Who hides disappointment the most? A series of *interpersonal perception questions* may be used to begin to develop a second-order cybernetic understanding: Does she notice whether you are beginning to have an erection or not? What does she usually think when you do not become physically aroused? What do you think she thinks is going on in your mind? Is that true? What exactly do you think he pays attention to when he is unable to get an erection? Whan you notice him becoming concerned, how do you feel and what do you do?

These circular questions are intended to help the therapist become oriented to the possible circular dynamics involved in the problem. Skills in circular hypothesizing are required to formulate these kinds of questions with ease. The answers provided may make it possible for the therapist to formulate a circular or cybernetic understanding of the problem. At the same time, the questions may have a liberating effect on the clients, since as they also begin to see the circular patterns they may free themselves from their original lineal understanding. They may begin to consider alternate explanations for their difficulty and formulate alternative actions on their own. In this way, circular questions are liable to have a therapeutic impact, even when they are not specifically intended to do so.

As therapists begin to recognize the therapeutic impact of certain questions, they usually start asking them intentionally to influence clients. In other words, statements can be introduced in the form of questions. Doing so adds complexity to the process of interviewing but enhances its therapeutic potential enormously. It also reduces the need for therapists to rely on instructions or to be directive. Whether a therapist's influencing questions are predominantly strategic or reflexive depends to a large extent on the degree to which a therapist is able to adopt and hold the conceptual posture of neutrality in his interviewing style. Reflexive questions require more acceptance of clients as autonomous persons. Strategic questions are driven primarily by a corrective intent and tend to reflect an urgency on the part of the therapist for clients to adopt his solutions. Because of this, these questions tend to have a constraining effect that limits clients to doing what the therapist thinks is good for them or not doing what the therapist thinks is bad for them. An example of each is, Why don't you spend some time together talking about your experiences of the day, before beginning to express sexual interest? and Why do you proceed to penetration when you notice that she is not yet aroused and lubricated? Such prescriptive and prohibitive questions can easily be heard as judgmental and blaming; consequently, using a large number of them could invite clients to experience their therapists as manipulating or controlling them.

Our preference is to use reflexive questions as much as possible. These questions are based on a facilitative intent and tend to have a generative effect on clients. Clients are invited to consider an issue from another perspective and generate an alternative point of view. (Several types of reflexive questions are described in Tomm, 1987b.) The earlier example of externalizing questions that invite clients to separate problems from person-hood are reflexive in intent. Other important groups of questions, derived from White's (1986) approach, that we use in a reflexive manner are dilemma, readiness, significance, and reconstructed-future questions. An example of a dilemma question is, Would you prefer to continue to drift in this direction of watching and worrying about your sexual performance, or would you prefer to confront and escape this spectator habit? A readiness question is, How ready are you to confront the performance expectations that have such a grip upon you? A significance question that could be used after an improvement has taken place is, Do you realize how significant your initiative in escaping those old expectations really is? Finally, an example of a reconstructed-future question is, Having turned a corner and embarked upon a new direction in your sexual relationship, in what way do you see your new future as different from your past?

It is important to note that these questions invite clients to make entirely new and novel distinctions. For instance, the dilemma question just given invites a new awareness of alternative possibilities and opens the choice for a new direction. The purpose of the readiness question is not for the therapist to determine the clients' objective state of readiness but to invite the client to reflect upon the issue and in so doing possibly generate greater readiness. The significance question brings forth and highlights constructive changes that have taken place, lessening likelihood that the therapeutic gains will be overlooked and lost. The reconstructed-future question invites further embedding of the constructive changes by connecting their significance to time. In these ways, reflexive questions enable self-healing processes that are more likely to endure. The questions invite clients to bring forth new heuristic distinctions. They open space for more options and facilitate the experience of personal agency. They invite clients to evolve toward a future-oriented, proactive lifestyle.

It is, of course, important to bear in mind that the therapist's intent in asking any particular question never guarantees its effect. Whatever impact it does have on clients, if any, will depend on their own organiza-tion and structure as observing systems. Generally, however, lineal questions are liable to have conservative effects; the clients answer them but remain unchanged. As already mentioned, circular questions may have liberating effects and strategic questions are liable to have constraining effects. Reflexive questions are, in our experience, the most likely to have healing effects, because they enable family members to generate new distinctions and to mobilize themselves into more constructive patterns of behavior, on their own. Thus, by becoming more observant of the assumptions and intent behind certain types of questions and making rigorous choices on the basis of ongoing client feedback in the circularity of the interview, the therapist may significantly enhance her therapeutic impact.

CONCLUSION

As clinicians we have evolved to the point where we now regard the interview itself as the major intervention when responding to problems of sexual dysfunction. We increasingly use second-order cybernetic theory to guide us in recognizing the importance of the distinctions we make and in understanding how we work together with our clients in co-creating therapeutic realities. In other words, while we have our theoretical preference, we are continuing to explore.

At the same time, we still value and use the more traditional domains of understanding and intervention. We quite often provide information, suggest experiments, and readily utilize behavioral directives. We also occasionally use formal end-of-session Milan-style interventions with paradoxical opinions and prescriptions. We feel that retaining this flexibility is important to avoiding becoming trapped within a single ideology and suffering from "therapist resistance."

PERSONAL RESPONSES: GARY SANDERS

Sex—such an all-encompassing word! To some, sex implies specific genital action, to others an unique experiential event, and to yet others a diverse set of markets for economic exploitation. Whatever one's view of sex and no matter how inclusive that view may be, it appears to take a central position in most people's experience.

I see myself as being like most others when it comes to past experiences of understanding and experiencing sexuality. I was raised in a quite traditional Canadian family of two parents and four children. I was surrounded in my family by an older brother and two younger sisters, one

16 years my junior. It was within this context that I began personally to appreciate sex.

At about age 8 or 9, I remember standing in the back alley with a group of boys and girls from the neighborhood, talking in conspiratorial tones about where babies came from. In the end, the group consensus was that they either came directly from the belly-button or out the anus. Either consideration was quite a shock, since I'd always believed that they had magically appeared on the day of delivery from that huge human factory called a hospital. A few years after this incident, at the age of 11 or 12, I remember pursuing girls for intimacy and sexual play. When the note from the teacher who found a girl and me in the nurse's room caressing each other was read by my parents, I was quite forcefully informed that this type of behavior was not permissible. At about the same time, through roughhousing with my group of boys, I found that sexual arousal could occur with the same sex as well, but I very quickly learned that this was not acceptable, either. It wasn't until my brother, in fact, showed me self-stimulation that I realized that there might be something that was acceptable only because no one else knew about it.

In my midteens, I became baffled by the neighborhood and peer reaction to a gay man who had moved in with his dying mother to look after her during her last days. The ridicule and abuse that this young man was subjected to, all the way from community centers to grocery stores, always perplexed me, for it appeared that he was doing such a benevolent and caring thing by looking after his widowed mother. It wasn't until I was in my late teens that I became more aware of women as an oppressed group, when in fact my mother became severely depressed and underwent chemical and electroconvulsive treatment for it. It seemed that all she really wanted was for her husband not to be out of town for half of the year and to value her openly as a complete and equal person.

It was from these rather inauspicious beginnings that I started to have a more academic interest in sex, compared to many of my peers. During my psychiatric residency training in family therapy, I found that child-oriented presenting problems would often quickly result in the marital subsystem alone receiving treatment. All too often, the marital concerns would revolve around those secret events that occurred behind the closed (one hoped) bedroom door. I seemed to become de-skilled when it came to such private events. However, being a good psychiatric resident, I quickly ran off to the medical library and read up on Masters and Johnson's and Helen Singer Kaplan's psychosexual treatments. Armed with brand-new cookbook solutions, I went back to my couples only to discover that the therapy fell absolutely flat.

It was when I realized that my therapeutic effectiveness appeared to be of little use, despite my interest and positive intent, that I elected to take a special training year at UCLA's Human Sexuality Program, under the auspices of Drs. Joe Golden and Susan Price. This was to be a pivotal year for me. Although the academic pursuit was very useful, it was the personal reflection afforded to me by living in a different culture—albeit not *obviously* all that dissimilar from my hometown of Calgary—that I found most useful. It was from this "stereo" view of sex, from holding a Southern Californian view and a Western Canadian view *simultaneously*, that I began to see sexuality from a more comprehensive view—a view that we are all limited by social restraints against acting on our sexually affiliative intent. It was my awareness of gay men and women, and the oppression they were subjected to simply for attempting to be loving and socially responsible, that seemed to me to be the most shocking of all. In addition, the treatment of human beings as property, whether men or women, was another shock to me. The notion of human property all too often was extended to include sexuality, such that individuals appeared to hold a belief that they had a *right* to the body of another for sexual purposes.

Overall, however, it has been my patients who have been most influential in my view of sexual issues. They have had more impact on how I understand sexuality and therefore on how I behave in relation to sexual issues than have my personal experiences—those successes and failures in my own intimate relationships. My clinical practice of usually seeing the couple as opposed to an individual has, I believe, helped me come to a very different perspective of human sexuality than I would have had otherwise.

For a number of years, I fancied myself a male feminist, but I can no longer claim such a title. In part, my throwing off the mantle of feminism had to do with a pragmatic reality. It appeared that no matter where I spoke, whether it was to a lesbian mothers' defense fund, a single fathers' support group, an early childhood services group in a rural or urban setting, or to academics, the use of feminist language and concepts was taken as an invitation to polarize that few could refuse. I was either instantly disqualified by the "true feminists" in the audience because I was male, or was classed as a "traitor" to the masculinists' cause, or, at best, was seen as a well-meaning but befuddled professional. Despite my good intent, the cloak of feminism didn't appear to fit me in the eyes of others. In addition to this, however, there was a more fundamental reason to abandon my feminist perspective: my experience with my patients. It appeared to me that the popular notion that is bantered about in Western culture, namely, that men are more interested in sex and women more interested in love, was in fact, a myth. Among the couples I met as patients, whether suffering directly from sexual concerns or from other problems, and those couples I counted simply as personal friends and acquaintances, both men and women appeared to want exactly the same thing: a mutually enjoyed, unique experience that defined their relationship as different than the others they were involved in. This most often included physical arousal, even to the point of orgasm, but, as important, it included emotional and physical vulnerability in the context of trust (what we usually perceive as intimacy). Because *both* partners in a relationship—whether heterosexual, male homosexual, or female homosexual—indicated to me that each wanted exactly the same thing that has led me to strive now for a more *mutualist* perspective. In other words, my patients have invited me to abandon feminism in favor of *mutualism*.

The effect that this has had for me, as well as for some of my patients, has been a liberation from the implicit adversarial nature of feminist or masculinist thinking. It helps put us all on the same side of the fence, all striving toward the same thing—an affiliative human event that is perceived mutually as positive and wanted.

It is these personal experiences that have shaped my influence on this chapter written by Karl Tomm and myself. The academic enlightenment that there is more to an event than the sum of its parts has also gone a long way toward liberating me from adversarial or dualistic thinking. However, I truly believe the biggest influence on my understanding and therapeutic actions has resulted from my patients. It is as if I *finally* accepted these people's invitation to realize more clearly their positive intent and purposeful striving toward a *mutual sexual relationship*, despite apparent gender differences and ill-fated methodologies.

As I look down the road and imagine training professionals, no matter from what discipline, in the area of sexuality, it's my belief that perhaps the greatest opportunity for these professionals to aid future sexual healing is by utilizing an accepting, comprehensive, reflective, and mutualistic perspective.

REFERENCES

de Shazer, S. (1982). *Patterns of brief family therapy: An ecosystemic approach*. New York: Guilford Press.

Heiman, J. R., LoPiccolo, M. S., & LoPiccolo, J. (1984). Treatment of sexual dysfunction. In A. S. Gurman & D. P. Kniskern (Eds.), *Handbook of family and marital therapy*. New York: Brunner/Mazel.

Hoffman, L. (1981). *Foundations of family therapy: A conceptual framework for systems change*. New York: Basic Books.

Hoon, E. F., Hoon, P. W., & Wincze, J. (1976). The SAI: An inventory for the measurement of female arousal. *Archives of Sexual Behavior, 5*, 208-215.

Hoon, P. W., Wirze, J., & Hoon, E. F. (1977). A test of reciprocal inhibition: Are anxiety and sexual arousal in women mutually inhibitory? *Journal of Abnormal Psychology, 85*, 65-74.

Kaplan, H. S. (1974). *The new sex therapy*. New York: Brunner/Mazel.

Kaplan, H. S. (1979). *Disorders of sexual desire and other new concepts and techniques in sex therapy*. New York: Brunner/Mazel.

Keeney, B. P. (1983). *The aesthetics of change*. New York: Guilford Press.

LoPiccolo, L. (1980). Low sexual desire. In S. Leiblum and L. Pervin (Eds.), *Principles and practice of sex therapy* (pp. 29-64). New York: Guilford Press.

Luckhurst, P. (1985). Resistance and the "new" epistemology. *Journal of Strategic and Systemic Therapies, 4*, 1-12.

Masters, W. H., & Johnson, V. E. (1970). *Human sexual inadequacy*. Boston: Little, Brown.

Morales, A., Surridge, D. H. C., & Marshall, P. G. (1981). Yohimbine treatment of impotence in diabetes. *New England Journal of Medicine, 305*, 1221.

Morales, A., Surridge, D. H. C., Marshall, P. G., & Fenmore, J. (1982). Nonhormonal pharmacological treatment of organic impotence. *Journal of Urology, 128*, 45-47.

Price, S. C., Heinrich, A. G., & Golden, J. S. (1980). Structured group treatment of couples experiencing sexual dysfunction. *Journal of Sex and Marital Therapy, 6*, 247-257.

Price, S. C., Reynolds, B. S., Cohen, B. D., Anderson, A. J., & Schochet, B. V. (1981). Group treatment of erectile dysfunction for men without partners: A controlled evaluation. *Archives of Sexual Behavior, 10*, 253-268.

Sanders, G. L., (1986). The interview as intervention in sexual therapy. [Special Edition on Interviewing.] *Journal of Strategic and Systemic Therapies, 5*(1 & 2).

Selvini Palazzoli, M., Boscolo, L., Cecchin, G., & Prata, G. (1978). *Paradox and counterparadox*. New York: Jason Aronson.

Selvini Palazzoli, M., Boscolo, L., Cecchin, G., & Prata, G. (1980). Hypothesizing-circularity-neutrality: Three guidelines for the conductor of the session. *Family Process, 19*, 3-12.

Tomm, K. M. (1984a). One perspective on the Milan systemic approach: Part I. Overview of development, theory and practice. *Journal of Marital and Family Therapy, 10*, 113-125.

Tomm, K. M. (1984b). One perspective on the Milan systemic approach: Part II. Description of session format, interviewing style and interventions. *Journal of Marital and Family Therapy, 10*, 253-271.

Tomm, K. M. (1987a). Interventive interviewing: Part I. Strategizing as a fourth guideline for the therapist. *Family Process, 26*, 3-13.

Tomm, K. M. (1987b). Interventive interviewing: Part II. Reflexive questioning as a means to enable self healing. *Family Process, 26*, 153-183.

Tomm, K. M. (1988). Interventive interviewing: Part III. Intending to ask lineal, circular, strategic, or reflexive questions? *Family Process, 27*, 1-15.

White, M. (1986). Negative explanation, restraint, and double description: A template for family therapy. *Family Process, 25*(2), 169-184.

AFTERWORD

David Kantor and Barbara F. Okun

Our thesis in this volume has been that there are indeed sexual and intimacy structures in families and that these determine the nature of intimate and sexual relationships. They appear to be less amenable to transformation by sociocultural changes and sexual practices than one would be likely to believe. For example, clients today have the same amount of sexual confusion and dysfunction as did clients prior to the "sexual revolution" of the 1960s and 1970s. Their expectations for heightened intimacy and sexuality have been influenced by sociocultural changes, but actual intimacy and sexual patterns of relating seem not to have changed accordingly. This implies that intergenerational influences have as powerful an effect on intimacy and sexuality as they have on other family structures and patterns. There also appear to be gender differences in the definition, expectations, and experience of intimacy and the interrelationship of caring, intimacy, and sexuality.

The major questions that underlie this volume are (1) Why and how have sexual and intimacy structures not been acknowledged and dealt with in family therapy theory and practice? (2) How and why do therapists respond or not respond to intimacy and sexual issues? (3) How does the gender of the therapist affect therapist responses?

The chapters in this book attest to the interest of family therapists in addressing or, more accurately, redressing issues pertaining to intimacy, sexuality, gender, and the person of the therapist, questions that have not been openly or widely acknowledged and discussed until very recently in our professional literature. These subjective issues involve feelings and thinking as well as doing. In different ways, our authors have presented their own thinking about these questions, their own views and approaches. In addition, many of our authors have been willing to acknowledge and reveal some aspects of how their personal experiences shape their professional views and vice versa.

Our involvement with this project has led us to the following thoughts and questions:

1. Family therapy ignores the reality of the mutual therapeutic relationship with clients. Do male therapists rely more on power and hierarchy than females in relating to clients? Are they more performance oriented and females more relational?

2. There are actually two therapy realities, not just one. The first therapy reality presumes that feelings of intimacy between therapist and clients are not a "real" intimacy, but an analogue. The second therapy reality presumes that feelings of intimacy between therapists and clients constitute real intimacy, albeit with clear differences regarding the development of intimate behaviors that accompany these feelings in mutual, bilateral, nonprofessional intimate relationship. Do male therapists fuse intimacy and sexuality more so than female therapists? Is that why sexual abuse in therapy most commonly involves male abusers and female victims?

3. If sexual structures exist in families, it follows that there are inevitably sexual structures in therapy. Could it be that family therapists have ignored the sexual structures in families, in order to avoid the threat of them in therapy?

4. Following this logic, these sexual structures are *both* real and imitation, within both the family and therapy systems.

5. Thus, the therapist's sexual and intimacy experiences in life do matter, in that they influence how the therapist responds (both consciously and unconsciously) to the sexual structures in client families and to both the real intimacy and pseudo-intimacy in the therapy system. Are there gender differences in therapist responses to sexual structures? Do males tend to act sexually on their feelings of closeness and caring more than females?

6. Given all of these questions and possibilities, the therapist's personal sexual and intimacy issues must be dealt with in training.

Once we redefine or reframe therapy to include both pseudo-intimacy and real feelings of intimacy in the therapeutic relationship—rather than having either no intimacy, pseudo-intimacy, or real intimacy—we need a new vocabulary to describe the therapy process. Perhaps a term such as *adjusted reality*, for example, will help us to describe what is really occurring in the therapy session. Many things are going on at once that are both real and imitations of reality. The therapist knowingly intervenes and can stand behind her intervention by acknowledging multiple realities and by identifying which reality an intervention is targeting.

The concept of therapist neutrality, which leads to the therapist distancing herself and retreating, and which denies the reality of the therapeutic relationship and the gendered person of the therapist, becomes an illusion rather than a reality. We believe that the family therapist can no longer hide behind the mask of detachment and omnipotence and focus only on what is seen, what technique is being used, and what is being done. Only by acknowledging the therapeutic relationship can it be used as both a cue and a model for addressing the intimacy and sexual structures within the family system, which are felt rather than seen.

We are not arguing for any one model of family therapy. We are suggesting that, as family therapy comes of age, we reassess and challenge our prevailing assumptions and models. What can family therapy models of the future become? What would be done differently? How would training be different? How would therapy be different?

In today's social, cultural, economic, and political climate, the imperative is toward brief, symptom-focused models of therapy. Is what we think we are dealing with in short-term therapy real or a convenient fiction? For some clients, we believe it is safe to think short-term therapy is real. For others, such a conclusion is a grave error. We hope that there will always be many different frameworks for assessing and treating different clients. We believe, however, that sexual structures, intimacy issues, and the person of the therapist exist and matter in all therapy situations, whether or not a particular case warrants their overt attention and consideration. A pluralistic paradigm can enable us to offer a wider array of treatment possibilities to a larger variety of clients, as well as to enrich the growth and capabilities of therapists.

We argue that our training criteria need revision. We need to bring under clinical control the specific effects of the therapist's nature on the therapy process and on different clients. By fostering therapist neutrality and technique, we have ignored and denied the influence of the therapist as a person. In addition to focusing our supervision on what therapists are doing, we need to consider what they are thinking and feeling, to "put the feeling back in family therapy." Techniques may be the only reality for the conventional family therapy view that the therapist relationship is not important and that any felt intimacy is simply an analogue. But, when we acknowledge the real intimacy component of the therapist relationship, the therapist's thinking and feeling become as critical as technique or doing. There is more danger of therapist crimes from denial and avoidance than from awareness and conscious attention.

Our discomfort with and reactivity to the psychodynamic model has resulted in our development of theoretical constructs and therapeutic stances that have created an artificial dualism of either internal or external influence, present or historical focus, doing or feeling, distance or intimacy, and a systemic or individual focus. A "both/and" approach seems to us to offer the likelihood of greater therapeutic effectiveness and therapist responsibility.

In midlife, we family therapists need to question our previous certainties and assumptions, to see what is currently real or illusory, and what new questions and thoughts can lead us toward expanding rather than restricting our views and practices.

INDEX

Abrams, J., 336
Absent father, 254-257
Acculturation, 132
Ackerman, Nate, 235, 236
Ackerman, Nathan, 103
Adamson, K., 334
Adamson, W., 334
Adequacy, tests of, 280-282
Age of therapist, 147-148
Age-discrepant marriages. *See* May-
    December marriages
Ahrons, C. R., 327
Albee, Edward, 115
Anderson, A. J., 353
Androgyny, 136, 230-231
Antilibidinal object, 3, 4
Attachment behavior, 78-79
Attraction, definition, 165
Autonomy, 136
    definition of, 200-201

B

Bateson, G., 41, 42, 56, 339
Batesonian approach, 348
Beavers, W. R., 156-157, 342
Being and doing, 126
Bellow, Saul, 260
Bem, S., 132
Benjamin, J., 39, 44
Bergman, A., 9, 79
Berman, E., 184, 292-319
Berryman, John, 258, 259
Bibliotherapy, 357
Biological aspects of sexuality, 355-356

Biological family, 113
Biological interventions, 356-357
Bion, W. R., 8-10
Biopsychosocial family, 108-110, 111, 113
Blame-guilt cycle, 361-362
Bloch, Donald A., 196-242
Bograd, M., 150, 163-194
Bolen, Jean Shinoda, 269
Boss, P., 181
Boszormenyi-Nagy, I., 82, 292, 294, 299,
    309, 331
Bowen, M., 294, 312, 308
Bowlby, J., 7, 78-79
Brazelton, T. B., 79
Breuer, J., 98, 99, 100
Brodsky, A., 181
Burr, Aaron, 210

C

Campbell, Joseph, 260, 261
Caretaking, definition, 164
Caring, definition, 164-165
Carter, E., 335
Children
    marital relationship after birth of, 84
    masturbation vs. physical
        expressiveness in, 76
    young. *See* Families with young
        children
Chodorow, N., 102, 134, 135
Class of therapist (socioeconomic), 148-
    149
Cohen, B. D., 353
Colapinto, Jorge, 50

Combrinck-Graham, Lee, 74-91
Commitment to patient, 122-123
Consultant, 118, 125
Cooper, B., 336
Co-therapist, 118
Co-transference, 117
Countertransference, 100, 167
Cowan, G., 321-322
Cross-generational coalition, 296
Cultivated intimacy, 113
Culture of abundance, 282-283
Culture of adequacy, 284
Culture of deprivation, 284-287
Culture myths, 206-212
Cybernetic-systemic approach, 346-379
    biological problems, 355-357
    blame-guilt cycle, 361-362
    client's knowledge about sex, 357
    clinical issues in, 364-376
    goal of therapy, 364
    moralistic injunctions, 365-366
    multiple domains of, 353-359
    mutual sexuality, 349
    negative feedback patterns, 360-361
    outsight vs. insight, 362-363
    performance anxiety, 358
    resistance, 358-359, 360
    self-healing, 362
    socially responsible sexual activity,
        351
    theoretical basis, 359-364
    therapist style and stance, 364-371
    use of questions, 371-376
    violence defined, 350-351

D

de Shazer, Steve, 358
Depressive position, 6
Detached stance, 185, 186
Developmental theorists, 102
Dicks, Henry, 7
Dimen, Muriel, 45
Dinnerstein, D., 134, 135
Disengaged stance, 185, 186
Divorce
    couples in process of, 296

following, 297
    in Updike, 93-94, 95, 97, 101, 103
Dominance, socialized, 131-134
Double standard, 268-270
Doyle, J., 293, 294
Duhl, F. J., 310

E

Eagle, M. N., 57
Economics of relationships, 213-214
Ecosystemic approach, 348
Edelwich, J., 181
Ehrhardt, A. A., 86
Eichenbaum, I., 135
Ellis, 75
Empathy in gender relations, 43-44
Empty nest in therapy, 122-123, 125
Engaged stance, 185-186
Enmeshment, 77
Ensminger, M. E., 83
Erikson, Eric, 80, 232
Evans, M., 55
Everett, C. A., 309

F

Fairbairn, W. R. D., 2, 3, 4, 5, 7, 8, 57
Falikov, C. J., 81
Families with young children, 74-91
    boundaries in intimacy and sexuality,
        88-89
    centripetal forces, 78-81
    child's contribution, 84
    exclusion of one parent, 84-85
    family-life spiral, 77-78
    masturbation vs. physical
        expressiveness, 76
    multigenerational contributions, 82
    other adults and, 83-84
    post-partum depression, 84
    role distinctions, 86-87
    sensuality and intimacy, 85-86
    sexuality and intimacy confused,
        75-77
    threats to, 82-85

Family. *See also* entries beginning Family
    biological, 113
    biopsychosocial, 108–110, 111, 113
    definition of, 108–110
    evolution of new, 111–112
    family-life spiral, 77–78
    life cycle of, sex and, 298–299
    psychosocial, 109, 113
    sexual development and, 10–15
    sexual differences in, 110–111
    sexuality in, 1
    social, 109–110, 113
    structure of, sex and, 295–298
    types of, 108–109
    with young children. *See* Families with
        young children
Family intimacy, 78–85
    causes of, 78–81
    threats to, 82–85
Family of origin, 292–319
    cross-generational coalition, 296
    divorce, 296–297
    incest, 297
    multigenerational family patterns, 304
    object relations theory, 301–304
    parent's sexual behavior, 295
    sex and family life cycle, 298–99
    theoretical issues, 295–304
    of therapist, 149–151, 178–179
    transmission of sexual loyalties, values,
        and concerns, 299–304
Family scripts, 309
Family therapy
    gender of therapist, literature on, 130–
        131
    sex therapy and, 305–308
    sexualization of, 123–126
Fantasy, sexual, 217–218, 237
Father
    absent, 254–257
    father-mothers, 87
    flight from, 259–260
    as primary nurturers, 87
Father-mothers, 87
Fay, A., 333
Feldstein, M., 166
Fenmore, J., 356
Ferenczi, Sandor, 105

Fischer, Helen, 213
Fisher, Charlie, 233
Fishman, H. C., 339
Fitting together, 79
Flight from father, 259–260
Foley, V. D., 309
Forced intimacy, 114
Ford, Ford Maddox, 103
Foster, D., 322
Framo, J., 292, 294, 299, 312
Freud, Sigmund, 2, 5, 11, 54, 57, 75–76,
    75, 98–100, 104–105, 106
Fuller, M., 166

G

Gagnon, J., 294
Game metaphor in sexual politics, 40, 41
Gartrell, N., 166
Gender and power. *See* Sexual politics
Gender contracts, 287–290. *See also*
    Sexual myths
Gender of therapist, 129–160, 220–233
    blind spots, 137–139, 144
    changing gender roles and, 140–143
    gender advantages, 144–146
    group process in dialoguing on, 233–
        238
    literature on, 130–131
    overlapping characteristics, 143–144
    power, 139–140
    socialized dominance, 131–134
    stereotypes about sexual relationships,
        144–146
Gender roles. *See also* Gender of
    therapist; Sexual politics
    in families with young children, 86–87
Generation gap in therapy, 118, 119
Generation of therapist, 147–148
Genogram
    creation of, 309–311
    introduction of concept of, 309
    sexual, 304, 308–318. *See also* Sexual
        genogram
Gestalt therapy, 105
Gilligan, Carol, 94–95, 102, 134, 135
Giordano, J., 147

Golden, J. S., 353, 378
Goldner, V., 28-52, 130
Gossett, J. T., 342
Greenberg, J., 57, 61
Greenblatt, C., 294
Grosser, G. H., 312
Guerin, P. J., 308, 310
Guntrip, 57

H

Haley, J., 41, 56, 102-103, 235
Hamilton, Alexander, 210
Hare-Mustin, R. T., 130, 145, 150
Hartman, 57
Hartnett, J., 322, 338
Heiman, J. R., 352
Heinrich, A. G., 353
Helen of Troy myth, 271-272
Hera and Zeus myth, 246, 269-270
Herman, J., 166
Hero's journey, 260-263
Hero's speech, 279-280
Hof, L., 177, 184, 292-319
Hoffman, L., 353
Hoon, E. F., 352
Hoon, P. W., 352
Horney, Karen, 57
Horton, Paul, 61
Hostile dependency, 7
Howard, K., 131, 134, 152

I

Ibsen, H. J., 333
Incest, 297
Infant attachment, 78-79
Informed stance, 185-186
Insight vs. outsight, 362-363
Intimacy
    activation of, 115-116
    boundaries in, 88-89
    cultivated, 113
    definition of, 74, 165, 198-203
    disruption of, 114-115
    family. See Family intimacy

forced, 114
models, 113-114
natural, 114
psychotherapy and, 116-119
sensuality and, 85-86
sex and love and, 112-113
sex vs., 133-134
as sexual intimacy, 82-83
sexual, 82-83
sexuality and, 203-205
sexuality vs., 75-77
therapist's empty nest, 122-123, 125
types of, 113-114
Introjective identification, 6

J

James, M., 293
Johnson, A. M., 12
Johnson, V. E., 10, 55, 63, 233, 352, 377
Jones, Ernest, 98
Jongeward, D., 293

K

Kafka, Franz, 259, 260
Kagan, J., 75
Kahn, M. D., 54-72
Kanter, R. M., 140
Kantor, D., 131, 183, 185, 196-242, 243-290, 381-384
Kaplan, A. G., 131
Kaplan, H. S., 55, 233, 294, 328, 339, 352-353, 377
Kardener, S., 166
Kaslow, F. W., 321-343, 325
Katz, R., 146
Keeney, Bradford, 348
Keith-Spiegel, P., 166, 182
Kellam, S. G., 83
Kennell, J. N., 80
Kernberg, O., 6, 57, 323, 325
Kerns, Lawrence, 74-91
Khan, M., 39, 44
Kingsbury, S. J., 154
Klaus, M. H., 80

Klaven, A., 261
Klein, Melanie, 2, 5-6, 323, 325
Klinger-Vertabedian, L., 322
Kohut, H., 58, 61-62, 65, 157
Koslowski, B., 79
Kramer, S., 79-80
Krasner, B., 82
Kraus, M. A., 84
Kunitz, Stanley, 257, 258, 259

L

Lackie, Bruce, 60
Laing, R. D., 103, 121
Lazarus, A. A., 333
Levinson, D., 155-156
Lewis, J., 342
Libidinal object, 3, 4
Lichtenstein, H., 8-10
Life script, 309
Lifton, Robert J., 249, 259
Localio, J., 166
Long-term relationships, 213, 216-220
LoPiccolo, L., 352
LoPiccolo, M. S., 352
Love
  definition, 75
  failure of modern psychology on, 104-
    105
  psychotherapy and, 116-119
  sex and intimacy and, 112-113
Luckhurst, P., 359

M

Magdoff-Singer, L., 331, 323, 325, 339,
  340
Mahler, M., 2, 9, 57-58, 79
Main, M., 79
Malone, P., 112
Maracek, J., 130
Margolin, G., 181
Marital relationship, after birth of child,
  84
Marital status of therapist, 125-126, 151,
  175-177

Marriage
  age-discrepant. See May-December
    marriages
  marital relationship after birth of child,
    84
  therapy's influence on, 94-97
Marshall, P. G., 356
Masters, W. H., 10, 55, 63, 233, 352, 377
Masturbation, 76
Maturana, 350
May-December marriages, 321-343
  case histories, 328-341
  clinical findings, 338-341
  factors conducive to, 325-328
  later marriages and, 326-327
  literature review, 321-324
  male longevity and, 327-328
  other couples vs., 324-325
McGoldrick, M., 147, 335
Mead, Margaret, 110
Mechanistic conceptions, 105
Mensh, I., 166
Mercouri, Melina, 211
Metachange, 364
Metaphor
  in Freud, 75
  game metaphor in sexual politics, 40,
    41
  sex as, 70
  for transcendence, 279
Milan systemic approach, 186, 348, 353,
  367
Miller, J. B., 133, 134, 136, 157
Miller, Michael, 93-106, 253
Miller, W. R., 310
Minuchin, P., 79
Minuchin, S., 292, 294, 295, 310, 339
Mitchell, S., 57, 61
Modell, A. H., 57
Money, J., 86
Monogamous relationships, 213-220
Morales, A., 356
Moralistic injunctions, 365-366
Moss, Howard, 258
Mutual sexuality, 349
Myths
  culture, 206-212
  Helen of Troy, 271-272

Myths (*continued*)
  importance of, 244-245
  Odysseus/Ulysses, 211-212, 246, 248-
    254, 279, 280, 282-283, 284
  Oedipus, 88-89, 209, 210
  Penelope, 211-212, 246, 279, 282-283
  in sexual contract. *See* Sexual myths
  Zeus and Hera, 246, 269-270

N

Napier, A. Y., 337
Natural intimacy, 114
Neal, J., 131, 183, 185
Negative feedback patterns, 360-361
Neutrality of therapist, 215-216, 367,
  368-371
Nichols, M. P., 63

O

Object relations theory/approach, 1-26,
  57, 135
  antilibidinal object, 3, 4
  antilibidinal system, 5
  assessment and treatment, 17-24
  case histories, 12-15, 17-24
  cycle of mutual influence, 24-26
  family interaction and sexual
    development, 16-17
  gender in, 135
  individual development in, 2-6
  libidinal object, 3, 4
  libidinal system, 5
  model of interaction, 7-10
  transmission of sexual loyalties, values,
    and concerns, 301-304
  unconscious structures, 5
Odysseus/ Ulysses myth, 211-212, 246,
  248-254, 279, 280, 282-283, 284
Oedipus complex and conflict, 88-89
Oedipus myth, 88-89, 209, 210
Offit, A. K., 55
Okun, Barbara F., 129-160, 196-242, 148,
  150, 381-384
Olarte, S., 166

O'Neill, G., 335
O'Neill, N., 335
Orbach, S., 135
Orlinsky, D., 131, 134, 152
Outsight, 362-363

P

Palazzoli, Selvini, 353, 366-367
Paranoid/schizoid position, 6
Parental sexuality, cycle of mutual
  influence on, 24-26
Parents' sexual behavior, 295
Passion, sex and, 270-274
Paternal connection, 256-257
Pathological certainties, 148
Pathological projective identification, 6
Patricidal obsession, 258-259
Paul, N. L., 157, 312
Pearce, J. K., 147
Pendagast, M. A., 308, 310
Penelope myth, Odysseus and, 211-212,
  246, 249, 252, 265, 267, 280, 282,
  283, 284
Penn, Peggy, 196-242
Peretz, A., 251
Performance anxiety, 358
Perry, Walter Copeland, 264-265
Person, Ethel, 216
Petry, R. A., 136
Phillips, V. A., 342
Pine, F., 9, 79
Pittman, Frank, 219
Pope, K., 166, 181, 182
Post-partum depression, 84
Power and gender. *See* Sexual politics
Pregnant teenagers, 80
Presser, H. B., 322
Price, S. C., 353, 378
Professional stance, 185, 187-188
Professional system, acculturation to, 154-
  156
Projection in transference, 120-122
Projection identification, 6
Pruett, K. D., 87
Psychoanalytic approach, in whole person
  treatment, 62-65

Psychosocial family, 109, 113
Psychotherapy. *See also* Therapy
  love and intimacy in, 116–119
  as parenting, 116

R

Raleigh, Sir Walter, 249
Rebellion vs. independence, 45
Reciprocity, 79
Redman, E. S., 84
Reid, Paul, 54
Reiss, D., 338
Resistance, 358–359, 360
Reynolds, B. S., 353
Rieff, Philip, 94
Riley, M. W., 325
Rodgers, R. H., 327
Rogerian therapy, 105
Rosen, F., 322, 338
Rubin, L., 133

S

Sager, C. J., 335, 337
Sander, F., 63
Sander, L. W., 79
Sanders, G., 185, 346–379
Sartre, J-P., 259, 260
Satir, Virginia, 139
Scantling, Sandra, 54
Scarf, M., 133–134, 196–242
Scharff, D., 1–26, 61, 63, 236, 302
Scharff, J. S., 5, 17, 26, 61, 63, 236, 302
Scheflen, A., 163
Schochet, B. V., 353
Schwartz, L. L., 327
Scripts
  family, 309
  life script, 309
  sexual, 293, 301
  sexual politics of control of, 49–50
Sensuality
  definition, 165
  intimacy and, 85–86
  sexuality vs., 89

Sex
  client's knowledge about, 357
  definition of, 348–351
  failure of modern psychology on, 104–
      105
  family life cycle and, 298–299
  family structure and, 295–298
  intimacy and love and, 112–113
  intimacy vs., 133–134
  as language, 103
  passion and, 270–274
  transference and, 98–101
Sex differences in families, 110–111
Sex life of therapist, 145, 146
Sex roles. *See* Gender of therapist; Sexual
      politics
  in families with young children, 86–87
Sex therapy
  as educational process, 306
  family therapist and, 305–308
  as low-priority item, 306–307
  as nonsystemic, 305
  reasons for reluctance to adopt, 305–
      308
  therapist discomfort with, 307
  as too medical, 305
Sexual desire, nature of, 245–248
Sexual development
  family influence on, 10–15
  family interaction and, 16–17
Sexual double standard, 268–270
Sexual dysfunction
  early approaches to, 352–353
  family-of-origin factors in, 292–293. *See
      also* Family of origin
Sexual fantasy, 217–218, 237
Sexual genogram, 304, 308–318
  case illustrations, 314–317
  contraindications to, 317–318
  creation of, 309–311, 311–312
  discussion with other family members,
      312–313
  indications for, 317–318
  introduction of concept, 309
  process, 308–314
  treatment plan with, 313–314
Sexual impasse, 243–244
Sexual interest, withdrawal of, 205–215

Sexual intimacy, 82-83
Sexual myths, 243-290
  absent father, 254-257
  culture of abundance, 282-283
  culture of adequacy, 284
  culture of deprivation, 284-287
  culture of waiting, 278-290
  disappointment, 287-290
  futile flight, 259-260
  hero's journey, 260-263
  hero's search, 279-280
  importance of myths, 244-245
  Odysseus-Penelope myth, 249-254,
      282-283
  paternal connection, 256-257
  patricidal obsession, 258-259
  sex and double standard, 268-270
  sex and passion, 270-274
  son's search, 257-263
  tests of adequacy, 280-282
  transcendence through work, 254
  types of, 245-248
  woman's dilemma, 263-278
  women's basic positions, 265-268
  women's power and work, 274-278
Sexual object, 44
Sexual politics, 28-52
  androgyny, 136, 230-231
  authorship of script, 49-50
  autonomy, 136
  bid for control in, 49-50
  complementary and symmetrical power
      arrangements, 41-42, 46
  economics in, 213-214
  empathy in, misuse of, 43-44
  game metaphor, 40, 41
  gender blind spots, 137-139
  gender of therapist, 129-160. See also
      Gender of therapist
  initial interview, 28-39
  male subject-female facilitator, 43
  mimicry in, escalating, 46
  mutual alienation, 44-45
  rebellion vs. independence, 45
  sexual objectifying in, 44
  sexual revolution casualties, 52
  sexuality as substitute for speech and
      independent action, 46

  social position and, 42
  socialized dominance, 131-134
  transference and, 101-103
  woman's dilemma, mythic perspective,
      263-278
  women therapists as sexual objects,
      179-180
Sexual response cycle, five phases of, 347,
    355-356
Sexual revolution, casualties of, 52
Sexual script, 293, 301
Sexual secrets, 219-220
Sexual shoulds, 365-366
Sexual values, transmission of, 299-304
Sexuality. See also Sexuality in therapy
  biological aspects of, 355-356
  boundaries in, 88-89
  definition, 75, 164, 164-165
  in family life, 1
  intimacy and, 203-205
  intimacy vs., 75-77
  mutual, definition of, 349
  parental, 24-26
  sensuality vs., 89
  as substitute for speech and
      independent action, 46
Sexuality in therapy, 163-194
  awareness of, 171-173
  countertransference and, 67
  ethical issues, 181-183
  family-of-origin issues in, 178-179
  objects of desire, 173-174
  personal vulnerability to, 175-177
  professional context as constraint, 168-
      169
  reactions to inquiry into, 171
  sexual contact with clients, 166-167
  sexualization of therapy, 123-126
  sexually exploitative therapy, 221-227
  theoretical issues, 183-188
  therapist stances, 185-188
  treatment unit and, 175-176
  voyeur vs. caregiver role and, 177-178
  women therapists as sexual objects,
      179-180
Sexually exploitative therapy, 221-227
Shapiro, Edward R., 148
Shlien, John, 100

Shumate, M., 322, 338
Simmel, 216
Simon, R., 177, 184
Siver, I., 164, 167
Slipp, S., 63, 323, 325
Sluzki, Carlos, 196-242
Smith, Valerie, 218
Social family, 109-110, 113
Social responsibility in sexual relations, 351
Socialized dominance, 131-134
Socioeconomic class of therapist, 148-149
Son's flight from father, 259-260
Son's search, 257-263
Spark, G., 292, 294, 299, 309, 331
Steiner, C. M., 293
Stern, D., 8, 9, 79
Stoller, Robert, 39, 40, 41, 244-245
Stolorow, R., 62
Strategic therapy, 102-103
Sullivan, H. S., 57
Surridge, D. H. C., 356
Sutherland, J., 3
Systemic, definition of, 348
Systemic therapy. See Cybernetic-systemic approach
Szurek, S. A., 12

T

Tabachnick, B., 166, 182
Teenagers, pregnant, 80
Tests of adequacy, 280-282
Therapeutic process, consultant in, 118, 125
Therapeutic relationship, 116-118
  gender of therapist in, 134
  sexuality in. See Sexuality in therapy
Therapeutic stance, 185-188, 364-371
Therapist
  age of, 147-148
  as caregiver, 177-178
  commitment and intimacy, 122-123
  empty nest, 122-123, 125
  family of origin of, 149-151, 178-179
  gender of. See Gender of therapist
  generation gap and, 118, 119
  generation of, 147-148

marital status of, 125-126, 151, 175-177
  maturity of, 119
  neutrality of, 215-216
  personal experiences of, 151-154
  professional system of, acculturation to, 154-156
  role of, 116-119
  sex lives of, 145, 146
  sexuality of, 178-179
  socioeconomic class, 148-149
  style of, 364-371
  as technician, 168
  unmarried, 125-126, 151
  as voyeur, 177-178
Therapist neutrality, 367, 368-371
Therapy. See also Psychotherapy;
    Therapist; entries beginning
    Therapeutic
  marriage and influence of, 94-97
  sexuality in. See Sexuality in therapy
  sexualization of, 123-126
Thomas, J. R., 136
Tomm, Karl, 346-379
Transactional Analysis, 293
Transcendence
  myth as metaphor for, 279
  through work, 254
Transference, 93-106
  bilateral, 120
  classical model, 101-102
  co-transference, 117
  countertransference, 67, 100
  projection in, 120-122
  sex and, 98-101
  sexual politics and, 101-103
  unilateral, 119-120
Turner, R. J., 83

U

Updike, John, 13, 93-94, 95, 97, 101

V

Victor, J., 294
Violence, 350-351
  definition of, 350

Visher, E. B., 335
Visher, J. S., 335

W

Wachtel, E. F., 308, 310
Walsh, F., 342
Weeks, 177
Weiner, J., 181
Weissman, Myrna, 231
Weitzman, L. J., 327
Whitaker, C., 60, 84-85, 103, 108-128, 151, 337
White, M., 61, 366, 375
Whole person, treating, 54-72
    case history, 65-71

psychoanalytic concepts in, 62-65
    theoretical influences, 56-60
Williams, William Carlos, 105-106
Williamson, D. S., 312
Wincze, J., 352
Winnicott, D. W., 4, 8-10, 13, 58-60
Wispe, L., 322
Wood, B., 77
Work, transcendence through, 254
Wyckoff, H., 293

Z

Zeus and Hera myth, 246, 269-270
Zilbergeld, B., 55
Zweig, Stefan, 98

93-107 Transference & Beyond

Whitaker 114-116

carrying unwanted feelings. of Collusion
definition p65

Belladona 30
Hepar
Sulphur
Ferrum